Chemotherapy-Induced Neuropathic Pain

Chemotherapy-Induced Neuropathic Pain

Edited by

Robert B. Raffa   Richard Langford   Joseph V. Pergolizzi, Jr.
Frank Porreca   Ronald J. Tallarida

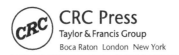

CRC Press
Taylor & Francis Group
Boca Raton London New York

CRC Press is an imprint of the
Taylor & Francis Group, an **informa** business

CRC Press
Taylor & Francis Group
6000 Broken Sound Parkway NW, Suite 300
Boca Raton, FL 33487-2742

First issued in paperback 2019

ISBN-13: 978-1-4398-6218-6 (hbk)
ISBN-13: 978-0-367-38102-8 (pbk)

Library of Congress Cataloging-in-Publication Data

Chemotherapy-induced neuropathic pain / editors, Robert B. Raffa ... [et al.].
   p. ; cm.
   Includes bibliographical references and index.
   ISBN 978-1-4398-6218-6 (hardcover : alk. paper)
   I. Raffa, Robert B.
   [DNLM: 1. Neuralgia--chemically induced--Review. 2. Neuralgia--therapy--Review. 3. Antineoplastic Agents--adverse effects--Review. 4. Chronic Pain--chemically induced--Review. 5. Chronic Pain--therapy--Review. 6. Pain Measurement--Review. WL 544]

616.99'4061--dc23   2012015721

Contents

Preface...vii
About the Editors ix
Contributors xi

Chapter 1   Chemotherapy-Induced Neuropathic Pain: Clinical Features 1

   Michael Husband and Richard Langford

Chapter 2   Assessment and Grading of Cancer Chemotherapy-Induced
   Neuropathic Pain.. 11

   Judith A. Paice

Chapter 3   Chemotherapy-Induced Peripheral Neuropathy: Review of
   Clinical Studies 19

   Joseph V. Pergolizzi, Jr. and Jo Ann LeQuang

Chapter 4   Orofacial Neuropathy and Pain in Cancer Patients............................ 95

   Yehuda Zadik, Noam Yarom, and Sharon Elad

Chapter 5   Cancer Chemotherapy-Induced Neuropathic Pain:
   The Underlying Peripheral Neuropathy 113

   Robert B. Raffa and Joseph V. Pergolizzi, Jr.

Chapter 6   Bedside to Bench: Research on Chemotherapy-Induced
   Neuropathic Pain.. 137

   Haijun Zhang, Juan P. Cata, and Patrick M. Dougherty

Chapter 7   *In Vivo* Models and Assessment of Pharmacotherapeutics for
   Chemotherapy-Induced Neuropathic Pain 147

   Sara Jane Ward

Chapter 8   Drug Treatment for Chemotherapy-Induced Neuropathic Pain:
   Amitriptyline as an Example 163

   Eija Kalso

Chapter 9   Experimental Design and Analysis of Drug Combinations
               Applicable to Chemotherapy-Induced Neuropathic Pain................. 169

               Ronald J. Tallarida

Chapter 10 Central Neuromodulation for Chemotherapy-Induced
               Neuropathic Pain.. 181

               Helena Knotkova, Dru J. Nichols, and Ricardo A. Cruciani

Chapter 11 Nerve Decompression for Chemotherapy-Induced
               Neuropathic Pain.. 195

               Michael I. Rose

Bibliography 205

Index... 211

Preface

There have been tremendous recent advances in the pharmacotherapy, dose regimens, and combinations used to treat cancer and for the treatment or prevention of spread of disease. As a direct result of these advances, there are an increasing number of cancer survivors. There are currently more than 25 million such survivors worldwide, and it is estimated that the number will grow to 75 million by 2030.

Each and every cancer survivor is forever thankful and appreciative of the advances in chemotherapy and other aspects of prevention, early detection, and treatment modalities that have contributed to the increasing percentage of patients who are surviving the disease. However, no drug, including chemotherapeutic drugs, is devoid of adverse effects. In the case of chemotherapeutic agents, the acute adverse effects are well known, and the chronic adverse effects are only now becoming known due to the increase in survival rates. For some types of cancer, in fact, patients live *decades* beyond their diagnosis.

It is becoming clear that a significant number of cancer survivors experience neuropathic pain, anxiety and depression, and cognitive (primarily memory) impairment. Together, these adverse effects negatively affect their quality of life and activities of daily living (functionality), and worse, might discourage a decision to receive chemotherapy.

A previous monograph addressed the decreased cognitive acuity (known as chemo-fog or chemo-brain).* This book is devoted to the adverse effects of neuropathic pain. The material that is presented here provides, we believe, the background, state-of-the-art clinical and basic research, and direction for future study.

The authors comprise an impressive list of clinical and basic science experts in the fields of pain mechanisms and pain management. Included are clinical directors of pain clinics and clinical research facilities, directors of large academic pain research laboratories, analgesic drug discoverers, experts in analysis of pain and analgesia clinical and preclinical studies, and presidents of the International Association for the Study of Pain and the British Pain Society. All are opinion leaders in the field of pain and analgesia. They have directed their collective experience and wisdom in this book to the underrecognized and underserved area of chemotherapy-induced neuropathic pain. The result is the first comprehensive coverage of the topic by so many experts in a single source. Through them, it is our goal and hope that this book provides the reader with an exceptional opportunity to acquire a fundamental understanding of the basic concepts related to this topic.

We asked the authors to write their chapters so that they can be read independently of the others and in any order desired. We believe that this best serves the readers' interest. As a result, there is some degree of overlap in background material, but we feel that this only enhances the experience and learning of the material.

---

* R.B. Raffa and R.J. Tallarida, eds., *Chemo-Fog: Cancer Chemotherapy-Related Cognitive Impairment*, Austin, TX: Springer/Landes Publishers, 2010.

Finally, we point out that the preparation of this book represents a further step in the work of the Forget-Me-Not Foundation, whose mission is fostering improved care for cancer survivors (http://fmnfoundation.org).

Robert B. Raffa, Ph.D.
Richard Langford, M.D.
Joseph V. Pergolizzi, Jr., M.D.
Frank Porreca, Ph.D.
Ronald J. Tallarida, Ph.D.

About the Editors

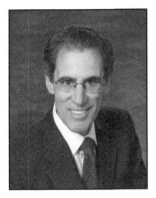

Robert B. Raffa, Ph.D., is professor of pharmacology in the Department of Pharmaceutical Sciences, Temple University School of Pharmacy, Philadelphia, Pennsylvania. He holds BChemE and B.S. degrees in chemical engineering and physiological psychology, M.S. degrees in biomedical engineering and toxicology, and a Ph.D. in pharmacology. He is the coauthor or editor of books on pharmacology and thermodynamics and over 225 articles in refereed journals. He is associate executive editor of *Life Sciences* and is active in National Institutes of Health (NIH)-funded research and professional society activities. Dr. Raffa is cofounder of the Forget-Me-Not Foundation, a nonprofit that is devoted to increasing the awareness, study, and treatment of medical needs of cancer survivors.

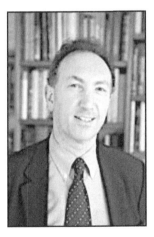

Richard Langford, M.D., is current president of the British Pain Society (BPS). He graduated in medicine from Middlesex Hospital, University of London, and trained in anaesthetics, pain medicine, and intensive care at St. Bartholomew's and University College Hospital, London. Since 2003, he has held the joint school and National Health Service (NHS) Trust posts of clinical director of Clinical Research Centres, and deputy director of Research and Development. In these roles, he contributed to the commissioning of new facilities for clinical research and gene therapy. Dr. Langford has played senior roles in training and education, and he established the Pain Research Group for development and evaluation of patient monitoring devices used during surgery and intensive care.

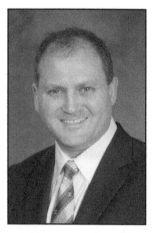

Joseph V. Pergolizzi, Jr., M.D., is adjunct assistant professor at Johns Hopkins University School of Medicine and senior partner in the Naples Anesthesia and Pain Associates Group of South West Florida. He holds a B.S. degree in physical chemistry in addition to his M.D. degree, with a residency at Georgetown University School of Medicine and fellowship at Johns Hopkins University School of Medicine. He has authored more than 100 publications and is editor in chief of *Clinical Researcher,* editor for the *International Journal of Pain Medicine and Palliative Care* and *Scientific World Journal of Anesthesia*, and invited feature editor of *Pain Medicine.* Dr. Pergolizzi is an internationally sought after lecturer at major medical schools, health systems, and national medical symposia.

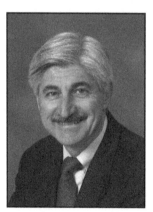

Frank Porreca, Ph.D., is professor of pharmacology and anesthesiology at the University of Arizona. His laboratory studies the mechanisms of chronic pain and opioid-induced hyperalgesia. His studies have addressed mechanisms of spontaneous and ongoing pain, and of neural plasticity in both the peripheral and central nervous systems. This work has resulted in over 400 publications. He is the executive editor in chief of *Life Sciences,* section editor for *Pain,* and the scientific organizer of the Spring Pain Research Conference. He has trained many students and postdoctoral fellows. Dr. Porreca is the recipient of the F.W. Kerr Award from the American Pain Society for studies in pain mechanisms.

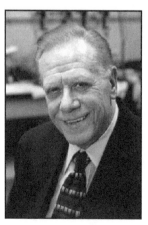

Ronald J. Tallarida, Ph.D., is professor of pharmacology in the Department of Pharmacology, Temple University School of Medicine, Philadelphia, Pennsylvania. He has B.S. and M.S. degrees in physics/mathematics and a Ph.D. in pharmacology. His work, primarily concerned with theoretical and quantitative aspects of pharmacology, is represented in more than 250 published works, including 8 books that he has authored or coauthored. Dr. Tallarida currently teaches, serves on editorial advisory boards, conducts NIH-funded research, and is active in professional societies, having served as president of the Mid-Atlantic Pharmacology Society. He is the cofounder of the Forget-Me-Not Foundation.

Contributors

Juan P. Cata, M.D.
Department of Pain Medicine
University of Texas M.D. Anderson
    Cancer Center
Houston, Texas

Ricardo A. Cruciani, M.D., Ph.D.
Institute for Non-Invasive Brain
    Stimulation
Research Division
Department of Pain Medicine and
    Palliative Care
Beth Israel Medical Center
New York, New York
and
Departments of Neurology and
    Anesthesiology
Albert Einstein College of Medicine
Bronx, New York

Patrick M. Dougherty, Ph.D.
Department of Pain Medicine
University of Texas M.D. Anderson
    Cancer Center
Houston, Texas

Sharon Elad, D.M.D., M.Sc.
Division of Oral Medicine
Eastman Institute for Oral Health
University of Rochester Medical Center
Rochester, New York

Michael Husband, M.D.
Barts and the London National Health
    Service (NHS) Trust
London, United Kingdom

Eija Kalso, M.D., Ph.D.
Faculty of Medicine
Institute of Clinical Medicine
Helsinki University and Pain Clinic
Helsinki University Central Hospital
Helsinki, Finland

Helena Knotkova, Ph.D.
Institute for Non-Invasive Brain
    Stimulation
Research Division
Department of Pain Medicine and
    Palliative Care
Beth Israel Medical Center
New York, New York
and
Department of Neurology
Albert Einstein College of Medicine
Bronx, New York

Jo Ann LeQuang
LeQ Medical Communications
Angleton, Texas

Dru J. Nichols, M.D.
Institute for Non-Invasive Brain
    Stimulation
Research Division
Department of Pain Medicine and
    Palliative Care
Beth Israel Medical Center
New York, New York

Judith A. Paice, Ph.D., R.N.
Cancer Pain Program
Division of Hematology-Oncology
Feinberg School of Medicine
Northwestern University
Chicago, Illinois

Michael I. Rose, M.D., FACS
Division of Hand Surgery
Division of Plastic and Reconstructive
    Surgery
Center for Treatment of Paralysis and
    Reconstructive Nerve Surgery
Jersey Shore University Medical Center
Neptune, New Jersey

Sara Jane Ward, Ph.D.
Department of Pharmaceutical Sciences
Temple University School of Pharmacy
Philadelphia, Pennsylvania
and
Center for Substance Abuse Research
    (CSAR)
Temple University
Philadelphia, Pennsylvania

Noam Yarom, D.M.D.
Department of Oral and Maxillofacial
    Surgery
Sheba Medical Center
Tel-Hashomer, Israel
and
Department of Oral Pathology and
    Oral Medicine
School of Dental Medicine
Tel-Aviv University
Tel-Aviv, Israel

Yehuda Zadik, D.M.D., M.H.A.
Department of Oral Medicine
Hebrew University–Hadassah School of
    Dental Medicine
Jerusalem, Israel
and
Department of Oral Medicine
The Oral and Maxillofacial Center
Medical Corps
Israel Defense Forces
Tel Hashomer, Israel

Haijun Zhang, M.D.
Department of Pain Medicine
University of Texas M.D. Anderson
    Cancer Center
Houston, Texas

1 Chemotherapy-Induced Neuropathic Pain
Clinical Features

Michael Husband and Richard Langford

CONTENTS

1.1 Introduction to Neuropathic Pain 1
1.2 Clinical Assessment.. 4
    1.2.1 Neuropathic Pain 4
    1.2.2 Chemotherapy-Induced Neuropathic Pain....................................... 5
1.3 Clinical Features—History 5
    1.3.1 Neuropathic Pain 5
    1.3.2 Chemotherapy-Induced Neuropathic Pain....................................... 6
1.4 Clinical Features—Examination 6
    1.4.1 Neuropathic Pain 6
    1.4.2 Chemotherapy-Induced Neuropathic Pain....................................... 7
1.5 Additional Tests and Investigations 8
References.. 8

1.1 INTRODUCTION TO NEUROPATHIC PAIN

Physiological pain arises as a consequence of the activation of primary nociceptive afferents by stimuli with the actual or potential ability to cause tissue damage (Treede et al., 2008). These stimuli are processed and modulated by the somatosensory system, with potential alterations in nociceptive thresholds, pain perception, and behavioral responses.

Pain may also arise by abnormal activity generated within the nociceptive pathways without adequate stimulation of the peripheral sensory endings and offers no benefit to the patient. For these clinical conditions, the term *neuropathic pain* has been introduced. The International Association for the Study of Pain (IASP) defines neuropathic pain as "pain initiated or caused by a primary lesion or dysfunction in the nervous system" (Merksey and Bogduk, 1994, 211). This definition has been criticized as lacking diagnostic specificity and anatomic precision; hence, another definition has been proposed that refers to identifiable disease processes or identifiable damage to the nervous system, namely: "pain arising as a direct consequence of a lesion or disease affecting the somatosensory system" (Treede et al., 2008, 1631).

TABLE 1.1

Neuropathic Pain Syndromes

Peripheral Neuropathic Pain Syndromes	Central Neuropathic Pain Syndromes
Chemotherapy-induced neuropathy	Central poststroke pain
Complex regional pain syndrome	Multiple sclerosis pain
HIV sensory neuropathy	Parkinson's disease pain
Neuropathy secondary to tumor infiltration	Spinal cord injury pain
Painful diabetic neuropathy	
Phantom limb pain	
Postherpetic neuralgia	
Postmastectomy pain	
Trigeminal neuralgia	
Spinal cord injury pain	

Source: Reprinted from *Clin J Pain*, Vol. 18, Dworkin, RH, An Overview of Neuropathic Pain: Syndromes, Symptoms, Signs, and Several Mechanisms, 343–349. Copyright 2002, with permission from Elsevier.

Neuropathic pain can arise from damage to the nerve pathways at any point from the terminals of the peripheral nociceptors to the cortical neurons in the brain. It is classified as central (originating from damage to the brain or spinal cord) or peripheral (originating from damage to the peripheral nerve, plexus, dorsal root ganglion, or nerve root). Neuropathic pain can also be classified by aetiology of the insult to the nervous system (Haanpää and Treede, 2010).

There are many central and peripheral processes that have the potential to cause neuropathic pain. Physical, infectious, metabolic, ischemic, toxic, neoplastic, degenerative, and immune mediated processes all have the potential to induce the somatosensory changes that can lead to ongoing neuropathic pain, although symptom development is not uniform among individuals (Callin and Bennett, 2008). Examples of neuropathic pain conditions are listed in Table 1.1.

Nociceptive and neuropathic pain may coexist and categorizing painful conditions as being either nociceptive or neuropathic may not reflect the true clinical picture (Callin and Bennett, 2008). Most patients with neuropathic pain have chronic symptoms with a significant impact on physical and psychological well-being; it is frequently difficult to treat and places substantial clinical and financial demands on society.

Neuropathic pain in the cancer population carries a high prevalence and is relatively resistant to symptom control interventions (Martin and Hagen, 1997). A recent systematic review analyzed a total of 13,683 cancer patients and conservatively estimated a neuropathic pain prevalence of around 20%, but when the investigators included patients with mixed nociceptive and neuropathic pain the prevalence rose to approximately 40% (Bennett et al., 2011). A variety of neuropathic pain syndromes have been described in the cancer patient population and some examples are listed in Table 1.2.

TABLE 1.2

Examples of Neuropathic Pain Syndrome Associated with Malignancy

Neuropathic Pain Syndromes in Cancer Patients	Mechanism of Action	Common Clinical Features	Common Examples
Cranial nerve neuralgias	Compression, bone destruction, tumor infiltration	Constant aching, neurological deficits, dysaesthesia	Bone or leptomeningeal metastases, e.g., from breast or prostate
Tumor-related mononeuropathy	Local compression, tumor invasion	Painful neuropathy	Rib metastases
Radiculopathy	Compression/invasion to dorsal nerve roots	Dermatomal pain, unilateral or bilateral	Epidural tumor mass, metastases
Brachial plexopathy	Tumor infiltration or compression	Pain and dysaesthesia, breast, apical lung tumors, and lymphomas	Pancoast tumor, lymph node metastases from breast and lymphoma
Paraneoplastic peripheral neuropathy	Inflammatory process involving dorsal root ganglion	Subacute sensory neuropathy, dysaesthesias, parasthesias, and sensory loss	Small cell carcinoma of the lung
Postsurgical neuropathic pain	Intercostobrachial nerve damage, neuroma formation	Burning, dysaesthesias, parasthesias	Postmastectomy, postthoracotomy
Chemotherapy-induced peripheral neuropathy	Dependent on class of chemotherapeutic agent	Painful peripheral dysaethesias, sensory (mild to moderate numbness), motor (taxane and vinca compounds), and autonomic deficits	Taxane, vinca alkaloid, and platinum compounds

Source: Reprinted from *J Pain Symptom Manage*, Vol. 14, Martin, LA, Hagen, NA, Neuropathic Pain in Cancer Patients: Mechanisms, Syndromes, and Clinical Controversies, 99–117. Copyright 1997, with permission from Elsevier.

In addition to the nerve damage and neuropathic pain arising from the cancer itself or treatment procedures (surgery or radiotherapy), patients may also develop chemotherapy-induced peripheral neuropathy (CIPN). CIPN results from toxic effects of chemotherapy drugs predominantly affecting the peripheral nervous system. This potentially treatment-limiting side effect may become a serious burden and is a common reason why cancer patients stop their treatment early (Moya del Pino, 2010). It persists in most cases, being at best only partially resolved (Pachman et al., 2011). A subset of these patients will develop painful CIPN that has a major impact on activities of daily living and their quality of life (Farquhar-Smith, 2011).

Painful CIPN is recognized as an area of unmet clinical need, which in a recent review article was attributed to five key reasons (Farquhar-Smith, 2011):

1. Poor recognition of the symptoms
2. Difficulties in diagnosis
3. Heterogenous assessment tools and interobserver variation
4. Reluctance of patients to report symptoms
5. Limited treatment and prevention options

Painful CIPN can be extremely disabling, with a marked impact on quality of life, functional ability, and risks of noncompliance with cancer treatments.

1.2 CLINICAL ASSESSMENT

1.2.1 Neuropathic Pain

Several steps are taken during the assessment of a patient with suspected neuropathic pain, all of which must be based on the foundations of a thorough history and examination to elucidate key characteristics and identify potential red flag features indicative of other pathologies. The pain history should include the location, radiation, intensity, quality, perceived triggers, and time course of the pain and any associated symptoms, such as numbness. Evoked or spontaneous pain can be distinguished by details in the history and attempts at eliciting the pain through stimuli such as touch to determine whether it is stimulus dependent or independent. The same principles are equally applicable in the assessment of patients with potential neuropathic pain as a result of CIPN or related to the malignancy itself, surgery, or radiotherapy. Potential consequences of the pain should also be noted, including impact on mood, sleep, quality of life, and social and physical functioning.

The IASP has highlighted several key steps required for a comprehensive clinical assessment: (1) recognizing neuropathic pain, (2) localization (whether it is peripheral or central), (3) diagnosing the causative disease or event, and (4) assessing the functional limitations that result from pain (Haanpää and Treede, 2010). The psychosocial features of the patients are necessary for a management strategy that is individually tailored (Haanpää and Treede, 2010). To confirm a diagnosis of neuropathic pain the following factors must be present (Kehlet et al., 2006):

1. Pain in a neuroanatomically defined area, corresponding to a peripheral or central innervation territory.
2. A history of relevant disease or lesion in the nervous system, which is temporally related to development of pain.
3. Partial or complete sensory loss in all or part of the painful area.
4. Confirmation of a lesion or disease by a specific test—for example, surgical evidence, imaging, clinical neurophysiology, biopsy.

Furthermore, the Initiative on Methods, Measurement and Pain Assessment in Clinical Trials (IMMPACT) collaborative group has published recommendations for the evaluation of neuropathic pain that include pain severity, physical and emotional functioning, ratings of improvement, and satisfaction with treatment, symptoms, and adverse effects (Turk et al., 2003). These recommendations are primarily proposed as key outcome measures in clinical trials, but they lend themselves to current clinical assessment and follow-up of patients with neuropathic pain or CIPN.

1.2.2 CHEMOTHERAPY-INDUCED NEUROPATHIC PAIN

The important goals during the assessment of CIPN are to confirm the diagnosis, rule out or establish other causes of neuropathic pain, confirm the severity of the patient's symptoms and effect on quality of life, and establish a therapeutic strategy. History, examination, and appropriate, supportive investigation are crucial in the early evaluation of CIPN. Quantitative tests of sensory and motor dysfunction are available but are not widely used in clinical decision making due to:

1. Lack of controlled studies assessing quantitative measurements as the primary outcome and poor correlation between quantitative measurements and severity of symptoms.
2. Quantitative measurements are unable to reliably monitor response to treatment (Cleeland et al., 2010).

Physician-based assessments are another tool with which to objectively assess neuropathic pain and CIPN. These include a variety of scores and rating scales that are in clinical use, but wide interobserver variation exists. They require patient and physician cooperation and training (Cleeland et al., 2010).

1.3 CLINICAL FEATURES—HISTORY

1.3.1 NEUROPATHIC PAIN

Symptoms and signs play an important role in identifying patients likely to suffer from neuropathic pain and may highlight an underlying mechanism of action. A feature of neuropathic pain is the combination of sensory loss with paradoxical hypersensitivity and a distinction between stimulus-evoked and spontaneous pain (Kehlet et al., 2006). Spontaneous pain occurs without any nociceptive stimulation and may be paroxysmal or continuous and vary in intensity. Different types of spontaneous pain are likely to be reported by the patient, suggesting that their pain has different qualities, for example, dysaesthesia—an unpleasant or abnormal sensation felt in the skin and parasthesias—abnormal sensations that are not unpleasant (Dworkin, 2002). Shooting, stabbing, or electric shock pains are terms that are frequently used by patients to describe these spontaneous phenomena. Stimulus or evoked pains represent the second broad type of symptoms in neuropathic pain sufferers. The different types of evoked pains generally produce unusual or exaggerated symptoms, for example, hyperalgesia and allodynia that can result from thermal, vibration, dynamic, and static (punctate and blunt) stimuli (Dworkin, 2002). Hyperalgesia is an increased response to a normally painful stimulus, and allodynia is pain due to a stimulus that does not normally provoke pain. Spontaneous and evoked pains fall under the category of positive phenomena. Negative phenomena that can occur with neuropathic pain syndromes include sensory loss, numbness, or hypoalgesia in the damaged nerve territory and corresponding motor deficits that lead the patient to complain of weakness. Pain intensity can be assessed verbally, numerically, or with a visual analogue scale (VAS), and the intensity of each painful symptom should be assessed.

It is important to establish the presence or absence of comorbidities as potential therapeutic strategies may be either contraindicated by existing medical conditions or fail to achieve the desired treatment outcomes. Additionally, a thorough psychosocial history and evaluation is paramount in all neuropathic pain sufferers, with work, sleep, and social functioning potentially adversely affected. Relationships with friends and family, as well as physical fitness and independence, are often severely affected in patients with neuropathic pain. To ensure the greatest chance of achieving therapeutic goals, an understanding of the psychosocial impact and expectations of the patient must be appreciated by the attending clinician.

1.3.2   CHEMOTHERAPY-INDUCED NEUROPATHIC PAIN

Sensory symptoms predominate in patients who suffer from CIPN and the type of symptom will depend on the sensory fibers affected; small fiber damage will likely result in alterations to pain and temperature perception (Farquhar-Smith, 2011). The most frequent symptoms caused by chemotherapeutic agents that commonly produce CIPN (paclitaxel, vincristine, and cisplatin) are numbness, tingling, and burning. Symmetry, with a glove and stocking type of distribution, often characterizes the pattern of sensory loss, and symptoms should be temporally related to the chemotherapeutic agent administered (Farquhar-Smith, 2011). The severity of the sensory symptoms frequently increases as the dose increases. Other symptoms of CIPN can include motor weakness, in particular the distal muscle groups and side effects that are unrelated to the neuropathy itself, such as nausea, arthralgia, and fatigue.

1.4   CLINICAL FEATURES—EXAMINATION

1.4.1   NEUROPATHIC PAIN

A thorough examination of the painful area and full neurological examination are other key steps in the clinical assessment. Simple bedside tests can help distinguish neuropathic pain from nonneuropathic pain, although individually they have low power to differentiate between the two (Callin and Bennett, 2008). Examination of the painful area needs to be compared with findings in a control area, such as a contralateral limb in unilateral limb pain. If the pain is bilateral, then comparison may be made against proximal or distal sites to the painful area. Tactile, thermoreceptive, and nociceptive sensory loss corresponds to the type of somatosensory pathway that has been damaged. Positive phenomena, such as hyperalgesia, are usually limited to nociceptive somatosensory pathways, while tactile or thermosensory

TABLE 1.3
Neuropathic Pain Syndromes

Summary of Tools Assessing Sensory Functions

Fiber Type	Sensation	Clinical Testing Instrument
Aβ	Touch	Cotton wool or soft brush
	Vibration	Tuning fork (64 or 128 Hz)
Aδ	Pinprick, sharp pain	23G needle in 2 ml syringe
	Cold	Cold object (20°)
C	Warmth	Warm object (40°)

Source: Haanpää M, Treede R, *Diagnosis and Classification of Neuropathic Pain. Pain: Clinical Updates*, Vol. XVIII, Issue 7, Seattle: IASP Press, 2010.

pathways rarely, if ever, cause sensory gain (Maier et al., 2010). Hyperalgesia should be specified with respect to the stimulus modality to which the patient exhibits an exaggerated pain response (Haanpää and Treede, 2010). While there are dedicated stimulus devices such as brushes, algometers, and electrical and thermal probes, there are also simple bedside approaches. One example is a standardized method of testing for hyperalgesia using pinprick stimuli by removing the plunger from a 2 ml syringe, inserting a 23G needle, and applying an equal pressure to the test site and control site and comparing the respective responses (Callin and Bennett, 2008). Allodynia can be demonstrated by lightly brushing a piece of cotton wool over the site to distinguish from hyperalgesia (resulting from a painful stimulus). The production of pain or an unpleasant sensation in the affected area, but not the control site, demonstrates allodynia (Callin and Bennett, 2008). Other tools that assess sensory functions are listed in Table 1.3.

Identifying the cause of neuropathic pain is based on the history of an underlying or preceding condition or localizing the lesion or disease process affecting the somatosensory system. The required thorough neurological examination should cover the sensory and motor systems, tendon reflexes, and cranial nerves, mindful of signs that correspond to any known or suspected disease processes. Skin changes, vasomotor signs, and sudomotor function are also important.

1.4.2 CHEMOTHERAPY-INDUCED NEUROPATHIC PAIN

Pertinent examination features to CIPN vary according to the therapeutic agent used, but common signs include sensory loss or altered sensory perception, particularly to the distal parts of the limbs. Areas of hyperalgesia or allodynia, if present, can be assessed in the same fashion as other neuropathic pain signs. Muscle weakness and reduced or absent deep tendon reflexes have been confirmed with several chemotherapeutic agents.

1.5   ADDITIONAL TESTS AND INVESTIGATIONS

When the diagnosis of neuropathic pain is not straightforward, the history and examination may be supplemented by additional investigations. Peripheral polyneuropathies can be assessed further with electroneuromyography in association with a full blood count, erythrocyte sedimentation rate, glucose, creatinine, liver function tests, and vitamin B12. Nerve conduction studies and somatosensory-evoked potentials assess large myelinated nerve fibers that can confirm neuropathy, but further quantitative sensory testing provides a powerful tool to analyze small fibers such as Aδ and C fibers. Nerve compression and infiltration may be assessed using neuro-imaging, for example, magnetic resonance imaging. When clinically indicated, additional diagnostic tests may include skin biopsy and cerebrospinal fluid analyses.

REFERENCES

Bennett MI, Rayment C, Hjermstad M, Aass N, Caraceni A, Kaasa S. (2011). Prevalence and etiology of neuropathic pain in cancer patients: A systematic review. *Pain*, doi:10.1016/ j.pain.2011.10.028.

Callin S, Bennett MI. (2008). Assessment of neuropathic pain. *Contin Educ Anaesth Crit Care Pain* 8:210–13.

Cleeland CS, Farrar JT, Hausheer FH. (2010). Assessment of cancer-related neuropathy and neuropathic pain. *Oncologist* 15:13–18.

Dworkin RH. (2002). An overview of neuropathic pain: Syndromes, symptoms, signs, and several mechanisms. *Clin J Pain* 18:343–49.

Farquhar-Smith P. (2011). Chemotherapy-induced neuropathic pain. *Curr Opin Support Palliat Care* 5:1–7.

Haanpää M, Treede R. (2010). *Diagnosis and classification of neuropathic pain: Clinical updates*. Vol. XVIII, Issue 7. Seattle: IASP Press.

Kehlet H, Jensen TS, Woolf CS. (2006). Persistent postsurgical pain: Risk factors and prevention. *Lancet* 367:1618–25.

Maier C, Baron R, Tölle TR, Binder A, Birbaumer N, Birklein F, Gierthmühlen J, Flor H, Geber C, Huge V, Krumova EK, Landwehrmeyer GB, Magerl W, Maihöfner C, Richter H, Rolke R, Scherens A, Schwarz A, Sommer C, Tronnier V, Uçeyler N, Valet M, Wasner G, Treede RD. (2010). Quantitative sensory testing in the German Research Network on Neuropathic Pain (DFNS): Somatosensory abnormalities in 1236 patients with different neuropathic pain syndromes. *Pain* 150:439–50.

Martin LA, Hagen NA. (1997). Neuropathic pain in cancer patients: Mechanisms, syndromes, and clinical controversies. *J Pain Symptom Manage* 14:99–117.

Merksey H, Bogduk N. (1994). *Classification of chronic pain. Descriptions of chronic pain syndromes and definitions of pain terms*, 2nd ed. Seattle: IASP Press, p. 211.

Moya del Pino B. (2010). Chemotherapy-induced peripheral neuropathy. http://www.cancer.gov/ aboutnci/ncicancerbulletin/archive/2010/022310/page6 (accessed November 16, 2011).

Pachman DR, Barton DL, Watson JC, Loprinzi CL. (2011). Chemotherapy-induced peripheral neuropathy: Prevention and treatment. *Clin Pharmacol Ther* 90:377–87.

Treede RD, Jensen TS, Campbell JN, Cruccu G, Dostrovsky JO, Griffin JW, Hansson P, Hughes R, Nurmikko T, Serra J. (2008). Neuropathic pain: Redefinition and a grading system for clinical and research purposes. *Neurology* 70:1630–35.

Turk DC, Dworkin RH, Allen RR, Bellamy N, Brandenburg N, Carr DB, Cleeland C, Dionne R, Farrar JT, Galer BS, Hewitt DJ, Jadad AR, Katz NP, Kramer LD, Manning DC, McCormick CG, McDermott MP, McGrath P, Quessy S, Rappaport BA, Robinson JP, Royal MA, Simon L, Stauffer JW, Stein W, Tollett J, Witter J. (2003). Core outcome domains for chronic pain clinical trials: IMMPACT recommendations. *Pain* 106:337–45.

2 Assessment and Grading of Cancer Chemotherapy-Induced Neuropathic Pain

Judith A. Paice

CONTENTS

2.1 Introduction 11
2.2 Assessment of Chemotherapy-Induced Peripheral Neuropathy (CIPN) 12
2.3 Grading of CIPN... 12
2.4 Physical Examination and Neurophysiologic Evaluation 12
2.5 Future Solutions.. 15
References... 16

2.1 INTRODUCTION

Toxicities to chemotherapy are common and skilled oncologists are trained to prevent, identify, and manage these adverse effects in a timely fashion. Unfortunately, chemotherapy-induced peripheral neuropathy (CIPN) presents several unique challenges that complicate effective prevention, early detection, and management (Paice, 2011). Risk factors for CIPN, aside from obvious comorbidities such as age, alcoholism, and diabetes, remain poorly understood. Additionally, like other pain syndromes, there is no simple laboratory value that can be frequently measured and monitored to detect CIPN. As a result, patient report remains vital, and yet, many of the existing assessment tools fail to capture early changes and, in general, do not adequately describe the patient experience of CIPN. Furthermore, existing grading scales are not sensitive and are of little assistance in guiding treatment for individual patients or in providing aggregate data about the experience of those receiving a particular agent or regimen.

This presents an extremely difficult clinical conundrum that can have long-term negative consequences for patients receiving chemotherapy. Some of the patients who develop CIPN will recover without long-term effects. Many may forgo potentially curative anticancer therapy due to the presence and intensity of CIPN. Others will experience persistent, painful neuropathy that will significantly impair their quality of life. Either way, the burden for individuals already facing a life-threatening illness is unacceptable.

2.2 ASSESSMENT OF CHEMOTHERAPY-INDUCED PERIPHERAL NEUROPATHY (CIPN)

Early clinical trials of chemotherapeutic agents often underestimated the prevalence of CIPN, largely due to lack of systematic assessment. This is complicated by the use of physician or observer-based instruments, rather than patient-reported outcomes. Many of the tools initially used to measure CIPN were validated in populations of patients with diabetic or postherpetic neuropathy. Although some sensations are similar, significant differences exist in the experiences reported by these patients when compared to those with CIPN. In the past few years, numerous tools to assess CIPN have been developed (Cavaletti et al., 2003, 2006; Cella et al., 2003; Hausheer et al., 2006; Huang et al., 2007; Leonard et al., 2005; Oldenburg et al., 2006; Postma et al., 2005; Shimozuma et al., 2009; Smith et al., 2011), yet limitations regarding these instruments exist. A number of the tools employed are lengthy, leading to respondent fatigue, and are more useful in research settings rather than demonstrating feasibility as a clinical screening tool. Many of the instruments currently employed have not yet undergone rigorous validity testing. In an excellent review of existing assessment tools, Cavaletti and colleagues (Cavaletti et al., 2010) conclude that none of the currently available tools are satisfactory (see Table 2.1). They recommend that valid and reliable instruments be developed that are simple, responsive, reproducible, and meaningful.

2.3 GRADING OF CIPN

Grading scales are designed to establish the degree of a particular toxicity. These provide information to guide individual care (e.g., when to reduce the dose of a chemotherapeutic agent or switch to an alternate drug) and to compare various agents or regimens when evaluating safety in clinical trials. The most commonly employed grading scales are the National Cancer Institute Common Toxicity Criteria (NCI-CTC), Ajani Sensory Scale, World Health Organization (WHO) scale, and Eastern Cooperative Oncology Group (ECOG) scale (Table 2.2) (Ajani et al., 1990, Miller et al., 1981; Trotti et al., 2003). These are all physician-based grading scales, grading CIPN from grade 0 (normal) to 4 (severe) or 5 (death—NCI-CTC). One study asked two neurologists to grade the severity of CIPN in 37 patients using these four scales. There was disagreement 80% of the time, with large variability in the interpretation of these scales (Postma and Heimans, 2000). Other studies support the high rate of interobserver disagreement, calling into question the sensitivity of these scales.

2.4 PHYSICAL EXAMINATION AND NEUROPHYSIOLOGIC EVALUATION

Examination should characterize the area(s) affected, as well as changes in deep tendon reflexes. Motor weakness should be assessed with particular attention to

TABLE 2.1

Chemotherapy-Induced Peripheral Neuropathy Assessment Tools

Tool	Attributes
European Organization of Research and Treatment of Cancer (EORTC) QLQ-CIPN20	Quality of life with CIPN subscale evaluating symptoms and functional limitations
Functional Assessment of Cancer Therapy/Gynecologic Oncology Group (GOG)-neurotoxicity (FACT/GOG-Ntx)	Quality of life and functional impairment associated with neuropathy in women with gynecologic cancers
Functional Assessment of Cancer Therapy–Taxane (FACT-Taxane)	Quality of life and same Ntx subscale as above with additional questions devoted to arthralgias, myalgias, and skin discoloration
Oxaliplatin-Associated Neuropathy Questionnaire	Symptoms in both upper and lower extremities; validity not assessed
Patient Neurotoxicity Questionnaire (PNQ)	Evaluates motor and sensory symptoms, including functional impairment
Peripheral Neuropathy Scale (PNS)	Functional status and impairment, symptoms of peripheral neuropathy
Scale for Chemotherapy-Induced Long-Term Neurotoxicity (SCIN)	Three subscales that assess neuropathy, Reynaud's phenomenon, and ototoxicity
Total Neuropathy Score (TNS)	Includes sensory, motor, and autonomic symptoms, as well as vibration sense and reflexes; sural and peroneal nerve conduction; abbreviated versions available

Sources: Data from Cavaletti G. et al., *Neurology* 61:1297–12300, 2003; Cavaletti G. et al., *J Peripher Nerv Syst* 11:135–141, 2006; Cella D. et al., *Cancer* 98:822–831, 2003; Hausheer FH. et al., *Sem Oncol* 33:15–49, 2006; Huang HQ. et al., *Int J Gynecol Cancer* 17:387–393, 2007; Leonard GD. et al., *BMC Cancer* 5:116–125, 2005; Oldenburg J. et al., *Qual Life Res* 15:791–800, 2006; Postma TJ. et al., *Eur J Cancer* 41:1135–1139, 2005; Shimozuma K. et al., *Support Care Cancer* 17:1483–1491, 2009.

gait. Autonomic symptoms, including hypotension, constipation, and decreased sexual function, are often neglected but should be assessed (Gutiérrez-Gutiérrez et al., 2010). Interestingly, foot deformities may be predictive of the risk for developing neuropathies. These include high arches or flat feet, as well as hammertoes (Stubblefield et al., 2009).

Quantitative sensory testing (such as vibration perception threshold), electromyography (EMG), and nerve conduction studies (NCS) are used in the evaluation of neuropathies, although poor correlation exists between findings obtained from these studies and the intensity of CIPN. Several other obstacles exist to the use of these tests. Patients may be reluctant to have an invasive procedure (i.e., EMG). Additionally, the cost of many of these tests may not be reimbursed by third-party payers (Hausheer et al., 2006).

Any diagnostic measure employed must be sensitive, yet practical, and reliable, so that the results would be reproducible across practitioners and time points.

TABLE 2.2
Grading Scales Used to Evaluate Sensory Component of Chemotherapy-Induced Peripheral Neuropathy

	0	1	2	3	4	5
Ajani Sensory Scale[a]	Normal	Paresthesia, decreased deep tendon reflexes	Mild objective abnormality, absence of deep tendon reflexes, mild to moderate functional abnormality	Severe paresthesia, moderate objective abnormality, severe functional abnormality	Complete sensory loss, loss of function	
ECOG Sensory Scale[b]	Normal	Mild paresthesia, loss of deep tendon reflexes	Mild or moderate objective sensory loss, moderate paresthesia	Severe objective sensory loss of paresthesia that interferes with function		
NCI-CTC 4.03 Peripheral Sensory Neuropathy[c]		Asymptomatic, loss of deep tendon reflexes or paresthesia	Moderate symptoms limiting instrumental activities of daily living (ADL)	Severe symptoms limiting self-care ADL	Life-threatening consequences, urgent intervention indicated	Death
WHO Scale Neuropathy—Sensory[d]	Normal	Decreased tendon reflexes or paresthesia	Severe paresthesia	Intolerable paresthesia		

[a] Data from Ajani JA. et al., *Cancer Invest* 8:147–159, 1990.
[b] Data from Eastern Cooperative Oncology Group, http://ecog.dfci.harvard.edu/general/common_tox.html (accessed March 31, 2012).
[c] Data from CTCAE Files, http://evs.nci.nih.gov/ftp1/CTCAE/About.html (accessed March 31, 2012).
[d] Data from Miller AB. et al., *Cancer* 47:207–214, 1981.

The physical examination and neurologic evaluation must be sufficiently specific to differentiate CIPN from other neurologic disorders, as treatment decisions regarding potentially curative therapy may be made based upon the results of these measures.

2.5 FUTURE SOLUTIONS

Chemotherapy-induced peripheral neuropathy is a potentially devastating complication of cancer treatment. However, it is one of many adverse effects of therapy. Oncologists must review a wide array of potential toxicities, often while managing physical and emotional symptoms in people with complex oncologic syndromes. This review and assessment must take place during what is typically a 15- to 20-minute clinic visit. Further complicating this care is the limited training provided to oncologists regarding pain management (Breuer et al., 2011), compounded by the upcoming predicted shortage of physicians specializing in oncology (Erikson et al., 2007). To incorporate a thorough assessment of CIPN will provide significant challenges in time and manpower.

Optimally, neurologists would be consulted to screen all patients who are scheduled to receive potentially neurotoxic chemotherapy. This might allow identification of patients at risk along with a strong neurologic assessment of the individual's baseline functioning that could be tracked sequentially during treatment. Neurologists might best discern whether the symptoms are due to peripheral neuropathy or another neurologic syndrome (Windebank and Grisold, 2008). However, there are several barriers to this approach in our current healthcare system. In some circumstances, there is an urgency to begin chemotherapy as soon as possible. An example of this might be the newly diagnosed patient with multiple myeloma experiencing severe bone pain, as chemotherapy can be particularly effective in providing reduction in tumor burden with resultant analgesia. Availability of neurologists, particularly those interested in neuropathy, may be limited in some areas. Additionally, the added cost to the patient of seeing another specialist may be overwhelming.

Given these barriers, a reasonable approach would be the development of a simple screening toolkit that could be used in the oncology clinic to reliably identify and stratify risk of CIPN prior to initiating chemotherapy. The toolkit would include valid and reliable assessment tools that include patient-reported outcomes while guiding clinical assessment and physical examination. Stratification of risk would result from these findings. Those patients with moderate to severe risk could be referred to a neurologist for more extensive screening and evaluation. In some cases, the chemotherapeutic regimen could be altered, particularly in the adjuvant setting when several alternative courses of therapy are available. In other cases, the oncologist informed by the neurologist's findings may recommend a reduced dose or altered schedule of administration of a potentially neurotoxic agent.

For those patients where prevention and early detection are not feasible, and persistent CIPN results, management of pain, maintenance of safety, and preservation of function are essential. Collaboration between oncologists, neurologists, rehabilitation experts, pain and palliative care practitioners, and patients is necessary to enhance oncology outcomes and improve quality of life.

REFERENCES

Ajani JA, Welch SR, Raber MN, Fields WS, Krakoff IH. (1990). Comprehensive criteria for assessing therapy-induced toxicity. *Cancer Invest* 8:147–59.

Breuer B, Fleishman SB, Cruciani RA, Portenoy RK. (2011). Medical oncologists' attitudes and practice in cancer pain management: A national survey. *J Clin Oncol* 29:4769–75.

Cavaletti G, Bogliun G, Marzorati L, Zincone A, Piatti M, Colombo N, Parma G, Lissoni A, Fei F, Cundari S, Zanna C. (2003). Grading of chemotherapy-induced peripheral Neurotoxicity using the Total Neuropathy Scale. *Neurology* 61:1297–300.

Cavaletti G, Frigeni B, Lanzani F, Mattavelli L, Susani E, Alberti P, Cortinovis D, Bidoli P. (2010). Chemotherapy-induced peripheral neurotoxicity assessment: A critical revision of the currently available tools. *Eur J Canc* 46:479–94.

Cavaletti G, Jann S, Pace A, Plasmati R, Siciliano G, Briani C, Cocito D, Padua L, Ghiglione E, Manicone M, Giussani G; Italian NETox Group. (2006). Multi-center assessment of the Total Neuropathy Score for chemotherapy-induced peripheral neurotoxicity. *J Peripher Nerv Syst* 11:135–41.

Cella D, Peterman A, Hudgens S, Webster K, Socinski MA. (2003). Measuring the side effect of taxane therapy in oncology. *Cancer* 98:822–31.

Erikson C, Salsberg E, Forte G, Bruinooge S, Goldstein M. (2007). Future supply and demand for oncologists: Challenges to assuring access to oncology services. *J Onc Pract* 3:79–86.

Gutiérrez-Gutiérrez G, Sereno M, Miralles A, Casado-Sáenz E, Gutiérrez-Rivas E. (2010). Chemotherapy-induced peripheral neuropathy: Clinical features, diagnosis, prevention and treatment strategies. *Clin Transl Oncol* 12:81–91.

Hausheer FH, Schilsky RL, Bain S, Berghorn EJ, Lieberman F. (2006). Diagnosis, management, and evaluation of chemotherapy-induced peripheral neuropathy. *Sem Oncol* 33:15–49.

Huang HQ, Brady MF, Cella D, Fleming G. (2007). Validation and reduction of FACT/GOG-Ntx subscale for platinum/paclitaxel-induced neurologic symptoms: A Gynecologic Oncology Group Study. *Int J Gynecol Cancer* 17:387–93.

Leonard GD, Wright MA, Quinn MG, Fioravanti S, Harold N, Schuler B, Thomas RR, Grem JL. (2005). Survery of oxaliplatin-associated neurotoxicity using an interview-based questionnaire in patients with metastatic colorectal cancer. *BMC Cancer* 5:116–25.

Miller AB, Hoogstraten B, Staquest M, Winkler A. (1981). Reporting results of cancer treatment. *Cancer* 47:207–14.

Oldenburg J, Fossa SD, Dahl AA. (2006). Scale for chemotherapy-induced long-term neurotoxicity (SCIN): Psychometrics, validation and findings in a large sample of testicular cancer survivors. *Qual Life Res* 15:791–800.

Paice JA. (2011). Chronic treatment-related pain in cancer survivors. *Pain* 152:S84–89.

Postma TJ, Aaronson NK, Heimans JJ, Muller MJ, Hildebrand JG, Delattre JY, Hoang-Xuan K, Lantéri-Minet M, Grant R, Huddart R, Moynihan C, Maher J, Lucey R; EORTC Quality of Life Group. (2005). The development of an EORTC quality of life questionnaire to assess chemotherapy-induced peripheral neuropathy: The QLQ-CIPN20. *Eur J Cancer* 41:1135–39.

Postma TJ, Heimans JJ. (2000). Grading of chemotherapy-induced peripheral neuropathy. *Ann Oncol* 11:509–13.

Shimozuma K, Ohashi Y, Takeuchi A, Aranishi T, Morita S, Kuroi K, Ohsumi S, Makino H, Mukai H, Katsumata N, Sunada Y, Watanabe T, Hausheer FH. (2009). Feasibility and validity of the patient neurotoxicity questionnaire (PNQ) during taxane chemotherapy in a phase III randomized trial of breast cancer: N-SAS BC 2. *Support Care Cancer* 17:1483–91.

Smith EM, Cohen JA, Pett MA, Beck SL. (2011). The validity of neuropathy and neuropathic pain measures in patients with cancer receiving taxanes and platinums. *Oncol Nurs Forum* 38:133–42.

Stubblefield MD, Burstein HJ, Burton AW, Custodio CM, Deng GE, Ho M, Junck L, Morris GS, Paice JA, Tummala S, Von Roenn JH. (2009). NCCN task force report: Management of neuropathy in cancer. *J Natl Comprehensive Cancer Network* 7:S1–26.

Trotti A, Colevas AD, Setser A, Rusch V, Jaques D, Budach V, Langer C, Murphy B, Cumberlin R, Coleman CN, Rubin P. (2003). CTCAE v3.0: Development of a comprehensive grading system for the adverse effects of cancer treatment. *Semin Radiat Oncol* 13:176–81.

Windebank AJ, Grisold W. (2008). Chemotherapy-induced neuropathy. *J Periph Nerv Syst* 13:27–46.

3 Chemotherapy-Induced Peripheral Neuropathy
Review of Clinical Studies

Joseph V. Pergolizzi, Jr. and Jo Ann LeQuang

CONTENTS

3.1 Introduction 22
3.2 Platinum Agents..22
   3.2.1 Carboplatin 22
      3.2.1.1 Combination Therapies..22
      3.2.1.2 Comparative Studies 25
   3.2.2 Cisplatin..27
      3.2.2.1 Combination Therapies..27
      3.2.2.2 Comparative Studies 29
   3.2.3 Oxaliplatin 30
      3.2.3.1 Combination Therapies..30
      3.2.3.2 Comparative Studies 35
3.3 Taxanes 36
   3.3.1 Paclitaxel...36
      3.3.1.1 Monotherapies...37
      3.3.1.2 Combination Therapies..38
      3.3.1.3 Comparative Studies 39
      3.3.1.4 Nanoparticle Albumin-Bound (Nab) Paclitaxel..................40
   3.3.2 Docetaxel 42
      3.3.2.1 Monotherapies...42
      3.3.2.2 Combination Therapies..42
      3.3.2.3 Comparative Studies 43
3.4 Vinca Alkaloids...44
   3.4.1 Vincristine 45
   3.4.2 Vindesine 45
   3.4.3 Vinflunine 46
   3.4.4 Vinorelbine 46
      3.4.4.1 Monotherapy...46
      3.4.4.2 Combination Therapies..46
      3.4.4.3 Comparative Studies 48
3.5 Bortezomib 49
   3.5.1 Monotherapy 50

    3.5.2   Combination Therapies...50
            3.5.2.1   Bortezomib Combined with Thalidomide and
                      Dexamethasone...50
            3.5.2.2   Bortezomib, Cyclophosphamide, Thalidomide, and
                      Dexamethasone...51
            3.5.2.3   Bortezomib and Dexamethasone and Pegylated
                      Liposomal Doxorubicin 52
            3.5.2.4   Bortezomib and Vincristine, Dexamethasone,
                      Pegylated L-Asparaginase, and Doxorubicin 52
            3.5.2.5   Bortezomib and Dexamethasone with Romidepsin.............52
            3.5.2.6   Bortezomib and Rituximab 52
            3.5.2.7   Bortezomib and Rituximab and Cyclophosphamide
                      and Dexamethasone...53
            3.5.2.8   Bortezomib and Tanespimycin 53
            3.5.2.9   Bortezomib and Temsirolimus..54
            3.5.2.10 Bortezomib and Tipifarnib 54
            3.5.2.11 Bortezomib and Dexamethasone Combined with
                      Itraconazole or Lansoprazole..54
    3.5.3   Comparative Studies...55
            3.5.3.1   Bortezomib and Dexamethasone with and without
                      Thalidomide...55
            3.5.3.2   Thalidomide and Dexamethasone with and without
                      Bortezomib..55
            3.5.3.3   Bortezomib with Melphalan and Prednisone versus
                      Bortezomib with Thalidomide and Prednisone...................56
            3.5.3.4   Bortezomib and Dexamethasone versus Vincristine,
                      Doxorubicin, and Dexamethasone 56
            3.5.3.5   Bortezomib and Dexamethasone versus Vincristine,
                      Pirarubicin, Dexamethasone, and Melphalan.....................57
            3.5.3.6   Melphalan and Prednisone with and without Bortezomib 57
            3.5.3.7   Melphalan and Prednisone with and without Bortezomib 57
            3.5.3.8   Rituximab with and without Bortezomib 58
    3.5.4   Dosing Frequency of Bortezomib...59
    3.5.5   Subcutaneous Bortezomib 60
    3.5.6   Bortezomib in Special Populations 60
3.6 Thalidomide.. 61
    3.6.1   Monotherapies 61
    3.6.2   Combination Therapies..66
            3.6.2.1   Thalidomide and Dexamethasone....................................66
            3.6.2.2   Thalidomide and Dexamethasone and
                      Cyclophosphamide 67
            3.6.2.3   Thalidomide and Bortezomib...67
            3.6.2.4   Thalidomide and Melphalan and Dexamethasone 67
            3.6.2.5   Thalidomide and Melphalan and Lenalidomide and
                      Prednisone...68

3.6.2.6 Thalidomide and Bortezomib with Chemotherapy (Cisplatin, Cyclophosphamide, Etoposide, and Dexamethasone)......68

3.6.2.7 Thalidomide and Bortezomib with Epirubicin and Dexamethasone......68

3.6.2.8 Thalidomide and a Combination of Bortezomib, Melphalan, and Dexamethasone......69

3.6.2.9 Thalidomide and Capecitabine......69

3.6.2.10 Thalidomide and Cyclophosphamide 70

3.6.2.11 Thalidomide, Cyclophosphamide, and Dexamethasone......70

3.6.2.12 Thalidomide and Dacarbazine......71

3.6.2.13 Thalidomide and Fludarabine......71

3.6.2.14 Thalidomide and Granulocyte Macrophage-Colony Stimulating Factor (GM-CSF) 71

3.6.2.15 Thalidomide and Interleukin-2 Plus Granulocyte Macrophage-Colony Stimulating Factor (GM-CSF) 72

3.6.2.16 Thalidomide and Rituximab......73

3.6.2.17 Thalidomide and Semaxanib......73

3.6.2.18 Thalidomide and Vincristine with Pegylated Doxorubicin and Dexamethasone......73

3.6.3 Comparative Studies......74

3.6.3.1 Carboplatin with and without Thalidomide......74

3.6.3.2 Carboplatin and Gemcitabine with and without Thalidomide......74

3.6.3.3 Carboplatin and Epotoside with and without Thalidomide 75

3.6.3.4 Dexamethasone with and without Thalidomide 75

3.6.3.5 Thalidomide and Dexamethasone with and without Bortezomib......75

3.6.3.6 Thalidomide with and without Interferon......76

3.6.3.7 Thalidomide and Dexamethasone versus Interferon-Alpha and Dexamethasone as Maintenance Therapy 76

3.6.3.8 Melphalan and Prednisone with and without Thalidomide 77

3.6.3.9 Vincristine, Liposomal Doxorubicin, and Dexamethasone with and without Thalidomide 77

3.6.4 Single Nucleotide Polymorphisms and Thalidomide-Induced Peripheral Neuropathy 78

3.7 Lenalidomide......78

3.8 Suramin 79

3.8.1 Monotherapy......79

3.8.2 Combination Therapy 80

3.8.2.1 Suramin and Epirubicin......80

3.8.2.2 Suramin and Mitomycin C......80

3.9   Epothilones 80
       3.9.1   Monotherapies 80
       3.9.2   Combination Therapies.. 82
3.10 Conclusion 83
References.. 83

3.1   INTRODUCTION

Chemotherapy-induced peripheral neuropathy is one of the most common treatment-limiting side effects of cancer therapy. Strategies to prevent or limit chemotherapy-induced peripheral neuropathy have not been generally effective. While peripheral neuropathy might resolve partially or completely when treatment is stopped, some cases of chemotherapy-induced peripheral neuropathy are irreversible. Peripheral neuropathy has been associated with particular chemotherapeutic drugs or classes: platinum agents, taxanes, vinca alkaloids, bortezomib, thalidomide, lanilomide, suramin, and epothilones. Chemotherapy-induced peripheral neuropathy can be complex to analyze, in that there is considerable interpatient variability, the condition does not consistently appear to be dose dependent, and it may be mistaken for neurological deficits associated with the malignancy. This review of recent clinical trials highlights the agents known to be associated with peripheral neuropathy along with the rates of treatment-emergent peripheral neuropathy.

3.2   PLATINUM AGENTS

The platinum chemotherapeutic agents, carboplatin, cisplatin, and oxaliplatin, have a well-established association with treatment-emergent peripheral neuropathy. In some cases, the peripheral neuropathy is reversible or at least improves after therapy is completed. There is some evidence that oxaliplatin-induced, but not cisplatin-induced, peripheral neuropathy is dose dependent (Brouwers et al., 2009). Preliminary evidence suggests that platinum-induced neuropathy in the hands is more likely to resolve or improve than similar neuropathy in the feet (Brouwers et al., 2009).

3.2.1   CARBOPLATIN

Carboplatin was first introduced in the 1980s and like its parent compound, cisplatin, is a chemotherapeutic agent that interacts with DNA. Although newer platinum agents have been developed, interest in carboplatin remains because of its widespread use, in that it has demonstrated effectiveness and a relatively favorable tolerability profile.

3.2.1.1   Combination Therapies

3.2.1.1.1   Carboplatin and Paclitaxel

Numerous studies have reported on the safety and efficacy of carboplatin and paclitaxel combination therapy in treating a variety of cancers. Both carboplatin and paclitaxel are associated with chemotherapy-induced peripheral neuropathy.

Carboplatin-paclitaxel chemotherapy was evaluated in 27 patients with recurrent or metastatic head and neck cancer in a phase II trial (Ferrari et al., 2009). Patients were treated on a 21-day cycle with 175 mg/m^2 paclitaxel and carboplatin (area under the curve = 5) for a maximum of four cycles. Disease control rate was 51.8% (95% confidence interval, 32.0 to 71.3) and overall response rate was 25.9% (95% confidence interval, 11.1 to 46.3). Median overall survival was 8.0 months (range, 2 to 27 months) with 1-year survival of 30.5%. The median progression-free survival was 1.0 month (range, 0 to 14 months). Peripheral neuropathy grade 1 or 2 occurred in 33.3% of patients, while 3.7% had grade 3, and there were no cases of grade 4.

The optimal doublet regimen of platinum agents for chemotherapy in elderly patients with non-small-cell lung cancer has yet to be defined. In a phase II trial of 82 geriatric patients (age ≥ 70 years) with advanced non-small-cell lung cancer, patients were randomized to receive weekly therapy (70 mg/m^2 paclitaxel on days 1, 8, and 15 and carboplatin (area under the curve = 6) on day 1) or standard therapy (200 mg/m^2 paclitaxel and carboplatin (area under the curve = 6) on day 1 only) (Sakakibara et al., 2010). The overall response rate was 55% with a median progression-free survival time of 6.0 months for the weekly patients versus 53% and 5.6 months for standard patients. Peripheral neuropathy occurred in none of the weekly patients and 25% of the standard therapy patients. This evidence suggests that the weekly regimen is similarly effective but less toxic than the standard regimen for elderly patients with non-small-cell lung cancer.

Twenty-five patients with ovarian or endometrial cancer with venous thrombosis taking warfarin received chemotherapy in the form of carboplatin (area under the curve = 2) and 80 mg/m^2 paclitaxel on days 1, 8, and 15 of a 21-day cycle (Tabata et al., 2008). The total number of courses administered was 115, with an average of 4.6 cycles per patients. The overall response rate was 62%. After chemotherapy, 76% of patients saw resolution of their venous thrombosis. Peripheral neuropathy ≥ grade 3 occurred in 4% of patients ($n = 1$). Weekly low-dose carboplatin combined with paclitaxel was effective with good tolerability in this population.

In a clinical trial that evaluated the activity and safety of non-anthracycline-containing paclitaxel combined with carboplatin to treat 107 consecutive breast cancer patients (85.2% had an initial diagnosis of stage III), patients received four cycles of 80 mg/m^2 non-anthracycline-containing paclitaxel and carboplatin (area under the curve = 2) on days 1, 8, and 15 of a 4-week cycle (Chen, Nie et al., 2010). The clinical response rate was 86.1% (complete response occurred in 32.4%). Peripheral neuropathy occurred in nearly half of the patients (47.7%) but was never more severe than grade 2. This suggests that non-anthracycline-containing paclitaxel combined with carboplatin is an effective and well-tolerated neoadjuvant therapy for breast cancer.

3.2.1.1.2 Carboplatin and Paclitaxel with Pegfilgrastim

Pegfilgrastim is the pegylated form of the recombinant human granulocyte colony stimulating factor (GCSF) analog filgrastim. Pegfilgrastam can be used to stimulate bone marrow to produce neutrophils that may help fight infections in chemotherapy patients and, as a result, may be used prophylactically in patients to allow for more aggressive chemotherapy regimens. In a phase I study of 43 patients with untreated stage III or IV epithelial ovarian (fallopian) tubal or primary peritoneal cancer, patients were treated with six 14-day cycles of carboplatin (area under the curve = 5) and 175 mg/m^2 paclitaxel on day 1 and 6 mg pegfilgrastim on day 2 (Tiersten et al., 2010). The overall response rate was 58%, and peripheral neuropathy ≥ grade 2 occurred in 30% of patients. Twelve patients (28%) discontinued treatment because of toxicities, including thrombocytopenia, supraventricular tachycardia, and neuropathy. While dose-dense carboplatin and paclitaxel appear to be effective from this study, the dose-limiting toxicities in six cycles, even with pegfilgrastim, preclude its clinical utility.

3.2.1.1.3   Carboplatin and Paclitaxel and Trastuzumab

Trastuzumab is a monoclonal antibody that interferes with the human epidermal growth factor receptor 2 (HER2 receptor), sometimes called the HER2/neu receptor. The HER2 gene becomes overexpressed or amplified in about 20 to 30% of patients with early-stage breast cancers. In a study of 32 patients with HER2-amplified metastatic breast cancer, patients were treated with 100 mg/m^2 albumin-bound paclitaxel and carboplatin (area under the curve = 2) on days 1, 8, and 15 of a 28-day treatment cycle. Trastuzumab was administered at 2 mg/kg weekly after a loading dose of 4 mg/kg. Hypersensitivity reactions in 4 of the first 13 patients caused the protocol to be amended, so that carboplatin was dosed at area under the curve = 6 on day 1 of each 28-day cycle. Patients were treated with six cycles and then could continue with all three drugs or only trastuzumab, if they were free of progression or if toxicity was unacceptable. The overall response rate was 62.5% (95% confidence interval, 45.7 to 79.3%), with 9% complete response. In this study, 13% of patients developed peripheral neuropathy (grades 2 and 3 only). Patients who received carboplatin every 4 weeks had a lower rate of peripheral neuropathy (3%) than those who received carboplatin weekly. While it appears that the dosing regimen of carboplatin at once every 4 weeks reduced hypersensitivity reactions and peripheral neuropathy rates (and resulted in similar antitumor activity rates), the study was not designed to evaluate the dosing regimens of carboplatin and should not be interpreted in that way.

3.2.1.1.4   Carboplatin Combined with Docetaxel and Trastuzumab

It was hypothesized from preclinical findings that there might be a synergistic benefit to combining trastuzumab with docetaxel and carboplatin for the treatment of breast cancer. In a human trial investigating the addition of carboplatin to a chemotherapeutic regimen of docetaxel and trastuzumab, 263 HER2-gene-amplified metastatic breast cancer patients received eight 21-day cycles of 100 mg/m^2 trastuzumab plus docetaxel (TH) or trastuzumab plus carboplatin (area under the curve = 2) and docetaxel 75 mg/m^2 (TCH). There was no significant difference between study arms in times to progression (median times were 11.1 months for TH and 10.4 months for TCH) or overall survival rates (37.1 versus 37.4 months, respectively). However, sensory neuropathy ≥ grade 3 occurred in 3% of TH versus 0.8% of TCH patients, although other adverse events (thrombocytopenia, anemia, fatigue, and diarrhea) were more common in TCH patients. The addition of carboplatin to trastuzumab and docetaxel appeared in this study not to improve efficacy.

3.2.1.1.5 Carboplatin and Thalidomide

Forty patients with stage Ic-IV ovarian cancer in a phase II trial received carboplatin (area under the curve = 7) intravenously every 4 weeks for up to six doses and were randomized as to whether or not they would also receive 100 mg oral thalidomide daily for 6 months (Muthuramalingam et al., 2011). The overall response rate at median follow-up duration of 1.95 years was 90% for carboplatin only and 75% for carboplatin-thalidomide ($p = 0.41$). Combination therapy patients exhibited more adverse events, including constipation, tiredness, dizziness, and peripheral neuropathy. While both treatments were effective, the combination of carboplatin and thalidomide increased side effects.

3.2.1.2 Comparative Studies

3.2.1.2.1 Carboplatin and Paclitaxel versus Carboplatin and Pegylated Doxorubicin

Carboplatin combined with paclitaxel has been a standard of care for patients with platinum-sensitive relapsed ovarian cancer. A newer therapy combines carboplatin with liposomal doxorubicin, which has been associated with less toxicity than paclitaxel. The CALYPSO study compared the safety and efficacy of pegylated liposomal doxorubicin and carboplatin (CD) to the standard treatment of carboplatin and paclitaxel (CP) in 976 patients with histologically proven ovarian cancer with recurrence more than 6 months after first- or second-line platinum/taxane therapy (Pujade-Lauraine et al., 2010). Patients in the CD group received carboplatin (area under the curve = 5) plus 30 mg/m^2 pegylated doxorubicin every 4 weeks. Patients in the CP group received carboplatin (area under the curve = 5) plus 175 mg/m^2 paclitaxel every 3 weeks. Patients were treated with at least six cycles. At median follow-up of 22 months, progression-free survival was 11.3 months for CD patients compared to 9.4 months for CP patients (hazard ratio, 0.821; 95% confidence interval, 0.72 to 0.94; $p = 0.005$). Sensory neuropathy occurred in 26.9% of CP patients versus 4.9% of CD patients. In a retrospective analysis of the CALYPSO study, investigators used multivariate analyses to determine whether chemotherapy-induced sensory neuropathy following CP versus CD therapy was associated with progression-free survival durations (Lee et al., 2011). For CP patients, there was a significant association between the presence of neuropathy and longer disease-free progression times. The median disease-free progression period was 11.5 months for CP patients with sensory neuropathy versus 10.1 months for those without sensory neuropathy (hazard ratio, 0.77; 95% confidence interval, 0.62 to 0.95; $p = 0.02$). However, in the CD patients, there was no significant difference in disease-free progression duration for patients with or without neuropathy (12.1 months versus 11.9 months, respectively; 95% confidence interval, 0.72 to 1.40; $p = 0.97$). Of all patients who did not develop sensory neuropathy, the benefits of CD versus CP were significantly greater (hazard ratio, 0.70; 95% confidence interval, 0.58 to 0.84; $p < 0.0001$), but there was no such difference among those with neuropathy (hazard ratio, 0.96; 95% confidence interval, 0.67 to 1.36; $p = 0.81$). This substudy also found that chemotherapy-induced leukopenia, as well as sensory neuropathy, was associated with improved prognosis in platinum-sensitive recurrent ovarian cancer patients treated with CP. Moreover, worsening chemotherapy-induced sensory neuropathy with CP in this population was associated with a 24% risk reduction in disease progression. While reasons underlying this remain unclear, this prognostic effect did not apply to patients treated with CD. It may be that patients with less toxicity have an insufficient drug exposure that, in certain chemotherapeutic regimens at least, manifests as a lack of sensory neuropathy. Further study is needed, but this at least suggests that toxicity-adjusted dosing may be a strategy to individualize chemotherapy for recurrent ovarian cancer.

3.2.1.2.2 Carboplatin and Paclitaxel as Maintenance Therapy

In a trial of 542 patients with stage Ia/b (grade 3 or clear cell) completely resected high-risk, early-stage ovarian cancer, intravenous carboplatin and pacli-taxel (175 mg/m^2 on day 1 of 21-day cycle, three cycles) were administered and patients were randomized to receive maintenance low-dose paclitaxel for 24 weeks (40 mg/m^2/week) or be observed without maintenance therapy (Mannel et al., 2011). The cumulative probability of the cancer recurring within 5 years was 20% for the pacl-itaxel maintenance group versus 23% for the control group (hazard ratio, 0.807; 95% confidence interval, 0.565 to 1.15), with 5-year survival rates of 85.4% versus 86.2%, respectively. Thus, maintenance paclitaxel added to standard carboplatin-paclitaxel chemotherapy conferred no significant increase in recurrence-free interval, but did worsen side effects. Peripheral neuropathy ≥ grade 2 occurred in 15.5% of paclitaxel maintenance patients versus 6% of control patients ($p < 0.001$).

3.2.1.2.3 Carboplatin and Paclitaxel with or without Trastuzumab

Patients with stage IIa/IIb breast cancer were treated with carboplatin (area under the curve = 6) every 4 weeks and 80 mg/m^2 paclitaxel weekly for 16 weeks; trastu-zumab weekly was added for patients with HER2-positive status (Sikov et al., 2009). Of the 55 patients enrolled, 43 had resectable disease; in these patients, the pathologic complete response rate was 45% (95% confidence interval, 28 to 58%). Patients with HER2-positive tumors exhibited higher pathologic complete response rates (76% versus 31% for HER2-negative tumors, $p = 0.003$). Pathologic complete response was higher in patients with estrogen-receptor-negative tumors (75% versus 27%, $p = 0.001$) and with triple-negative tumors (67% versus 12%, $p = 0.002$). At a median of 28 months following surgical resection, the recurrence-free survival rate was 88.7%. Of all patients, 3.6% developed peripheral neuropathy ≥ grade 3.

3.2.1.2.4 Carboplatin or Paclitaxel Plus Belinostat

Belinostat is a novel hydroxamic acid-type histone deacetylase (HDAC) inhibitor observed to have antineoplastic activity. Belinostat targets HDAC enzymes, which in turn inhibit tumor cell proliferation, induce apoptosis, promote cellular differen-tiation, and inhibit angiogenesis. A phase I study designed to evaluate dose-limiting toxicities of belinostat combined with carboplatin or paclitaxel enrolled 23 patients (Lassen et al., 2010). Maximum doses were 1,000 mg/m^2 belinostat per day for days 1 through 5, and on day 3, patients received carboplatin (area under the curve =5) or 175 mg/m^2 paclitaxel. Investigators observed that the pharmacokinetic properties of the agents were not affected by their concurrent administration. Overall, there was a

9% partial response rate and one patient (4%) showed a complete CA-125 response. Peripheral neuropathy ≥ grade 3 occurred in 9% of patients.

3.2.2 Cisplatin

Cisplatin is associated with a relatively high rate of peripheral neuropathy that appears to be related to the total cumulative dose. Neuroprotection may be conferred by vitamin E supplementation, which was shown to reduce the relative risk of neurotoxicity in cisplatin chemotherapy, in terms of both incidence and severity (Pace et al., 2010).

3.2.2.1 Combination Therapies

3.2.2.1.1 Cisplatin and Docetaxel

Esophageal cancer is a relatively common cancer with a 5-year survival rate of 16%. Many patients present with unresectable or metastatic disease and have a poor prognosis. In a study of 38 male patients with metastatic or recurrent esophageal squamous cell carcinoma previously treated with 5-fluorouracil and cisplatin chemotherapy or chemoradiotherapy, patients were administered 70 mg/m^2 docetaxel and 75 mg/m^2 cisplatin intravenously for 1 hour on day 1 of a 21-day cycle. In this study, the median number of cycles delivered was 3.5 (range, 1 to 9). The overall response rate was 34.2% (95% confidence interval, 19.6 to 51.3%), with 2.6% ($n = 1$) achieving complete response. The median progression-free survival time was 4.5 ± 1.3 months (95% confidence interval, 4.1 to 4.9%) and the overall survival times were 7.4 ± 0.4 months (95% confidence interval, 7.3 to 7.5 months). Six patients (15.8%) developed peripheral neuropathy ≥ grade 3.

3.2.2.1.2 Cisplatin and Paclitaxel

While both paclitaxel and cisplatin are known to have dose-limiting toxicities in high-dose monotherapeutic chemotherapy, investigators conducted a 10-year follow-up of a phase II dose-intense study combining cisplatin and paclitaxel in an effort to analyze, among other things, the potential of this combination for additive toxicity (Sarosy et al., 2010). Sixty-two patients with newly diagnosed, advanced-stage epithelial ovarian cancer were enrolled and received a dose-intense chemotherapy: 750 mg/m^2 cyclophosphamide followed by a 24-hour infusion of 250 mg/m^2 paclitaxel and 75 mg/m^2 cisplatin on day 2 and 10 µg/kg filgrastim on day 3 in a total of six 9-day cycles. Complete remission occurred in 89% of patients; median progression-free survival was 18.9 months with median survival 5.4 years. Peripheral neuropathy developed in most patients: rates of peripheral neuropathy were 37% grade 1, 31% grade 2, 19% grade 3, and no cases of grade 4. Improvement in neuropathy was observed when paclitaxel was decreased or discontinued; this is counterintuitive, as it might have been assumed that peripheral neuropathy would be more closely associated with cisplatin. Neuropathy resolved in 41% of patients at a median time of 11 months (range, 3 to 36) after treatment stopped. Peripheral neuropathy and other toxicities were not exacerbated by the combination of cisplatin and paclitaxel relative to the monotherapeutic use of these agents.

In a study of 47 outpatients with epithelial ovarian carcinoma, patients received 100 mg/m² intraperitoneal cisplatin combined with 175 mg/m² intravenous paclitaxel in a 3-hour infusion administered every 21 days (Chin et al., 2009). Patients received a total of 238 intraperitoneal/intravenous therapy cycles with six cycles as median (range, 1 to 6). Peripheral neuropathy occurred in 57% of patients and was ≥ grade 3 in 9%. Patients were followed 9 to 30 months and at last follow-up, residual peripheral neuropathy was reported in 41% ($n = 11$) of the patients who reported neuropathy during the study. Of the 11 patients with residual peripheral neuropathy at last follow-up, 6 (54.5%) had received six cycles of treatment.

In a study of 49 advanced gastric and gastroesophageal cancer patients, 100 mg/m² paclitaxel was administered intravenously for 1 hour on days 1 and 8 of a 21-day cycle; 30 mg/m² cisplatin was also administered along with a program of forced diuresis that included at least 2,000 ml of fluids following paclitaxel infusion over 30 minutes on days 1 and 8 (Sun et al., 2009). Patients received up to nine cycles. The overall response rate was 42.9% (95% confidence interval, 29.0 to 56.8%), median time to progression was 5.9 months (range, 1.6 to 9.1), and overall survival was 11.2 months (range, 6.1 to 21.3). Grade 3 peripheral neuropathy occurred in 4.3% of patients.

3.2.2.1.3   Cisplatin and Paclitaxel Plus Etoposide

In a phase II study of 63 patients with previously untreated limited-stage, small-cell lung cancer, patients were treated with four cycles of chemotherapy (Horn et al., 2009). In cycles 1 and 2, patients were administered 170 mg/m² paclitaxel intravenously on day 1, 80 mg/m² etoposide intravenously on days 1 through 3, and 60 mg/m² cisplatin intravenously on day 1, followed by 5 μg/kg filgrastim subcutaneously on days 4 through 13. Cycles 3 and 4 reduced paclitaxel to 135 mg/m² on day 1, maintained the same doses of etoposide and cisplatin, and applied 1.8 Gy concurrent thoracic radiation therapy in 35 fractions (total 63 Gy) over 7 weeks. The overall response rate was 79% and 1-year survival was 64%. Median overall survival was 15.7 months, with median progression-free survival of 8.6 months. Fourteen percent of patients developed grade 3 peripheral neuropathy. The investigators stated that compared to historical control studies, this particular combination of cisplatin, etoposide, and paclitaxel with concurrent, delayed radiation therapy offered no survival advantages.

3.2.2.1.4   Cisplatin and Paclitaxel Plus 5-Fluorouracil

Forty-six patients with advanced or recurrent and inoperable gastric cancer were treated in 28-day cycles with weekly 60 mg/m² paclitaxel on days 1, 8, and 15 combined with 500 mg/m² 5-fluorouracil by continuous intravenous infusion on days 1 through 5, and 75 mg/m² intravenous cisplatin for 3 days (Gu et al., 2009). The overall response rate was 50.0% (95% confidence interval, 34.9 to 65.1%), with median progression-free survival of 24 weeks and overall survival of 46 weeks. The 1-year survival rate of patients in this study was 41.3% (95% confidence interval, 27.0 to 56.8%). Peripheral neuropathy grade 1 occurred in 15.2% of patients, while grade 2 occurred in 6.5%. There were no cases of more severe peripheral neuropathy.

In a phase II study of this same chemotherapeutic combination, 41 patients with histologically confirmed metastatic gastric adenocarcinoma were treated with 175 mg/m² paclitaxel and 75 mg/m² cisplatin as a 1-hour infusion on day 1, followed by 750 mg/m^2 5-fluorouracil as a 24-hour continuous infusion for 5 days in a 21-day cycle (Hwang et al., 2008). About 30 minutes before the paclitaxel infusion, patients were given 20 mg dexamethasone, 50 mg ranitidine, and 5 mg chlorpheniramine maleate intravenously to help prevent hypersensitivity reactions. The cisplatin dose was reduced to 75% of the original dose in the next cycle if any of these conditions were met: patients had grade 3 neutropenia or infection, grade 4 neutropenia, grade 3 thrombocytopenia with bleeding that required platelet transfusion, any sensory neurotoxicity greater than grade 3, or nephrotoxicity greater than grade 2. If further such reactions occurred, then the paclitaxel dose was reduced to 75% of the original dose in the next cycle. The overall response rate was 51.2% (95% confidence interval, 35 to 67), with a median response duration of 23 weeks. Grade 1 or 2 peripheral neuropathy occurred in 72% of patients, peripheral neuropathy grade 3 occurred in 5% ($n = 2$), and there we no cases of grade 4.

3.2.2.2 Comparative Studies

3.2.2.2.1 *Liposomal Cisplatin versus Cisplatin in Combination with Paclitaxel*

Liposomal cisplatin is a novel agent developed to help reduce systemic toxicities associated with conventional cisplatin. It was hypothesized that liposomal cisplatin might improve targeting of the drug to the primary tumor and metastases by increasing its circulation time in the body fluids. In a phase III study of 236 chemotherapy-naïve patients with inoperable non-small-cell lung cancer, patients were randomized to receive either 200 mg/m^2 liposomal cisplatin with 135 mg/m^2 paclitaxel (arm A) or 75 mg/m^2 cisplatin and 135 mg/m^2 paclitaxel (arm B) once every 2 weeks (Stathopoulos et al., 2010). All therapy was administered on an outpatient basis. Both treatment regimens were similarly effective. Arms A and B exhibited no significant difference in median survival times (9 and 10 months, respectively) and time to progression (6.5 and 6 months, respectively). Grade 1 or 2 neurotoxicity occurred in 44.7% of arm A and 50.4% of arm B patients, while grade 3 neurotoxicity occurred in 0.9% of arm A and 4.3% of arm B; there were no cases of grade 4 neurotoxicity. This study suggests that liposomal cisplatin is not superior to conventional cisplatin in terms of efficacy, but found that it may be better tolerated in terms of nephrotoxicity. In terms of neurotoxicity, there was no statistically significant difference between study arms.

3.2.2.2.2 *Cisplatin versus Carboplatin in Combination with Paclitaxel*

Non-small-cell lung cancer often presents in geriatric patients. In a randomized phase II clinical trial, cisplatin was compared to carboplatin in combination with paclitaxel for the treatment of non-small-cell lung cancer in 81 patients ≥ 70 years of age (Chen et al., 2006). All patients received 160 mg/m^2 paclitaxel on day 1 of a 21-day cycle and patients were randomized to also receive either carboplatin (area under the curve = 6) on day 1 or 60 mg/m^2 cisplatin on day 1. A total of 152 carboplatin-paclitaxel chemotherapeutic cycles compared to 172 cycles of cisplatin-paclitaxel were administered in this study. The median number of cycles per patient was four in both study arms. Overall response rates were similar, namely, 40% for carboplatin-paclitaxel versus 39% for cisplatin-paclitaxel; each study arm had one patient with a complete response. However, peripheral neuropathy occurred significantly more often in the cisplatin-paclitaxel arm ($p = 0.017$) along with alopecia and fatigue. Median times to disease progression were 6.6 months (carboplatin-paclitaxel arm) and 6.9 months (cisplatin-paclitaxel arm), and median survival times were 10.3 and 10.5 months, respectively. In this geriatric population, carboplatin and paclitaxel were effective and associated with lower toxicity than cisplatin and paclitaxel, particularly in terms of significantly reduced rates of peripheral neuropathy.

3.2.3 OXALIPLATIN

Oxaliplatin is a platinum compound used in chemotherapeutic applications that was first discovered in 1976 but not approved in the United States by the Food and Drug Administration until 2002. Oxaliplatin is frequently combined with fluorouracil and leucovorin in a chemotherapeutic regimen called FOLFOX, known to be effective in the treatment of colorectal cancers. Oxaliplatin-induced neuropathy is common and often includes a sensitivity to cold.

3.2.3.1 COMBINATION THERAPIES

3.2.3.1.1 Oxaliplatin and 5-Fluorouracil and Leucovorin (FOLFOX)

The chemotherapeutic regimen known as FOLFOX (infusional 5-fluorouracil and leucovorin with oxaliplatin) is a standard chemotherapy regimen for patients with pretreated colorectal cancer. FOLFOX regimens are sometimes designated FOLFOX4, FOLFOX6, FOLFOX7, and so on, in which the final numeral designates which variation of the FOLFOX protocol is used. FOLFOX4, for example, uses a 22-hour infusion of 5-fluorouracil, while FOLFOX6 uses a 46-hour infusion. Patients who receive FOLFOX4 therapy must visit the hospital twice weekly. These treatment regimens are well established for colorectal cancers.

FOLFOX6 potentially offers greater convenience to patients than other FOLFOX protocols, in that it requires a hospital visit once every other week. In a study of 49 metastatic colorectal cancer patients who failed to respond to first-line chemotherapy, patients were administered 100 mg/m^2 oxaliplatin, 200 mg/m^2 1-leucovorin intravenously over 2 hours, followed by a bolus of 400 mg/m^2 intravenous 5-fluorouracil with a 46-hour infusion of 2,400 mg/m^2 of the same (FOLFOX6) (Kato et al., 2011). The response rate was 14.3% (95% confidence interval, 5.9 to 27.2%); overall survival was 11.4 months. The rate of peripheral neuropathy ≥ grade 3 was 41.2%. Investigators reported that FOLFOX6 has an acceptable safety and efficacy profile for pretreated colorectal patients.

FOLFOX6 was the subject of a multicenter trial that compared toxicities in younger versus older patients. Adverse events were examined retrospectively in 14 non-elderly patients (age < 70 years) and 8 similar but older patients (age ≥ 70 years) with unresectable advanced or recurrent colorectal therapy who had received FOLFOX6 therapy (Sugimoto et al., 2009). The most frequent adverse events in elderly patients were neutropenia grade ≥ 3 (62.5%) and peripheral neuropathy ≥ grade 1 (87.5%). Younger patients had a lower rate of neutropenia grade ≥ 3 (28.6%) and a similar rate of peripheral neuropathy ≥ grade 1 (86.4%), both of which were not statistically significant. From this study, it appears that the risk of peripheral neuropathy in FOLFOX6 chemotherapy is not exacerbated by advanced age.

In a study of 46 geriatric patients (age ≥ 65 years) with advanced gastric cancer, patients were administered first-line FOLFOX6 therapy (85 mg/m^2 oxaliplatin intravenously over 2 hours on day 1, together with 400 mg/m^2 leucovorin over 2 hours, followed by a 46-hour infusion of 2,600 mg/m^{2}5-fluorouracil) every 2 weeks (Zhao et al., 2009). Patients received a median of seven cycles. Overall response rate was 45.6% (95% confidence interval, 31 to 61%). Median time to progression was 6.2 months (range, 4.6 to 7.8 months) and median overall survival was 9.8 months (range, 8.2 to 11.4). Peripheral neuropathy was observed in 43.5% of patients, and was never more severe than grade 2. This study further adds to the evidence that FOLFOX6 therapy, in particular with relatively low doses of oxaliplatin, is effective and well tolerated in older gastric cancer patients.

Since FOLFOX therapies in general have been associated with relatively high rates of peripheral neuropathy, a study randomized 27 patients with colorectal cancer to receive FOLFOX4 adjuvant chemotherapy and either 1,500 mg/m^2 glutathione (GSH) or saline before the oxaliplatin infusion to investigate whether or not GSH affected the pharmacokinetics of the drugs used and, moreover, if GSH conferred any neuroprotective effect (Milla et al., 2009). The GSH regimen showed no statistically significant difference in the main pharmacokinetic parameters of the two regimens except for the area under the plasma concentration-time curve and a smaller steady-state volume of distribution with GSH. Investigators reported that this difference might be explained by the natural function of GSH in detoxifying oxaliplatin and its ability to remove platinum-bound plasma proteins. At the conclusion of therapy, GSH patients had significantly less neurotoxicity than the placebo ($p = 0.0037$). This study suggests that coadminstration of GSH may reduce oxaliplatin-induced neurotoxicity without adversely impacting the pharmacokinetics of oxaliplatin.

3.2.3.1.2   FOLFOX and Erlotinib

In a study of therapy for previously untreated, advanced, or metastatic esophagus or gastroesophgaeal junction cancer, 33 patients were treated with 85 mg/m^2 oxaliplatin and 400 mg/m^2 leucovorin (LV) on day 1, then 2,400 mg/m^2 5-fluorouracil (FU) over 48 hours, and then 150 mg oral erlotinib daily in a 14-day treatment cycle. The objective response rate for therapy was 51.5% (95% confidence interval, 34.5 to 68.6%), with 6% achieving a complete response (Wainberg et al., 2011). Eight percent of patients had peripheral neuropathy grade ≥ 3.

3.2.3.1.3   FOLFOX and Gemcitabine

Gemcitabine is a nucleoside analog approved as monotherapy for the treatment of pancreatic cancer. Although gemcitabine chemotherapy improves both survival and quality of life, research is ongoing to find combination therapeutic regimens for pancreatic cancer that may be more effective and better tolerated. Forty-five patients with advanced pancreatic carcinoma were administered oxaliplatin, infusional fluorouracil, and leucovorin combined with gemcitabine (Ch'ang et al., 2009). Patients were treated every 2 weeks with fixed-dose rates of 10 mg/m^2/minute infusion of 800 mg/m² gemcitabine, followed by a 2-hour infusion of 85 mg/m² oxaliplatin and then a 48-hour infusion of 3,000 mg/m² fluorouracil and 300 mg/m² leucovorin. Patients received a median of seven cycles. The overall response rate was 33.3% (95% confidence interval, 4 to 48.0%), and the disease control rate was 68.9% (95% confidence interval, 54.8 to 83.0%). Median time to tumor progression was 5.1 months (range, 4.0 to 6.3) and overall survival rate was 8.7 months (range, 6.1 to 11.3). Peripheral sensory neuropathy grade 3 occurred in 15.6% of patients; there were no instances of grade 4 neuropathy.

3.2.3.1.4   Oxaliplatin and Gemcitabine and Fluoropyramidine S-1

Twenty-two patients with advanced pancreatic cancer refractory to gemcitabine and oral fluoropyrimidine S-1 received second- or third-line chemotherapy (82% and 18%, respectively) of 1,000 mg/m² gemcitabine over 30 minutes and 85 mg/m² oxaliplatin over 120 minutes on days 1 and 15 of a 15-day cycle repeated every 4 weeks (Isayama et al., 2011) The disease control rate was 59%, but tumor response did not occur in any of the patients. Median overall survival and time to progression were 6.8 months (95% confidence interval, 2.8 to 11.5 months) and 2.6 months (95% confidence interval, 1.5 to 3.8 months), respectively. The most frequent adverse events ≥ grade 3 were anorexia (23%), peripheral neuropathy (14%), and neutropenia (14%).

3.2.3.1.5   Oxaliplatin and Gemcitabine and Cetuximab

There is no standard palliative chemotherapy for patients with biliary tract cancer. Investigators evaluated 30 patients with unresectable locally advanced or metastatic biliary tract cancer to be treated for 12 14-day cycles of 500 mg/m² intravenous cetuximab on day 1, 1,000 mg/m² gemcitabine on day 1, and 100 mg/m² oxaliplatin on day 2 (Gruenberger et al., 2010). The objective response rate was 63% (95% confidence interval, 46.2 to 59.8%), with complete response in 10% (range, 3.2 to 16.8). In nine patients (30%), their response to chemotherapy allowed them to undergo potentially curative secondary resection. Peripheral neuropathy occurred in 13% of patients.

3.2.3.1.6   Oxaliplatin and Gemcitabine and Bevacizumab

Bevacizumab is a humanized, monoclonal antibody that inhibits vascular endothelial growth factor A and blocks angiogenesis. In a phase II study of 35 patients with advanced biliary tract cancer, patients were administered a 28-day cycle chemotherapy regimen consisting of 10 mg/kg bevacizumab followed by 1,000 mg/m² gemcitabine (10 mg/m² per minute) and 85 mg/m² oxaliplatin (2-hour infusion) on days 1 and 15 (Zhu et al., 2010). Median progression-free survival was 7.0 months (95% confidence interval, 5.3 to 10.3 months). Fourteen percent of patients developed peripheral neuropathy ≥ grade 3.

3.2.3.1.7   Oxaliplatin and Doxorubicin

Treatment of hepatocellular carcinoma is often limited by the underlying hepatic disease or intrahepatic dissemination of the tumor. Monotherapy with doxorubicin, a topoisomerase II inhibitor, has not been particularly effective in patients with inoperable hepatocellular cancers. However, it was hypothesized that doxorubicin combination therapy might be effective. In a phase II study of 40 patients with inoperable metastatic hepatocellular cancer, patients received 130 mg/m^2 intravenous oxaliplatin over a 2-hour infusion and then received 60 mg/m^2 intravenous doxorubicin over a 30-minute infusion on day 1 of a 21-day cycle (Uhm et al., 2009). A total of 82 treatment cycles were administered in this study for a median of 2 cycles per patient (range, 1 to 6). The overall response rate was 15.6% (95% confidence interval, 3.3 to 28.7%), with 1-year survival of 29.4% (95% confidence interval, 13.6 to 45.2%). The median progression-free survival was 12 weeks (95% confidence interval, 5 to 19 weeks). Grade 1 peripheral neuropathy occurred in 22.5% of patients, and 2.5% ($n = 1$) had grade 3 peripheral neuropathy, which was treatment limiting.

3.2.3.1.8   Oxaliplatin and Etoposide, 1-Leucovorin, and Fluorouracil

Etoposide, 1-leucovorin, and fluorouracil (ELF) is a chemotherapeutic regimen typically administered for the treatment of advanced gastric cancer. In a study of 69 patients, patients were administered a 21-day cycle of 100 mg/m^2 oxaliplatin intravenously for 2 hours on day 1, 200 mg/m^2 calcium folinate intravenously for half an hour on days 1 to 3, 500 mg/m^2 5-fluorouracil intravenously for 2 hours on days 1 to 3, and 100 mg/m^2 etoposide intravenously for 3 hours on days 1 to 3 (Lou et al., 2009). Of the patients, 60.9% had newly diagnosed disease, while 39.1% had undergone previous chemotherapy. The total response rate was 51.6%, and median time to progression was 5.7 months, with a median overall survival of 9.2 months. About half of patients (47.1%) developed peripheral neuropathy (all grades).

3.2.3.1.9   Oxaliplatin and Dexamethasone and Cytarabine and Rituximab

In a study of 22 relapsed or resistant patients with CD20-positive non-Hodgkin's lymphoma, patients were treated in a 21-day cycle with 375 mg/m^2 rituximab on day 1, 40 mg/day dexamethasone on days 1 through 4, 130 mg/m^2 oxaliplatin on day 1, and 2,000 mg/m^2 cytarabine every 12 hours on day 2 (Machover et al., 2010). Patients received eight cycles. Most patients (95%) experienced a complete response and one patient (5%) had a partial response. Progression-free survival plateaued at 84% at 38.2 months. At a median follow-up time of 58.3 months, two of the complete responders (2/22) relapsed. Sensory peripheral neuropathy occurred in 86% of patients (14% grade 1, 18% grade 2, 50% grade 3, no cases of grade 4). In six patients (28%), grade 3 peripheral neuropathy caused discontinuation of treatment. Of the 11 patients who experienced grade 3 peripheral neuropathy, 8 reported complete resolution of all symptoms within 2 years of cessation of treatment, while 3 patients had only partial resolution of symptoms between 3 and 40 months after cessation of treatment. Patients received a median dose of oxaliplatin at 797 mg/m^2. Oxaliplatin-induced sensory peripheral neuropathy does not appear to be exacerbated by this chemotherapeutic regimen, although toxicity was high. Much of the oxaliplatin-induced sensory peripheral neuropathy resolved, at least partially, over time. Other toxicities included grade 4 granulocytopenia (46%) and grade 4 thrombocytopenia (55%).

3.2.3.1.10   Oxaliplatin and Irinotecan

Non-small-cell lung cancer is the most common type of lung cancer, which is the main cause of cancer death worldwide. Platinum-based chemotherapy, including combination therapies, is currently the main course of treatment. A trial enrolled 18 non-small-cell cancer patients at stage IIIb/IV with recurrent disease deemed unsuitable for primary resection and no palliative therapies (chemotherapy, radiotherapy, chest, or immunotherapy). Patients were administered 65 mg/m^2 irinotecan on days 1 and 8 and 130 mg/m^2 oxaliplatin on day 1 of a 21-day cycle (Chang et al., 2009). Patients underwent a median of four cycles (range, 1 to 6) and the overall response rate was 27.7% (95% confidence interval, 7 to 48.4%), with a median overall survival of 14 months and median time to progression of 4.2 months. Peripheral neuropathy occurred in only two patients (12%) and was grade 3 in 6%.

3.2.3.1.11   Oxaliplatin and Vinorelbine

In a study of 55 chemotherapy-naïve patients with stage IV non-small-cell lung cancer treated on an outpatient basis, patients received vinorelbine 25 mg/m^2 intravenously on day 1 and 60 mg/m^2 orally on day 8 and 85 mg/m^2 oxaliplatin intravenously on day 1 (Mir et al., 2009). A total of 288 cycles was administered; the mean cycle number was four (range, 1 to 11). The objective response rate was 26% (95% confidence interval, 14.4 to 37.6%). In the patient population, 40% had two or more metastatic sites and 25% had central nervous system metastases. The median progression-free survival time and overall survival were 3.5 and 9.5 months, respectively. Peripheral neuropathy ≥ grade 3 occurred in 15% of patients.

3.2.3.1.12   Oxaliplatin and Capecitabine

Capecitabine is an oral form of fluorouracil that may have similar efficacy in treating colon cancer as 5-fluorouracil/calcium folinate, but with lower rates of toxicity. A study of 33 chemotherapy-naïve patients with advanced gastric cancer was designed to assess the efficacy and toxicity of the use of oxaliplatin and capecitabine as first-line chemotherapy (Dong et al., 2009). Patients received a 2-hour intravenous infusion of 130 mg/m^2 oxaliplatin on day 1 and 2,000 mg/m^2 oral capecitabine in two daily doses on days 1 through 14 in a 21-day cycle. Patients completed a median of five cycles with a maximum of eight cycles allowed. Of the 31 evaluable patients, the overall response rate was 54.8% (95% confidence interval, 37.3 to 72.3%), with a rate of 3.2% complete response ($n = 1$). The median time to progression was 5.9 months (95% confidence interval, 4.7 to 7.1 months) and overall survival was 10.4 months (95% confidence interval, 7.9 to 12.9 months). Peripheral neuropathy was frequent but mild; 36.4% and 18.2% of patients developed grade 1 or 2 peripheral neuropathy, respectively. No more severe cases of treatment-emergent peripheral neuropathy were observed.

Adenocarcinoma of the small bowel and ampulla of Vater is a relatively rare form of cancer. In a phase II study of oxaliplatin combined with capecitabine to treat 30 patients for advanced, unresectable adenocarcinoma of the small bowel and ampulla of Vater, 30 patients received 130 mg/m^2 oxaliplatin on day 1 and 750 mg/m^2 capecitabine twice daily on days 1 through 14 of a 21-day cycle (Overman et al., 2009). No patient had undergone prior systemic chemotherapy for advanced disease. The overall response rate was 50%. Three patients with metastatic disease achieved a complete response (10%). The median time to progression was 11.3 months, with median overall survival of 20.4 months. Peripheral neuropathy occurred in 10% of patients. The results from this study suggest that oxaliplatin and capecitabine are effective and ought to be more widely used as a standard regimen for adenocarcinomas of the small bowel and ampulla of Vater.

Radiotherapy is often administered to colorectal cancer patients prior to surgery and concomitant with chemotherapy. Oxaliplatin and capecitabine are thought to work synergistically with radiotherapy against colorectal neoplasms. In a study of 46 patients with rectal cancer, two cycles of 50 mg/m^2 oxaliplatin on days 1 and 8 and 825 mg/m^2 capecitabine twice daily on days 1 through 14 were administered on a 21-day cycle concomitantly with pelvic conformal radiotherapy (45 Gy) (Carlomagno et al., 2009). Pathologic complete response occurred in 20.9% of patients (95% confidence interval, 8.7 to 33.1%). Hematological toxicities were rare, and 13% of patients experienced peripheral neuropathy.

3.2.3.1.13   Oxaliplatin and Capecitabine with Epirubicin

In a phase II study of oxaliplatin-capecitabine-epirubicin (EXE) chemotherapy for first-line treatment of 54 patients with nonresectable gastric cancer, patients received 50 mg/m^2 epirubicin on day 1, 1,000 mg/m^2 capecitabine on day 1, and 130 mg/m^2 oxaliplatin on day 1 of a 21-day cycle (Schonnemann et al., 2008). Patients could be treated with a maximum of eight cycles; the median number of treatment cycles in this study was 6 (range, 1 to 8). The overall response rate was 45% and median progression-free survival was 6.8 months (range, 5.2 to 7.9), with a median survival of 10.1 months (range, 7.9 to 10.1). Peripheral neuropathy (exclusively grades 1 and 2) occurred in 36% of patients.

3.2.3.2   Comparative Studies

3.2.3.2.1   FOLFOX4 with and without Oxaliplatin

In the MOSAIC trial, 2,246 patients who had undergone resection in an attempt to cure stage II or III colon cancer had been randomized to receive either bolus plus continuous infusion fluorouracil plus leucovorin (LV5FU2) or that same therapy plus oxaliplatin (FOLFOX4). FOLFOX4 patients had a significantly improved 3-year disease-free survival rate of 78.2% (95% confidence interval, 75.6 to 80.7%) versus 72.9% (95% confidence interval, 70.2 to 75.7%) in the LV5FU2 group ($p = 0.002$) (Andre et al., 2004). A subsequent report of 5-year disease-free survival rates of the MOSAIC population showed values of 73.3% for FOLFOX and 67.4% for LV5FU2 (without oxaliplatin) groups (hazard ratio, 0.80; 95% confidence interval, 0.68 to 0.93; $p = 0.003$). Six-year disease-free survival rates were 78.5% and 76.0%, respectively, (hazard ratio, 0.84; 95% confidence interval, 0.65 to 0.97%; $p = 0.023$) (Andre et al., 2009). Peripheral sensory neuropathy ≥ grade 3 was reported by 12.5% of FOLFOX and 0.2% of LV5FU2 patients during the course of therapy. Twelve months after treatment, the overall rate of peripheral neuropathy was 1.3%. Four years post-treatment, the rate of peripheral neuropathy was 0.7%.

The addition of oxaliplatin to the chemotherapeutic regimen for patients following a curative gastrectomy in 80 gastric adenocarcinoma patients was evaluated in a study that randomized patients into two groups (Zhang et al., 2011). In the FOLFOX 4 group, patients were administered intravenous oxaliplatin (85 mg/m^2) 2 hours on day 1, bolus injection of leucovorin (200 mg/m^2) on days 1 and 2, bolus injection of

5-fluorouracil (400 mg/m^2) on days 1 and 2, and continuous intravenous infusion of 5-fluorouracil (600 mg/m^2) for 22 hours on days 1 and 2. Chemotherapy was administered on an outpatient basis using disposable pumps and central venous catheters. Cycles were repeated at 2-week intervals. In the control group, patients were treated with 5-fluorouracil and leucovorin, but not given oxaliplatin. Median follow-up was 36.2 months (range, 10 to 42) with a median cumulative dose of oxaliplatin in the active treatment arm of 550 mg/m^2. The 3-year recurrence-free survival rate and the 3-year overall survival rate were significantly better in the FOLFOX4 group than in the control (30.0 versus 16.0 months, respectively; $p < 0.05$; and 36.0 versus 28.0 months, respectively; $p < 0.05$). Using COX multivariant analysis, oxaliplatin was determined to be the independent prognostic factor for improved survival rates. Peripheral neuropathy was significantly more frequent in the FOLFOX4 group, with 19% of FOLFOX4 patients versus no control patients reporting peripheral neuropathy ($p < 0.05$). Three (3.8%) of the FOLFOX4 patients withdrew from the study because of neuropathy.

3.2.3.2.2   Oxaliplatin and Fluoropyrimidine with and without Cetuximab

In the COIN trial, 1,630 patients with previously untreated advanced colorectal cancer received either continuous oxaliplatin and fluoropyrimidine (arm A), continuous chemotherapy plus cetuximab (arm B), or intermittent chemotherapy (arm C). In arms A and B, treatment continued until one of three things occurred: the disease progressed, cumulative toxic effects occurred, or the patient opted to stop chemotherapy (Adams et al., 2011). In arm C, patients who had not progressed at their 12-week examination and scan started a chemotherapy-free interval until there was evidence of disease progression, at which point chemotherapy was resumed. When comparing arms A and C, median survival was 15.8 months (range, 9.4 to 26.1) in arm A versus 14.4 months (range, 8.0 to 24.7) in arm C (hazard ratio, 1.084; 80% confidence interval, 1.008 to 1.165). Peripheral neuropathy ≥ grade 3 occurred in 27% of arm A versus 5% of group C; hand-foot syndrome ≥ grade 3 occurred in 4% of arm A versus 3% of arm B. Overall, peripheral neuropathy and hand-foot syndrome were more frequent in patients on continuous rather than intermittent treatment. Subgroup analysis in this study suggests that patients with normal baseline platelet counts could experience reduced toxicity and improved quality of life with intermittent rather than continuous chemotherapy without sacrificing survival benefits.

3.3   TAXANES

Taxanes, primarily paclitaxel and docetaxel, are well-established chemotherapeutic agents. Taxanes get their name from the fact that they were originally derived from plants of the genus *Taxus* (yew). Taxanes can be effective agents both as monotherapy or in combination with other drugs (particularly platinum agents) but have been associated with peripheral neuropathy.

3.3.1   PACLITAXEL

Paclitaxel and docetaxel are considered standard of care for treating metastatic breast cancer. These agents are also frequently used in adjuvant chemotherapy for patients with early-stage breast cancer. In a study of comparing doses of paclitaxel for treating metastatic breast cancer, higher doses were associated with increased toxicity but not necessarily increased efficacy (Winer et al, 2004). In a head-to-head comparison study of paclitaxel versus docetaxel in treating metastatic breast cancer, docetaxel was associated with both greater efficacy and higher toxicity (Jones et al., 2005). Taxane-induced peripheral neuropathy can be so severe it is treatment limiting. Effective neuroprotective regimens remain to be determined. Glutamate supplementation has been explored but has not been shown to protect against paclitaxel-indeuced peripheral neuropathy (Loven et al., 2009).

Preclinical studies have suggested that the toxic effects of paclitaxel may owe more to its vehicle substance (Cremophor EL) than the active agent itself (Mielke et al., 2006). However, paclitaxel itself is known to have an adverse effect on axons and glia. New formulations of paclitaxel eliminating the solvent still report dose-limiting instances of peripheral neuropathy. Thus, cremophor may contribute to paclitaxel-induced peripheral neuropathy, but it is does not appear that it is its sole cause.

Patients ($n = 94$) who took weekly paclitaxel (70 to 90 mg/m^2) were surveyed about paclitaxel-associated acute pain syndromes and chronic neuropathy (Loprinzi et al., 2011). This syndrome, sometimes called paclitaxel-induced arthralgia or myalgia, occurs in about half of patients who take the drug. Paclitaxel-induced arthralgia or myalgia can have an immediate and severe onset. Acute pain of ≥5 on an 11-point scale (0 to 10, with 10 the worst pain imaginable) occurred with the first dose of paclitaxel in 20% of patients. In total, 71% of these patients reported some degree of pain ≥ 1 associated with paclitaxel. Sensory neuropathy symptoms were more prominent than motor neuropathy or autonomic neuropathy. The most prominent sensory neuropathy symptoms were numbness and tingling, in contrast to shooting pains or burning sensations. Higher pain scores with the first dose of paclitaxel were associated with a higher rate of chronic neuropathy. This study suggests that paclitaxel-associated acute pain syndrome may actually be more of a nerve pathology than arthralgia or myalgia.

3.3.1.1 Monotherapies

Paclitaxel in a 1-hour infusion at a dose of 100 mg/m^2 weekly for 6 weeks in a 7-week cycle was administered to 74 patients with recurrent or metastatic head or neck cancer (Tahara et al., 2011). Patients received a median number of two cycles with median dose intensity of 84.2 mg/m^2/week. Overall response rate was 29.0% and median duration of response was 7.4 months. The median time to progression and survival time were 3.4 and 14.3 months, respectively. Peripheral neuropathy occurred in 5.6% of the patients.

A phase I study of hepatic arterial infusion of paclitaxel was conducted in 26 pretreated patients with liver metastases (Tsimberidou et al., 2011a). Patients were administered 150 to 275 mg/m^2 paclitaxel and 15,000 IU heparin intra-arterially every 28 days. The study was set up on a 3 + 3 design. Patients had diagnoses of colorectal, breast, and other cancers and poor prognoses. The median number of prior therapies was four (range, 0 to 10). The maximum tolerated dose of hepatic arterial infusion paclitaxel was 225 mg/m^2. Dose-limiting toxicities were grade 3 neuropathy (one out of five patients), which occurred at a dose of 275 mg/m^2 hepatic arterial infused paclitaxel.

Patients with advanced or recurrent gastric cancer who had previously been treated with fluoropyrimidine-based chemotherapy were included in a study of second-line biweekly chemotherapy with paclitaxel (Koizumi et al., 2009). The trial enrolled 40 patients who were treated with 140 mg/m^2 intravenous paclitaxel on days 1 and 15 of a 28-day cycle. Patients received a median of 3.5 cycles (range, 1 to 14). The overall response rate was 17.5% (95% confidence interval, 7.3 to 32.8%) with a 70.0% disease control rate. The median progression-free survival time was 111 days and median overall survival time was 254 days. Grade 3 or 4 peripheral neuropathy occurred in 2.5% of patients.

3.3.1.2 Combination Therapies

3.3.1.2.1 Paclitaxel and Lapatinib

Lapatinib is an orally active dual-tyrosine kinase inhibitor. It inhibits the tyrosine kinase activity associated with two oncogenes, epidermal growth factor receptor (EGFR) and HER2/neu (human EGFR type 2), which is overexpressed in a subset of breast cancer patients. Lapatinib has been used in treating breast cancer as monotherapy and is now being studied in combination therapies. In a phase II study of lapatinib combined with paclitaxel in first-line therapy of previously untreated patients with HER2-overexpressing metastatic breast cancer, 57 patients were treated (Jagiello-Gruszfeld et al., 2010). Patients received 80 mg/m^2 paclitaxel intravenously weekly for 3 weeks in a 28-day cycle plus 1,500 mg/day lapatinib daily. Patients underwent six cycles unless disease progression or withdrawal from the study intervened. Dose delays of up to 2 weeks of lapatinib were permitted for hematologic and nonhematologic toxicities; in cases of cardiac toxicity, a 3-week delay was permitted. The overall response rate was 51%, the median duration of response was 39.7 weeks, and the median progression-free survival was 47.9 weeks. Peripheral sensory neuropathy occurred in 25% of patients.

3.3.1.2.2 Paclitaxel and Tosedostat

Tosedostat is a novel aminopeptidase inhibitor shown to induce an amino acid deprivation response, which is selectively toxic to certain types of cancer cells. Preclinical studies suggest that tosedosat may be effective in both monotherapeutic and combination applications. Tosedosat may confer synergistic benefits when combined with paclitaxel and possibly other chemotherapeutic agents. A phase Ib dose-escalating study in 22 patients administered 135 to 175 mg/m^2 intravenous paclitaxel once every 21 days for up to six cycles with oral tosedostat (90 to 240 mg) daily (van Herpen et al., 2010). Paclitaxel infusion reactions occurred frequently in the second administration (59%) and interrupted oral tosedosat for 5 days. The study could not determine the maximum tolerable dose of tosedostat because of paclitaxel-associated adverse events. Peripheral sensory neuropathy occurred in 59% of patients.

3.3.1.2.3 Paclitaxel with Cyclophosphamide and Cisplatin

A phase II study evaluated 62 patients with stage III/IV epithelial ovarian cancer, all of whom had a poor prognosis (Sarosy et al., 2010). Patients received 760 mg/m^2 cyclophosphamide followed by a 24-hour infusion of 250 mg/m^2 paclitaxel and

75 mg/m^2 cisplatin on day 2. On day 3, patients received 10 µg.kg filgrastim daily for 9 days. Patients received six cycles of all agents. Based on an intention-to-treat analysis, 89% of patients had a clinical complete remission. This was a long-term study that followed patients for a median of 11.4 years. Median progression-free survival was 18.9 months and median survival was 5.4 years. Peripheral neuropathy occurred frequently. During treatment, patients exhibited grade 1 (37%), grade 2 (31%), or grade 3 (19%) peripheral neuropathy, but there were no cases of grade 4. Neurological improvement was observed when the dose of paclitaxel was reduced or treatment discontinued. This was somewhat surprising to investigators, as it was assumed that neuropathy rates were more associated with cisplatin than paclitaxel. This finding suggests that the addition of cisplatin to high-dose paclitaxel chemotherapy does not worsen the incidence of treatment-emergent peripheral neuropathy. In many instances, this chemotherapy-induced peripheral neuropathy proved to be reversible. At 14 months, 41% of patients with peripheral neuropathy during treatment reported complete resolution of their symptoms.

3.3.1.2.4 Paclitaxel and Cisplatin plus Doxorubicin

It had been determined in a clinical study that when paclitaxel was added to the chemotherapy combination of cisplatin and doxorubicin for the treatment of advanced endometrial cancer, it increased toxicity without conferring additive benefits (Lincoln et al., 2003). A subanalysis of that study ($n = 659$) found that the patients treated with cisplatin, doxorubicin, and paclitaxel (CDP) scored worse, on average, for neuropathy than similar patients treated with cisplatin and doxorubicin without paclitaxel (CD), namely, 5.2 points lower (95% confidence interval, 4.0 to 6.5; $p < 0.001$) (Cella et al., 2010). The neuropathy mostly involved a sensory component. The gap between CDP and CD in terms of sensory neuropathy closed somewhat at 6 months, but remained statistically significant (difference, 1.6 points; 95% confidence interval, 0.3 to 2.8; $p = 0.014$).

3.3.1.3 Comparative Studies

3.3.1.3.1 Paclitaxel and Gemcitabine versus Gemcitabine and Pemetrexed

In a phase II study of 105 patients with stage IIIb/IV non-small-cell lung cancer, randomization assigned patients to receive either 1,250 mg/m^2 gemcitabine on day 1 and 500 mg/m^2 pemetrexed followed by 1,250 mg/m^2 gemcitabine on day 8 of a 21-day cycle (GA group), or 120 mg/m^2 paclitaxel followed by 1,000 mg/m^2 gemcitabine both given on days 1 and 8 of a 21-day cycle (PG group) (Comella et al., 2010). The response rate was 20% (95% confidence interval, 10 to 33%) in the GA group compared to 32% (95% confidence interval, 20 to 46%) in the PG group. Median progression-free survival was also better among paclitaxel patients: 5.1 months (95% confidence interval, 3.7 to 6.5 months) for GA compared to 8.3 months (95% confidence interval, 5.9 to 10.7 months) for PG patients. Severe neutropenia and febrile neutropenia were more common in GA patients than PG patients (36% versus 22%, and 14% versus 7%, respectively), while peripheral neuropathy (any grade) occurred more frequently in the PG group (2% in GA versus 31% in PG patients).

3.3.1.3.2 *Paclitaxel with Epirubicin and Vinorelbine versus Cyclophosphamide, Methotrexate, and 5-Fluorouracil*

A comparative study was conducted in 244 patients with breast cancer involving more than three nodes (Boccardo et al., 2010). Patients were treated with chemotherapy (CT) alone or chemotherapy combined with endocrine therapy (ET). Patients were randomized to receive either four 21-day cycles of epirubicin (100 mg/m^2) on day 1 followed by four 4-week cycles of 600 mg/m^2 cyclophosphamide, 40 mg/m^2 metho-trexate, and 600 mg/m^2 5-fluorouracil on days 1 and 8 (ECMF group), or to receive four 21-day cycles of 175 mg/m^2 paclitaxel on day 1 followed by four 21-day cycles of 75 mg/m^2 epirubicin and 25 mg/m^2 vinorelbine on days 1 and 8 (T-EV group). At the conclusion of chemotherapy, tamoxifen (plus an LH-RH analog in menstru-ating women) was given to all hormone-receptor-positive patients for 5 years. At a median follow-up interval of 102 months (range, 3 to 146 months), the overall survival rate was similar (ECMF versus T-EV; hazard ratio, 0.94; 95% confidence interval, 0.59 to 1.48; $p = 0.8$) and the recurrence-free survival time was likewise not significantly different by group (hazard ratio, 0.86; 95% confidence interval, 0.57 to 1.29; $p = 0.45$). Multivariate statistical analysis further confirmed that there was no difference in efficacy between the ECMG and T-EV study arms. However, there were differences in toxicity. Patients in the T-EV (paclitaxel) group had a signifi-cantly higher incidence of peripheral neuropathy ($p < 0.0001$) and musculoskeletal disorders ($p < 0.0001$), while patients in the E-CMF group had a significantly greater rate of stomatitis ($p = 0.001$). All side effects were evaluated by investigators as being moderate and manageable.

3.3.1.4 Nanoparticle Albumin-Bound (Nab) Paclitaxel

Nanoparticle albumin-bound (nab) paclitaxel is a novel taxane formulation of paclitaxel requiring no solvent for delivery. Nab paclitaxel was developed in order to help reduce the risk of hypersensitivity reactions to paclitaxel administered in solvent (cremophor) and possibly reduce or eliminate the need for steroid or antihistamine premedication. In a randomized phase II clinical trial of 302 patients with previously untreated metastatic breast cancer by Gradishar and colleagues (2009), patients were treated in one of four arms: 300 mg/m^2 nab paclitaxel every 3 weeks (q3w), 100 mg/m^2 nab paclitaxel weekly, 150 mg/m^2 nab paclitaxel weekly, or 100 mg/m^2 docetaxel q3w. In contrast to the pacli-taxel, docetaxel was administered in its solvent-based formulation. The 150 mg/m^2 weekly nab paclitaxel was shown to offer significantly longer progression-free sur-vival times than docetaxel when assessed by an independent radiologist (12.9 versus 7.5 months, respectively; $p = 0.0065$) and an investigator (14.6 versus 7.8 months, respectively; $p = 0.012$) (Gradishar et al., 2009). The overall response rate was higher for both 150 mg/m^2 and 100 mg/m^2 nab paclitaxel (49 and 45%, respectively) than for docetaxel (35%), but this difference was not statistically significant. While fatigue, neutropenia, and febrile neutropenia were more frequent in docetaxel than any of the nab paclitaxel groups, the rate of peripheral neuropathy was similar in all four study arms. Sensory neuropathy resolved more rapidly in patients who received nab paclitaxel (any dose) compared to those who received docetaxel. The median time to improvement of grade 3 sensory neuropathy was 22, 22, and 19 days for those who

TABLE 3.1

Rates of Peripheral Neuropathy by Study Arm in Study by Gradishar et al.

Peripheral Neuropathy Grade	Nanoparticle Albumin-Based (Nab) Pacitaxel			Docetaxel
	300 mg/m² q3w (n = 76)	100 mg/m² weekly (n = 76)	150 mg/m² weekly (n = 74)	100 mg/m² q3w (n = 74)
1	34%	38%	28%	30%
2	22%	12%	26%	19%
3	17%	8%	14%	12%
4	0	0	0	0

Source: Adapted from Gradishar, WJ. et al., *J Clin Oncol* 27(22):3611–3619, 2009.

received nab paclitaxel 300 mg/m² q3w, 100 mg/m² weekly, and 150 mg/m² weekly, respectively, compared to 37 days for docetaxel patients. This study suggests that nab paclitaxel may be both more effective and less likely to induce peripheral neuropathy than docetaxel. Peripheral neuropathy was frequent but often mild (see Table 3.1).

The interest in nab paclitaxel therapies involves finding a safe but effective dose range. In a study of 106 women heavily pretreated with taxane agents for meta-static breast cancer, it was found that 100 mg/m² nab paclitaxel administered weekly demonstrated similar antitumor activity as 125 mg/m² nab paclitaxel, but with better tolerability (Blum et al., 2007). Overall response rates were 14% and 16% for the 100 mg/m² and 125 mg/m² groups, respectively, with median progression-free survival times of 3.0 and 3.5 months, respectively. Sensory neuropathy was the reason for treat-ment discontinuation for 6% of 100 mg/m² and 9% of the 125 mg/m² patients. Nine patients (8%) in the 100 mg/m² group developed treatment-related grade 3 sensory neu-ropathy, of which one-third (n = 3) had preexisting neuropathy. Neuropathy occurred after a median of five treatment cycles (range, 1 to 23). In the 125 mg/m² group, 19% of patients (n = 14) developed grade 3 sensory neuropathy, three of whom had preexisting neuropathy. In this group, the onset of neuropathy occurred after a median of three cycles (range, 2 to 6). Of all 23 patients (both arms) who developed grade 3 sensory neuropathy, 4 continued treatment with no modifications, 15 restarted treatment at a reduced dose, and 4 discontinued treatment. The presence of preexisting neuropathy in some patients in this population may have a confounding effect on the incidence of peripheral neuropathy observed over the course of the study.

3.3.1.4.1 Nab Paclitaxel Combined with Bevacizumab and Gemcitabine

In an open-label study of 29 patients with HER2-negative metastatic breast cancer, patients were administered 1,500 mg/m² gemcitabine, 160 mg/m² nab paclitaxel, and 10 mg/kg bevacizumab intravenously on days 1 and 15 of a 28-day cycle (Lobo et al., 2010). The overall response rate was 75.9% with 27.6% complete responses. The median progression-free survival time was 10.4 months (95% confidence interval, 5.6 to 15.2 months). The clinical benefit rate was 93.1% (27/29) in the overall group and 84.6% in the triple-negative group (11/13). The 18-month survival rate was 77.2% (95% confidence interval, 51.1 to 90.5%). Peripheral neuropathy ≥ grade 3 occurred in 3% of patients.

3.3.1.4.2   Nab Paclitaxel Combined with Carboplatin and Trastuzumab

In a phase II trial of 32 women with HER2-overexpressing metastatic breast cancer, patients were treated with 100 mg/m^2 nab paclitaxel and carboplatin (area under the curve = 2) on days 1, 8, and 15 of a 28-day cycle as first-line therapy (Conlin et al., 2010). Trastuzumab (2 mg/kg per week) was administered after a loading dose of 4 mg/kg. Sensitivity reactions caused the protocol to be amended to reduce the dose of carboplatin (area under the curve = 6) for 1 day each cycle rather than weekly; no premedications were used. The overall response rate was 62.5% (95% confidence interval, 45.7 to 79.3%); complete response occurred in three patients (9%). Grades 2 and 3 peripheral neuropathy occurred in 13 and 3% of patients, respectively. Hematologic toxicities were the only grade 4 toxicities observed and were considered rare.

3.3.2   DOCETAXEL

Docetaxel is a semisynthetic analog of paclitaxel that differs from paclitaxel at two positions in its chemical structure. Docetaxel has a hydroxyl group on carbon 10, while paclitaxel has an acetate ester; a tert-butyl carbamate ester is on the phenyl-propionate side chain in docetaxel instead of the benzyl amide in paclitaxel. Docetaxel is more water soluble than paclitaxel and does not require a solvent. It is disputed as to whether docetaxel is more effective than paclitaxel in certain chemotherapeutic regimens.

3.3.2.1   Monotherapies

In a phase II trial of 45 patients with disease progression after initially responding to docetaxel chemotherapy for the treatment of castration-resistant prostate cancer, patients were retreated with docetaxel (Di Lorenzo et al., 2011). The endpoint was assessed as >50% decline in prostate-specific antigen (PSA). Partial PSA responses occurred in 24.5% of patients; 25% of patients exhibited an objective response. Median progression-free survival was 5 months and median overall survival was 13 months. Grades 1 and 2 peripheral neuropathy occurred in 13.3% of patients, while 4.4% had grade 3 peripheral neuropathy.

3.3.2.2   Combination Therapies

3.3.2.2.1   Docetaxel and Dexamethasone

Docetaxel has shown promise in the treatment of advanced gastric cancer. In a phase II study, 49 patients with unresectable adenocarcinoma of the stomach who had previously been treated with fluoropyrimidine or related agents (capecitabine, doxifluridine, and others) and a platinum agent (cisplatin or oxaliplatin) were enrolled (Lee et al., 2008). Most of these patients (82%) had suffered cancer progression within 4 months after withdrawal of first-line chemotherapy. The median treatment-free interval for the patients in this study was 28.0 days. Patients were administered 75 mg/m^2 intravenous docetaxel every 3 weeks with dexamethasone as prophylaxis. Patients received a median of three cycles (range, 1 to 9), and a total of 182 cycles of docetaxel were given. The objective response was 16.3% (95%

confidence interval, 6.0 to 26.6%) and the median response duration was 4.7 months. The median time to disease progression was 2.5 months (95% confidence interval, 2.3 to 2.7 months). Sensory neuropathy was common but generally not severe. Grades 1, 2, and 3 sensory neuropathy occurred in 61.2, 14.3, and 8.2% of patients, respectively, and no patients were observed to have grade 4 sensory neuropathy.

3.3.2.2.2 Docetaxel and Gemcitabine

Non-small-cell lung cancer frequently occurs in geriatric patients. A study evaluated the treatment of 80 mg/m^2 docetaxel and 1,000 mg/m^2 gemcitabine on days 1 and 14 of a 28-day cycle in a total of 38 patients of ≥65 years of age (median age, 72 years) (Syrigos et al., 2005). Partial response was observed in 58.8% of patients and median time to disease progression was 3 months (range, 1 to 11), with a mean survival period of 7 months (range, 1 to 29). Peripheral neuropathy was common (76.3%) but mostly mild (grades 1 and 2). In this study, peripheral neuropathy occurred significantly more often in patients over the age of 70 ($p = 0.048$).

3.3.2.2.3 Docetaxel and Mitomycin

In a phase II trial of 38 patients with locally advanced or metastatic non-small-cell lung cancer, patients had all been previously treated with a platinum-based chemotherapy (Feliu et al., 2006). Patients were treated with 75 mg/m^2 docetaxel followed by 8 mg/m^2 mitomycin C on day 1 in a 21-day cycle. Patients received at least three cycles of treatment unless the disease progressed. A median of five cycles per patient was administered (total, 190), with 8% of patients having a partial response (95% confidence interval, 2.6 to 21.6%), with median time to progression of 3.6 months and median overall survival of 10.4 months. Peripheral neuropathy ≥ grade 3 occurred in 3% of patients ($n = 1$).

3.3.2.2.4 Docetaxel and Cisplatin

In a phase II study of 35 male patients with metastatic or recurrent esophageal squamous cell carcinoma previously treated with 5-fluorouracil and cisplatin or chemoradiotherapy, 70 mg/m^2 docetaxel and 75 mg/m^2 cisplatin were administered in a 1-hour intravenous infusion on day 1 of a 21-day cycle (Shim et al., 2010). Patients received a median of 3.5 cycles (range, 1 to 9) with a total of 162 cycles delivered in the population. The overall response rate was 34.2% (95% confidence interval, 19.6 to 51.3%), with one patient (2.6%) achieving a complete response. Peripheral neuropathy ≥ grade 3 developed in 15.8% of patients. Four patients (10.5%) had grade 4 peripheral neuropathy, all of whom required a dose reduction of cisplatin.

3.3.2.3 Comparative Studies

3.3.2.3.1 Docetaxel versus Vinflunine

Docetaxel was compared to vinflunine in 551 stage IIIb/IV non-small-cell lung cancer patients who had experienced treatment failure with first-line chemotherapy using a platinum agent (Krzakowski et al., 2010). In this phase III trial, patients were randomized to receive either 320 mg/m^2 vinflunine or 75 mg/m^2 docetaxel every 21 days until the disease progressed or serious toxicity occurred. Median progression-free survival was 2.3 months in each study group (hazard ratio, 1.004; 95% confidence interval, 0.841 to 1.199). The overall response rate was 4.4% for vinflunine compared to 5.5% for docetaxel; median overall survival times were 6.7 and 7.2 months, respectively. There were no significant differences in patient benefits or quality-of-life assessments. Vinflunine patients had a 10.7% rate of peripheral neuropathy, while docetaxel patients had a rate of 15.0%. On the other hand, vinflunine patients had higher rates of anemia (82.1% versus 79.8%), neutropenia (49.3% versus 39.0%), thrombocytopenia (30.6% versus 14.3%), constipation (39.2% versus 11.7%), injection site reaction (31.9% versus 0.7%), nausea (26.7% versus 23.7%), vomiting (23.8% versus 14.2%), stomatitis (19.4% versus 12.4%), abdominal pain (20.1% versus 3.6%), and myalgia (14.7% versus 6.6%). Investigators reported that the adverse events were not unexpected and could be clinically managed.

3.3.2.3.2 Docetaxel and Trastuzumab with and without Carboplatin

Docetaxel and trastuzumab (TH) are known to be effective in treating HER2-amplified metastatic breast cancer. Preclinical studies have suggested there might be a synergistic effect between trastuzumab and carboplatin. A multicenter phase III clinical trial was designed in order to compare docetaxel and trastuzumab with docetaxel, trastuzumab, and carboplatin. A total of 263 patients with HER2-gene-amplified metastatic breast cancer enrolled and were randomized to receive eight 21-day cycles of TH (trastuzumab plus 100 mg/m^2 docetaxel) or TCH (trastuzumab plus carboplatin at area under the curve = 6 and 75 mg/m^2 docetaxel) (Valero et al., 2011). Trastuzumab was administered with a loading dose of 4 mg/kg followed by a weekly dose of 2 mg/kg during chemotherapy, and then 6 mg/kg once every 3 weeks until progression. The primary endpoint of the study was time to progression. There was no significant difference between TH and TCH arms in terms of the primary endpoint (time to progression, 11.1 and 10.4 months, respectively; hazard ratio, 0.914; 95% confidence interval, 0.694 to 1.203; $p = 0.57$), nor were there significant differences for response rate (72% in both arms) and overall survival (median 37.1 versus 37.4 months, respectively; $p = 0.99$). Sensory neuropathy ≥ grade 3 occurred in 3% of TH and 0.8% of TCH patients. Of adverse effects, neutropenic-related complications, sensory neuropathy, and peripheral edema were more common in the TH group, while thrombocytopenia, anemia, fatigue, and diarrhea were more common in the TCH group.

3.4 VINCA ALKALOIDS

The vinca alkaloid agents are antimitotic and antimicrotubule agents originally derived from the periwinkle plant (*Catharanthus roseus*). Vinca alkaloid agents include vincristine, vindesine, vinflunine, and vinorelbine. Peripheral neuropathy associated with vinca alkaloid therapy may develop late, and has been observed in some instances to worsen after treatment is discontinued (Verstappen et al., 2005). For that reason, clinical trials reporting immediate or short-term results may not fairly capture the true rate of vinca-alkaloid-induced peripheral neuropathy.

3.4.1 VINCRISTINE

Vincristine is available as a vincristine sulfate liposomes injection (VSLI), a sphingomyelin/cholesterol nanoparticle encapsulated formulation, designed to improve the agent's pharmacokinetic profile without exacerbating its toxicity. Vincristine-induced peripheral neuropathy is one of the agent's most common adverse effects and can be treatment limiting. In a phase I trial, 36 patients with relapsed or refractory acute lymphoblastic leukemia were treated with intravenous VSLI at 1.5, 1.825, 2.0, 2.25, or 2.4 mg/m^2 to determine the maximum tolerated dose of VSLI (Thomas et al., 2009). Based on dose-limiting toxicities, the maximum tolerated dose of VSLI was determined to be 2.25 mg/m^2. The most common toxicities observed in this study were peripheral neuropathy, which occurred in 55% of patients, and constipation (53%). Based on an intention-to-treat analysis, complete response was achieved by 19% of patients ($n = 7$); four of those seven patients were then able to undergo allogeneic stem cell transplantation in remission.

3.4.2 VINDESINE

A trial of 139 patients with metastasized melanoma following complete metastasectomy evaluated the safety and efficacy of vindesine therapy (Eigentler et al., 2008). Patients had metastatic spread to regional sites, lymph nodes, and distant sites and were randomized either to be treated with vindesine for 2 years or to be observed (no treatment) over the same period. In the vindesine group, patients were administered 3 mg/m^2 intravenous vindesine biweekly for 26 weeks, then every 3 weeks for the next 26 weeks, and then every 4 weeks for the following 52 weeks. Median follow-up in this study was 45 months. There was no significant difference in median recurrence free survival or 3-year overall survival between the vindesine group or the observation group (7.9 months versus 7.6 months, and 55.0% versus 43.6%, respectively). Vindesine patients were found to have two main adverse effects: alopecia and peripheral neuropathy. No cases of grade 4 peripheral neuropathy were determined, but 10 patients discontinued treatment because of grade 3 peripheral neuropathy. In most cases, peripheral neuropathy was persistent, whereas alopecia was typically reversible.

Sequential chemotherapy may hold promise for certain types of cancer. In a pilot study, 30 evaluable, chemotherapy-naïve patients with locally advanced or metastatic non-small-cell lung cancer received three treatment sequences (Rixe et al., 2005). Sequence A involved four 21-day cycles of 100 mg/m^2 docetaxel on day 1. Sequence B was four 28-day cycles of 120 mg/m^2 cisplatin on day 1 and 3 mg/m^2 vindesine on days 1, 8, 15, and 22. Those patients responding to therapy then received three 21-day cycles of 100 mg/m^2 docetaxel on day 1 as consolidation therapy; this was considered sequence C. The objective response rate was 16.7% and median survival time (based on intent-to-treat analysis) was 11 months (95% confidence interval, 8.0 to 15.4 months), with a 1-year survival rate of 47%. Median time to progression was 17.6 weeks. Grade 3 peripheral neuropathy was observed in 17% ($n = 5$) during sequence B.

3.4.3 VINFLUNINE

A study of 551 patients with stage IIIb/IV non-small-cell lung cancer who had experienced treatment failure with first-line platinum-agent chemotherapy randomized patients to receive either 320 mg/m² vinflunine or 75 mg/m² docetaxel on day 1 of a 21-day cycle to continue until disease progression or serious toxicity occurred (Krzakowski et al., 2010). Vinflunine was shown to be noninferior to docetaxel in this patient population, which was the primary endpoint of the study. Median progression-free survival was 2.3 months for each arm (hazard ratio, 1.004; 95% confidence interval, 0.841 to 1.199). Peripheral neuropathy grade ≥ 1 was reported in 10.7% of vinflunine versus 15.0% of docetaxel patients. Other adverse events, including anemia, abdominal pain, constipation, and fatigue, were higher in vinflunine patients.

3.4.4 VINORELBINE

3.4.4.1 Monotherapy

In a phase II trial of 26 patients with metastatic breast cancer previously treated with anthracycline and taxane agent chemotherapy, patients were treated with intravenous 25 mg/m² vinorelbine monotherapy on days 1, 8, 15, and 22 of a 28-day cycle (Seo et al., 2011). The overall response rate was 20.8%, with a median response duration of 2.8 months and median time to progression of 3.7 months (range, 0.5 to 22.6). The median overall survival duration was 10.4 months (range, 1.3 to 57.6). Peripheral neuropathy was common but not severe; 42.3% of patients were observed to have peripheral neuropathy grade 1 or 2; there were no cases of higher-grade peripheral neuropathy.

3.4.4.2 Combination Therapies

3.4.4.2.1 Vinorelbine and Cisplatin

In a phase II trial combining vinorelbine with cisplatin in the treatment of 37 patients with advanced squamous cell carcinoma of the cervix, patients were administered 30 mg/m² vinorelbine on days 1 and 8 and 100 mg/m² cisplatin on day 1 of a 28-day cycle (Goedhals et al., 2005). The objective response rate was 64.8% with median duration of response and time to progression of 17.6 and 13.2 months, respectively. The median survival was 20.6 months (range, 0.4 to 55). While nausea and vomiting were common side effects (50%), peripheral neuropathy was less frequent. Peripheral neuropathy occurred in 5% of patients and was never more severe than grade 2.

The role of cisplatin-based chemotherapy for treating non-small-cell lung cancer in elderly patients remains controversial. A pilot phase I/II trial treated patients aged 70 years and older with newly diagnosed non-small-cell lung cancer (Pereira et al., 2004). Patients were then stratified by age and defined as younger (≤75 years) and older (>75 years) patients. All patients were administered cisplatin-based chemotherapy with 25 mg/m² vinorelbine on days 1 and 8 and cisplatin on day 1 of a 28-day cycle. Younger patients received moderate doses of cisplatin (80 or 90 mg/m²), while older patients received lower doses (60 or 70 mg/m²). Global median time to progression was 27.0 weeks (95% confidence interval, 10.1 to 43.7 weeks) and overall survival was 30.1 weeks (95% confidence interval, 24.4 to 35.8 weeks). The 1- and 2-year survival rates were 36.3 and 13.2%, respectively. The overall response rate was 50.0% (95% confidence interval, 35.4 to 64.5%). The main grade 3 or 4 toxicities were neutropenia, anemia, alopecia, and fatigue. Peripheral neurotoxicity was reported in 2% of patients. This study suggested that elderly non-small-cell lung cancer patients could be safely and effectively treated with cisplatin and vinorelbine.

Peripheral neuropathy occurred in 19% of patients in a study of vinorelbine and cisplatin chemotherapy for treating recurrent or metastatic carcinoma of the uterine cervix (Gebbia et al., 2002). In this study, 42 patients were treated with 80 mg/m^2 cisplatin on day 1 and 25 mg/m^2 vinorelbine on days 1 and 8 of a 21-day cycle. Patients included in this study were treatment naïve (38%), had prior surgery (7%), had prior radiotherapy (31%), or had both prior radiation and surgery (24%). The overall response rate was 48% (95% confidence interval, 22 to 52%). In subanalysis, patients with recurrent disease and prior radiation therapy had a lower overall response rate, namely, 28%. Median time to progression was 5.6 months (range, 2.0 to 14) and median overall survival was 9.1 months. Peripheral neuropathy (19%) was exclusively grades 1 and 2.

3.4.4.2.2 Vinorelbine and Oxaliplatin

Many patients with non-small-cell lung cancer are not suitable candidates for cisplatin chemotherapy because of renal dysfunction or other comorbidities. In a feasibility study of 55 chemotherapy-naïve patients with stage IV non-small-cell cancer and considered unsuitable candidates for cisplatin, patients were treated with 25 mg/m^2 intravenous vinorelbine and 85 mg/m^2 oxaliplatin on day 1 and 60 mg/m^2 oral vinorelbine on day 8 of a 14-day cycle (Mir et al., 2009). Of these patients, 40% had two or more metastatic sites and 25% had central nervous system metastases. The objective response rate in this study was 26% (95% confidence interval, 14.4 to 37.6%), with median progression-free survival and median overall survival of 3.5 and 9.5 months, respectively. The 1-year survival rate was 24% (95% confidence interval, 12.7 to 35.3%). Peripheral neuropathy ≥ grade 3 occurred in 15% of patients.

3.4.4.2.3 Vinorelbine and Paclitaxel

In a phase II study, 34 patients with stage IIIb non-small-cell lung cancer were treated with 175 mg/m^2 paclitaxel in a 3-hour infusion on day 1 and 25 mg/m^2 vinorelbine in a 10-minute infusion on days 1 and 8 of a 21-day cycle (Ginopoulos et al., 2002). The overall response rate was 67.7%, with 16.1% having a complete response ($n = 5$). The overall median survival time was 10 months (range, 3 to 18) and median disease-free survival time was 9 months (range, 3 to 9) with a 1-year survival rate of 45.1%. Leukopenia and anemia were the most frequent adverse events (48.4% and 45.4%, respectively). Peripheral neuropathy ≥ grade 3 occurred in 6% of patients.

3.4.4.2.4 Vinorelbine and Gemcitabine

About half of all breast cancer patients treated with curative intent will develop metastatic disease. Combination therapy with vinorelbine and gemcitabine has been shown to be effective in the treatment of metastatic breast cancer. In a phase II trial designed to investigate the safety and efficacy of prolonged gemcitabine infusion

TABLE 3.2

Peripheral Neuropathy Rates with Vinolrelbine with and without Cisplatin from a Study by Chen et al.

Grades	Vinorelbine and Gemcitabine			Vinorelbine and Gemcitabine with Cisplatin		
	1	2	3 and 4	1	2	3 and 4
Peripheral neuropathy	27.9%	7%	0	20.9%	39.5%	0

Source: Adapted from Chen, Reury Perng et al., *Lung Cancer* 47(3):373–380, 2005.

versus shorter administration, 26 previously treated patients (anthracycline or taxane) with metastatic disease were administered 350 mg/m^2 gemcitabine as a 4-hour infusion and 25 mg/m^2 vinorelbine on days 1 and 8 of a 21-day cycle (Schmid et al., 2005). Patients were treated for up to six cycles. The overall response rate was 30.4% and a clinical benefit rate of 47.8% was determined. Median duration of response and time to progression were, respectively, 7.3 and 4.6 months. Median overall survival was 14.5 months. Peripheral neuropathy of grades 1, 2, and 3 occurred in 15.4, 3.8, and 3.8% of patients, respectively; there were no cases of peripheral neuropathy grade 4. In this study, all patients with grade 2 and 3 neuropathy had preexisting neuropathy at the onset of treatment.

3.4.4.2.5   *Vinorelbine and Gemcitabine with and without Cisplatin*

In the treatment of non-small-cell lung cancer, phase II studies suggest that vinorelbine and gemcitabine combination chemotherapy achieves a response rate similar to that of cisplatin-based combination chemotherapy but with an improved toxicity profile. In a study (Chen, Reury Perng et al., 2005) of 86 chemotherapy-naïve patients with non-small-cell lung cancer, patients were randomized to receive 20 mg/m^2 intravenous vinorelbine plus 800 mg/m^2 gemcitabine on days 1, 8, and 15 with or without 60 mg/m^2 intravenous cisplatin on day 15 of a 28-day cycle. The median number of cycles was three in the vinorelbine-gemcitabine arm compared to five in the cisplatin arm (total treatments were 125 and 178, respectively). Partial response occurred in 23.3% of the vinorelbine-gemcitabine group compared to 46.5% in the vinorelbine-gemcitabine-cisplatin group ($p = 0.022$), and there was one complete response in the latter group. The adverse effects of neutropenia, nausea, vomiting, and peripheral neuropathy were all significantly more frequent in the group with added cisplatin. Peripheral neuropathy rates are shown in Table 3.2. No cases of grade 3 or 4 peripheral neuropathy occurred in either study arm.

3.4.4.3   **Comparative Studies**

3.4.4.3.1   *Vinorelbine and Gemcitabine Compared to Carboplatin and Paclitaxel*

A phase II trial of advanced (stage IIIb/IV) non-small-cell lung cancer randomized 165 chemotherapy-naïve patients to one of two treatment regimens (Lilenbaum et al., 2005). One group was treated with vinorelbine-gemcitabine (VG) and the other with carboplatin-paclitaxel (CP). The VG patients received 25 mg/m^2 vinorelbine intravenously and 1,000 mg/m^2 gemcitabine on days 1 and 8 of a 21-day cycle. The CP patients received 200 mg/m^2 intravenous paclitaxel plus carboplatin (area under the curve = 6) on day 1 of a 21-day cycle. Treatment continued for six cycles or until disease progression was observed. Both groups received a median of four cycles. Efficacy was similar between arms with overall response rates of 14.6% (VG) and 16.9% (CP). Median time to progression was 3.9 months for VG patients (95% confidence interval, 3.0 to 4.8 months) and 4.8 months for CP patients (95% confidence interval, 3.3 to 6.5 months). The 1-year survival rates were 38.4% (VG) and 31.9% (CP), a difference that was not statistically significant. Patients taking carboplatin and paclitaxel had a higher rate of all grades of peripheral neuropathy, which did not achieve statistical significance (13.3% versus 4.9%, $p = 0.06$).

3.4.4.3.2 *Epirubicin with and without Vinorelbine*
Epirubicin is an anthracycline drug that seems to have fewer side effects than a similar agent, doxorubicin. In a phase III study, 387 patients with advanced breast cancer were randomized for front-line treatment. The active group was administered 90 mg/m^2 intravenous epirubicin on day 1 and 25 mg/m^2 vinorelbine on days 1 and 8, while the control group received 90 mg/m^2 epirubicin on day 1 of a 21-day cycle (Ejlertsen et al., 2004). Treatment continued for up to 1 year or until a cumulative dose of 1,000 mg/m^2 of epirubicin was achieved or until disease progressed. Overall response rates were similar in the active and control group (50% versus 42%, respectively; $p = 0.15$), but complete response rate was significantly superior for the combination therapy of vinorelbine and epirubicin (17% versus 10%, respectively; $p = 0.048$). Median survival times were similar (19.1 versus 18.0 months, respectively; $p = 0.050$). Peripheral neuropathy $\geq$ grade 3 was significantly more frequent in the vinorelbine-epirubicin group ($n = 3$) than the epirubicin-alone group ($n = 0$), but was infrequent in both arms.

3.5 BORTEZOMIB

Immunomodulatory drugs such as bortezomib are increasingly used as frontline agents in hematological cancers, particularly multiple myeloma. Bortezomib may be administered in monotherapy or in combination therapies with one, two, three, or more other agents. Multiple myeloma is typically treated with induction chemotherapy, followed by autologous stem cell transplantation, whereupon consolidation therapy begins, followed by maintenance treatments. Bortezomib is a proteasome inhibitor that has been shown to be effective in treating both newly diagnosed and relapsed or refractory multiple myeloma, but it has been associated with adverse events, including a painful and potentially dose-limiting peripheral neuropathy. Bortezomib-induced peripheral neuropathy occurs in 37 to 44% of clinical trial multiple myeloma patients, with cumulative dose as its most significant predictor (Cavaletti and Jakubowiak, 2010). However, evaluation of peripheral neuropathy in multiple myeloma patients is complicated by the fact that some degree of peripheral neuropathy may be related to the disease itself, rather than the treatment. Moreover, the literature suggests that, in rare instances, bortezomib may be associated with an inflammatory autoimmune neuropathy that is superficially similar to bortezomib-induced peripheral neuropathy

(Schmitt et al., 2011) but requires different treatment (Nakano et al., 2011). The incidence of peripheral neuropathy in multiple myeloma patients treated in clinical studies *with any agents* ranges from 37% to 88% (Richardson et al., 2010b). Combination therapy as well as dose adjustments may play a role in reducing chemotherapeutic toxicities, including peripheral neuropathies. It is unclear if combination therapy offers better tolerability than bortezomib monotherapy.

Much remains to be learned about bortezomib-induced neuropathy. It is generally considered reversible, but a recent study suggests that in some instances, at least, bortezomib may be associated with permanent impairment of nerve fibers, resulting in a persistent painful syndrome (Boyette-Davis et al., 2011). Recovery from bortezomib-induced peripheral neuropathy may take as long as 1.7 years (Cavaletti and Jakubowiak, 2010). Elderly patients, in particular, are thought to be more susceptible to bortezomib-induced peripheral neuropathy than similar younger patients (Palumbo et al., 2011).

The incidence of bortezomib-induced peripheral neuropathy does not seem to vary when used in the treatment of previously untreated versus pretreated patients. In a retrospective study of 55 patients who received bortezomib as frontline therapy for multiple myeloma compared to 70 patients who received bortezomib for the first time for relapsed or refractory multiple myeloma, there was no statistically significant difference in the rate of peripheral neuropathy (55% for untreated and 52% for pretreated patients), the severity of the peripheral neuropathy (9% of untreated and 14% of pretreated had ≥ grade 3 peripheral neuropathy), or outcome (peripheral neuropathy improved or resolved in 90% of untreated and 91% of pretreated patients) (Corso et al., 2010). The main risk factors for bortezomib-induced peripheral neuropathy are male gender (3.035; confidence interval, 1.356 to 6.793; $p = 0.0069$) and lack of coadministration with dexamethasone (0.455; confidence interval, 0.208 to 0.955; $p = 0.0376$) (Kanbayashi et al., 2010). A high number of chemotherapy cycles—a risk factor for peripheral neuropathy with taxanes, vincristine, and oxaliplatin—does not appear to be a risk factor for bortezomib-induced peripheral neuropathy.

3.5.1 MONOTHERAPY

In a study of 49 multiple myeloma patients who underwent autologous peripheral blood stem cell transplant and high-dose mephalan without complete response, patients were administered 1.3 mg/m² bortezomib on days 1, 4, 8, and 11 of a 21-day cycle (Rifkin et al., 2010). Responders were permitted up to four additional cycles. Eight percent of patients had complete response to treatment, and 14% were observed to have peripheral neuropathy ≥ grade 3.

3.5.2 COMBINATION THERAPIES

3.5.2.1 Bortezomib Combined with Thalidomide and Dexamethasone

Thalidomide in combination with dexamethasone has been a common induction therapy for multiple myeloma. Recently, treatment protocols have added bortezomib.

While bortezomib-thalidomide combination therapies have improved outcomes in multiple myeloma patients, they are likewise associated with treatment-limiting and potentially persistent peripheral neuropathy (Delforge et al., 2010).

In a phase II study, the combination of bortezomib and thalidomide was evaluated in 34 patients with recently diagnosed multiple myeloma. Bortezomib (1.3 mg/m^2) was administered intravenously on days 1, 4, 8, and 11 of a 21-day cycle, along with 100 mg oral thalidomide every day (Chen et al., 2011). The complete response rate was 30.8% after eight cycles, with 23.1% achieving a near-complete response. The estimated continuous remission rate at 12 months was 62%. In this study, mild to moderate (grades 1 and 2) peripheral neuropathy occurred in 38.0% of patients.

In a 3-year study (Ghosh, 2011), 27 newly diagnosed multiple myeloma patients were administered 1.3 mg/m^2 bortezomib on days 1, 4, 8, and 11 and 150 mg oral thalidomide daily in a 21-day cycle (maximum eight cycles), with no steroids permitted. The overall response rate was 81.5%, with a complete or near-complete response of 25.8%. Peripheral neuropathy occurred in 22% of patients and completely resolved in 80% of those patients upon completion of therapy.

In a study of 34 patients with recently diagnosed multiple myeloma, 1.3 mg/m^2 bortezomib was administered in a 21-day cycle on days 1, 4, 8, and 11 of a 21-day cycle along with 100 mg oral thalidomide daily for up to eight cycles (Chen, Jiang et al., 2010). The overall response rate was 100%, broken down as 31% complete response, 23% near-complete response, 42% partial response, and 4% minimal response. In this study, 38% of patients developed peripheral neuropathy. One patient (3%) developed grade 3 peripheral neuropathy that improved with bortezomib and thalidomide dose reduction.

3.5.2.2 Bortezomib, Cyclophosphamide, Thalidomide, and Dexamethasone

A four-drug combination therapy for multiple myeloma consisting of bortezomib, cyclophosphamide, thalidomide, and dexamethasone was evaluated in 70 patients with relapsed or refractory multiple myeloma (Kim et al., 2010). Patients received 1.3 mg/m^2 bortezomib and 20 mg/m^2 dexamethasone intravenously on days 1, 4, 8, and 11 of a 21-day cycle; 150 mg/m^2 oral cyclophosphamide was administered on days 1 through 4; and patients received 50 mg oral thalidomide every day. The overall response rate was 88% (46% complete response), with a median 12.6 months follow-up. Grade 3 or 4 peripheral neuropathy occurred in 3% of patients, suggesting this combination is an effective and well-tolerated salvage therapy.

In a study of sequential three-drug chemotherapeutic regimens for treating newly diagnosed multiple myeloma, 44 patients were administered 1.3 mg/m^2 bortezomib and 40 mg dexamethasone on days 1, 4, 8, and 11 and 300 mg/m^2 cyclophosphamide on days 1 and 8 of a 21-day therapeutic cycle (Bensinger et al., 2010). After three cycles, treatment shifted to 1.0 mg/m^2 bortezomib, 40 mg dexamethasone, and 100 mg/day thalidomide daily for three cycles. The overall response rate for evaluable patients was 95% (19% complete response), with an estimated 81% 1-year event-free survival. Eighty-two percent of patients in the study completed all six cycles. The most commonly reported grade 3 or 4 adverse event was peripheral neuropathy, which occurred in 11% of patients.

3.5.2.3 Bortezomib and Dexamethasone and Pegylated Liposomal Doxorubicin

In a retrospective study of 28 patients with relapsed or refractory multiple myeloma (83% of whom had been previously treated with bortezomib), patients were treated with 40 mg dexamethasone intravenously, 1.0 mg/m^2 bortezomib, and 5.0 mg/m^2 pegylated liposomal doxorubicin (PLD) on days 1, 4, 8, and 11 of a 28-day cycle for a maximum of eight cycles (Waterman et al., 2011). The overall response rate was 61% (4% complete response, $n = 1$). Six patients (21%) exhibited a worsening of their baseline peripheral neuropathy during this treatment, and one patient discontinued treatment because of grade 2 peripheral neuropathy. Peripheral neuropathy observed over the course of this trial was reversible in most cases.

In a study of multiple myeloma patients administered 40 mg dexamethasone intravenously, 1 mg/m^2 bortezomib, and 5 mg/m^2 PLD on days 1, 4, 8, and 11 of a 4-week cycle (maximum eight cycles), patients achieved an 86% response rate to therapy, with peripheral neuropathy (any grade) occurring in 34% (Berenson et al., 2011). Peripheral neuropathy was relatively mild (five patients had grade 1, five grade 2, two grade 3, and no cases of grade 4). This study suggests that appropriate dosing regimens may allow for effective treatment while reducing the rate of chemotherapy-induced peripheral neuropathy.

3.5.2.4 Bortezomib and Vincristine, Dexamethasone, Pegylated L-Asparaginase, and Doxorubicin

In a study of 15 pediatric patients with acute lymphoblastic leukemia (five in first bone marrow relapse, five in second relapse), escalating doses of bortezomib were administered on days 1, 4, 8, and 11 of a four-drug induction chemotherapy regimen (vincristine, dexamethasone, pegylated L-asparaginase, and doxorubicin) (Messinger et al., 2010). Four patients were enrolled at dose level 1 (1 mg/m^2 bortezomib). Six and thereafter five more patients were enrolled at dose level 2 (1.3 mg/m^2 bortezomib). There was one instance in the study of a dose-limiting adverse event (hypophosphatemia and rhabdomyolysis). Complete response was achieved by 67% of patients and two patients developed mild (grade 1 and 2) peripheral neuropathy.

3.5.2.5 Bortezomib and Dexamethasone with Romidepsin

A study of previously treated multiple myeloma patients now treated with romidepsin, bortezomib, and dexamethasone found the maximum tolerated doses to be 1.3 mg/m^2 bortezomib, 20 mg dexamethasone, and 10 mg/m^2 romidepsin every 28 days (Harrison et al., 2011). Peripheral neuropathy occurred in 76% of patients in this study, with 8% of patients experiencing peripheral neuropathy $\geq$ grade 3.

3.5.2.6 Bortezomib and Rituximab

Preclinical studies suggest that bortezomib combined with rituximab may offer synergistic activity (Hideshima et al., 2001; Rose et al., 2002; Wang et al., 2008). In a study of 16 chemotherapy refractory patients with mantle cell lymphoma, treatment with bortezomib (1.3 mg/m^2 on days 1, 4, 8, and 11 of a 21-day cycle; six cycles), rituximab (375 mg/m^2, day 1), and oral dexamethasone (40 mg, days 1 through 4) was administered (Lamm et al., 2011). Patients designated as responders received four consolidating doses of rituximab. The overall response was 81.3%, with 43.8% achieving complete response. Peripheral neuropathy occurred in 12.5% of patients and was the cause for discontinuation of the study for two patients (2/16).

Waldenström macroglobulinemia (WM) is a lymphoproliferative disorder with a 5-year survival rate ranging from 36% to 87%. In a study of 37 relapsed or refractory WM patients, patients received 1.6 mg/m^2 intravenous bortezomib on days 1, 8, and 15 every 28 days for six cycles and 376 mg/m^2 rituximab weekly during cycles 1 through 4 (Ghobrial et al., 2010). Peripheral neuropathy occurred in only 5% of patients ($n = 2$) and both cases were grade 2. Minimal response to treatment or better occurred in 81% of patients, with two patients in complete remission.

3.5.2.7 Bortezomib and Rituximab and Cyclophosphamide and Dexamethasone

Twelve chemotherapy-naïve patients with low-grade non-Hodgkin's lymphoma were treated with a combination therapy of bortezomib, rituximab, cyclophosphamide, and dexamethasone for a median of 22 months before the study was closed for lack of funding (Nabhan et al., 2011). Despite the fact that the study was not completed, results were published, and the overall response rate was 90%, with a complete response rate of 54%. In this study, no cases of grade 3 or 4 peripheral neuropathy were observed.

3.5.2.8 Bortezomib and Tanespimycin

Tanespimycin (17-allylamino-17-demethoxygeldanamycin (17-AAG)) is an anticancer agent currently in development. Tanespimycin disrupts the heat shock protein 90 (HSP90), a molecular chaperone for the signal transduction proteins (and other client proteins) known to be crucial to myeloma growth, survival, and drug resistance. Tanespimycin binds to the ATP-binding site of HSP90, blocks ATPase activity, and degrades the HSP90 proteins via the ubiquitin-protease pathway. In an open-label phase II study, 1.3 mg/m^2 bortezomib and three doses of tanespimycin (50, 175, and 340 mg/m^2) were administered to 22 pretreated patients with relapsed, refractory multiple myeloma (Richardson et al., 2010a). Although all patients (100%) reported at least one adverse event, peripheral neuropathy was not a common side effect and occurred in 18% of patients (compared to 73% who reported fatigue, 68% nausea, 64% diarrhea, 50% constipation, and 45% vomiting). Of the 18% ($n = 4$) who developed peripheral neuropathy in this study, half had preexisting peripheral neuropathy. No patients discontinued treatment on account of peripheral neuropathy. Although this study was closed prematurely owing to resource shortages, investigators published that the overall response rate to this therapy was 14%. This study hints that tanespimycin may offer some sort of neuroprotective benefit, although that remains to be elucidated. Further study is warranted.

An open-label dose escalation study of 63 patients with relapsed or relapsed and refractory multiple myeloma evaluated the safety and efficacy of 100 to 340 mg/m^2 tanespimycin combined with 0.7 to 1.3 mg/m^2 bortezomib administered on days 1, 4,

8, and 11 in a 21-day cycle (Richardson et al., 2011). In the second phase of the study, doses were increased; the highest tested doses were 340 mg/m^2 tanespimycin and 1.3 mg/m^2 bortezomib. The objective response rate was 27% (3% complete response, 12% partial response, and 12% minimal response), with no cases of severe peripheral neuropathy observed.

3.5.2.9 Bortezomib and Temsirolimus

Temsirolimus is a kinase inhibitor approved for the treatment of renal cell carcinoma; temsirolimus may also be effective in other anticancer treatments. Bortezomib and temsirolimus combination therapy has been studied in the treatment of multiple myeloma. Twenty patients with relapsed or refractory multiple myeloma were administered 1.6 mg/m^2 bortezomib on days 1, 8, 15, and 22 in combination with 25 mg temsirolimus on days 1, 8, 14, 22, and 29 of a 35-day cycle in an open-label study (Ghobrial et al., 2011). This was the first phase of this trial; in the second phase, doses were escalated until dose-limiting adverse effects were observed in two out of three in the dose cohort. Steroids were not permitted in this trial. The maximum tolerated doses were 1.6 mg/m^2 of bortezomib combined with 25 mg of temsirolimus. Four patients (20%) in the first phase and 11 patients (55%) in the second phase experienced sensory peripheral neuropathy ($\leq$ grade 2), whereas seven patients (35%) exhibited motor peripheral neuropathy (one patient had grade 3; all others had $\leq$ grade 2).

3.5.2.10 Bortezomib and Tipifarnib

Tipifarnib is a farnesyltransferase inhibitor and has been tested in combination therapy with bortezomib in patients with advanced acute leukemia. Its use in combination therapy is based on the fact that tipifarnib and bortezomib act on nonoverlapping targets and may have synergistic antitumor effects. In one study, 27 patients were enrolled to be treated with escalating doses of tipifarnib (days 1 through 14) and bortezomib (days 1, 4, 8, and 11) in a 21-day cycle until the maximum tolerated dose was achieved (Lancet et al., 2011). The study used a 3 + 3 design, meaning that if a dose-limiting adverse effect was observed in one out of three patients, the group was expanded to six patients. If no further toxicity was observed, three patients were enrolled at the next higher incremental dose level. The maximum tolerated dose, defined as the dose level below the one at which two or more dose-limiting toxicities occurred, was not achieved in the study. Three patients in the study experienced a dose-limiting toxicity, and the maximum tolerated dose levels were not achieved over the course of the 21-day study. The dose-limiting toxicities were diarrhea (one patient), severe fatigue (one patient), and grade 3 sensorimotor neuropathy (one patient), which started on day 21 of the study, improved within 2 months after the study, but never completely resolved.

3.5.2.11 Bortezomib and Dexamethasone Combined with Itraconazole or Lansoprazole

Combination pharmacological therapy may result in additive effects, which is the sum of the agents, or synergistic effects, where the net effect is greater than the sum of its parts. Such additive or synergistic interactions may apply to adverse events as well as drug effectiveness. A retrospective analysis was conducted on six adult relapsed multiple myeloma patients to explore a potential drug interaction between bortezomib and itraconazole, a cytochrome (CYP) P450 inhibitor, or lansoprazole, a CYP2C19 inhibitor (Iwamoto et al., 2010). All patients received intravenous bortezomib and oral dexamethasone as the first course of a 21-day cycle. Four of the six patients also received concomitant therapy with itraconazole ($n = 2$), lansoprazole ($n = 1$), or both ($n = 1$). All three itraconazole patients experienced new or worsening peripheral neuropathy as well as grade 4 thrombocytopenia. The patient who received lansoprazole exhibited no changes in adverse effects. Using the Horn drug interaction probability score, investigators found that the increased severity of chemotherapy-induced peripheral neuropathy was probably related to itraoconazole in combination with bortezomib. The exact mechanisms of this interaction are unknown, and it is unclear if other CYP3A4 inhibitors might have a similar effect.

3.5.3 Comparative Studies

3.5.3.1 Bortezomib and Dexamethasone with and without Thalidomide

One hundred ninety-nine patients with newly diagnosed multiple myeloma awaiting autologous stem cell transplantation were randomized to receive either bortezomib plus dexamethasone or reduced doses of bortezomib and thalidomide plus dexamethasone (Moreau et al., 2011a). Patients in the bortezomib-dexamethasone group received four 21-day cycles of 1.3 mg/m² bortezomib on days 1, 4, 8, and 11 and 40 mg dexamethasone on days 1 through 4 (all cycles) and days 9 through 12 (cycles 1 and 2 only). The bortezomib-thalidomide-dexamethasone group received lower doses of bortezomib, namely, 1 mg/m² on days 1, 4, 8, and 11 of the same 21-day cycle with 100 mg oral thalidomide administered daily and dexamethasone on the same schedule as the bortezomib-dexamethasone group. After four cycles of treatment, both groups had similar rates of complete response (14% versus 13%, respectively; not significant [NS]), but the bortezomib-thalidomide-dexamethasone patients scored significantly higher in terms of good partial response (49% versus 36%, respectively; $p = 0.02$) than the bortezomib-dexamethasone patients. The bortezomib-thalidomide-dexamethasone patients had a significantly lower incidence of peripheral neuropathy than the bortezomib-dexamethasone patients ≥ grade 2 (14% versus 34%, $p = 0.001$). The combination of three agents (bortezomib, thalidomide, dexamethasone) with reduced bortezomib dose resulted in better partial response rates with significantly reduced rates of peripheral neuropathy.

3.5.3.2 Thalidomide and Dexamethasone with and without Bortezomib

Four hundred seventy-four treatment-naïve myeloma patients received three 21-day cycles of 100 mg/day thalidomide for the first 14 days and 200 mg/day thereafter together with dexamethasone (40 mg/day for 8 of the first 12 days, but not consecutively, for a total of 320 mg per cycle) (Cavo et al., 2010). Patients were randomized to receive treatment with or without 1.3 mg/m² bortezomib on days 1, 4, 8, and 11. Following double autologous stem cell transplantation procedures, patients received two 35-day cycles of the drug regimen (with or without bortezomib) as consolidation therapy. Complete or near-complete response occurred significantly more frequently among bortezomib than nonbortezomib patients (31% versus 11%, respectively; $p < 0.0001$). Bortezomib patients had a higher incidence of all types of adverse events ≥ grade 3 (56% versus 33%, respectively; $p < 0.0001$). Peripheral neuropathy occurred significantly more often in bortezomib patients (10% versus 2%, respectively; $p = 0.0004$). Of the patients with severe peripheral neuropathy, improvement or resolution was observed in 78% of bortezomib patients (18/23) compared to 60% of the nonbortezomib patients (3/5).

3.5.3.3   Bortezomib with Melphalan and Prednisone versus Bortezomib with Thalidomide and Prednisone

Combination induction therapy with melphalan, prednisone, and bortezomib is now a well-recognized induction therapy for geriatric multiple myeloma (Palumbo and Gay, 2009). A randomized clinical trial of elderly patients (≥65 years) with untreated multiple myeloma received either six cycles of bortezomib plus mephalan and prednisone or bortezomib plus thalidomide and prednisone as induction therapy, in the form of one cycle of bortezomib twice weekly for 6 weeks (1.3 mg/m² on days 1, 4, 8, 11, 22, 25, 29, and 32) plus either melphalan (9 mg/m² on days 1 through 4) or 100 mg thalidomide daily and prednisone (60 mg/m² on days 1 through 4) (Mateos et al., 2010). The first cycle was followed by five more cycles of weekly bortezomib for 5 weeks (1.3 mg/m² on days 1, 8, 15, and 22) plus the same doses of melphalan-prednisone or thalidomide-prednisone. Patients who completed this phase ($n = 178$) were then randomized to maintenance therapy with bortezomib-prednisone or bortezomib-thalidomide. Partial responses or better in the induction phase were similar between groups (81% for patients receiving bortezomib-mephalan-prednisone versus 80% for those receiving bortezomib-thalidomide-prednisone). Patients treated with bortezomib-thalidomide-prednisone had significantly more adverse events overall (41% versus 15%, respectively; $p = 0.01$) and discontinuations of therapy (17% versus 12%, respectively; $p = 0.03$). However, the rates of peripheral neuropathy were similar (7% versus 9%, respectively). This study suggests that bortezomib may be safely used as an effective chemotherapy for elderly patients.

3.5.3.4   Bortezomib and Dexamethasone versus Vincristine, Doxorubicin, and Dexamethasone

In a study that found the bortezomib-dexamethasone combination chemotherapy to be more effective than vincristine-doxorubicin-dexamethasone chemotherapy prior to autologous stem cell transplantation in 482 newly diagnosed multiple myeloma patients, the rate of peripheral neuropathy was higher in the bortezomib-dexamethasone group (Harousseau et al., 2010). Patients were randomized to receive vincristine-doxorubicin-dexamethasone or bortezomib-dexamethasone, or one of those treatments plus cyclophosphamide, etoposide, and cisplatin, as induction therapy to be followed by autologous stem cell transplantation. Patients who did not achieve a good partial response received a second transplantation. Postinduction overall response rates were significantly higher with bortezomib-dexamethasone than vincristine-doxorubicin-dexamethasone (14.8% versus 6.4%, respectively; $p = 0.004$).

Three-year survival rates were 81.4% compared to 77.4% (median follow-up, 32.2 months). Patients in the vincristine-doxorubicin-dexamethasone group exhibited higher hematologic toxicities and toxicity-related mortality rates than bortezomib-dexamethasone patients, but the latter had higher rates of peripheral neuropathy. A total of 20.5% of bortezomib-dexamethasone patients had $\geq$ grade 2 peripheral and 9.2% had $\geq$ grade 3 neuropathy compared to 10.5% and 2.5%, respectively, of vincristine-doxorubicin-dexamethasone patients.

3.5.3.5 Bortezomib and Dexamethasone versus Vincristine, Pirarubicin, Dexamethasone, and Melphalan

In a retrospective analysis, 24 patients with newly diagnosed multiple myeloma receiving bortezomib and dexamethasone were compared to 30 matched patients who received combination therapy of vinctristine-pirarubicin-dexamethasone-melphalan (Li et al., 2009a). Response rates were not significantly different (87.5% in bortezomib-dexamethasone group versus 76.7% in vincristine-pirarubicin-dexamethasone-melphalan combination group, $p = 0.483$), although bortezomib-dexamethasone patients had a significantly shorter median time to response. Adverse events were similar in both groups, but peripheral neuropathy was among the five most-reported adverse events only in the bortezomib-dexamethasone group (54.2%).

3.5.3.6 Melphalan and Prednisone with and without Bortezomib

High-dose melphalan (200 mg/m^2) is considered to be a conditioning regimen in newly diagnosed or relapsed/refractory multiple myeloma patients awaiting autologous stem cell transplant. However, prolonged treatment with melphalan may have an adverse effect on the harvesting of peripheral blood stem cells. For that reason, combining melphalan with bortezomib may help prepare a patient for autologous stem cell transplantation by shortening the course of therapy and truncating the patient's duration of exposure to melphalan. Moreover, synergistic interaction between melphalan and bortezomib has been reported *in vitro* (Mitsiades et al., 2003) and *in vivo* (San Miguel et al., 2008). In a study of 54 previously untreated multiple myeloma patients who were administered bortezomib and high-dose mephalan (200 mg/m^2) as conditioning therapy, 70% had a very good or better partial response rate (complete response, 32%) (Roussel et al., 2009). In this study, one case of peripheral neuropathy $\geq$ grade 3 was observed.

In a study of 44 patients with previously untreated multiple myeloma, patients received up to six 28-day cycles of 1.3 mg/m^2 bortezomib on days 1, 4, 8, and 11 plus 6 mg/m^2 melphalan and 60 mg/m^2 prednisone on days 1 through 7 (Gasparetto et al., 2010). After two to six cycles, consenting patients underwent autologous stem cell transplantation, which was successful in 100% of patients. The overall response rate was 95% (18% complete response) and 38% of patients experienced peripheral neuropathy $\geq$ grade 2; five patients (11%) discontinued treatment because of peripheral neuropathy. In most cases, the peripheral neuropathy was reversible.

3.5.3.7 Melphalan and Prednisone with and without Bortezomib

The VISTA clinical trial evaluated 682 multiple myeloma patients who were not considered appropriate candidates for autologous stem cell transplant (San Miguel et al.,

2008). Standard therapy for such patients is chemotherapy with melphalan and prednisone. All patients in this study were treated with mephalan and prednisone, and randomized as to whether or not bortezomib was administered (Spicka et al., 2011). Patients received nine 6-week cycles of 9 mg/m² oral melphalan and 60 mg/m² prednisone on days 1 through 4, either alone or with 1.3 mg/m² intravenous bortezomib on days 1, 4, 8, 11, 22, 25, 29, and 32 during the first four cycles and thereafter on days 1, 8, 22, and 29 for the remainder of the course of therapy. Response was significantly better in the bortezomib group, with 71% showing partial or better response compared to 35% of the melphalan-prednisone group ($p < 0.001$), and complete response rates were 30% versus 4%, respectively ($p < 0.001$). While hematological adverse events were not statistically different between groups, bortezomib patients were statistically significantly more likely to exhibit grade 3 adverse events (53% versus 44%, $p = 0.02$), including peripheral sensory neuropathy (13% of all study patients had grade 3 neuropathy and less than 1% had grade 4). While bortezomib patients were more likely to experience grade 3 adverse events, the risk of grade 4 adverse events was similar in both groups (28% versus 27%, NS).

A subanalysis of the VISTA trial ($n = 682$) found that 47% of the newly diagnosed multiple myeloma patients who received the following therapy developed peripheral neuropathy: nine 6-week cycles of 1.3 mg/m² bortezomib on days 1, 4, 8, 11, 22, 25, 29, and 32 in cycles 1 through 4 and on days 1, 8, 22, and 29 of cycles 5 through 9, along with 9 mg/m² melphalan on days 1 through 4 of all nine cycles and 60 mg/m² prednisone on days 1 through 4 of all cycles (Dimopoulos et al., 2011). It should be noted here that 19% of the patients ($n = 63$) had neuropathy at baseline, which was shown through multivariate analysis to be a risk factor for treatment-emergent peripheral neuropathy. The median time to onset of peripheral neuropathy in this study was 2.3 months (range, 0.03 to 10.8). The severity of peripheral neuropathy in this study depended on the cumulative dose of bortezomib. The median cumulative dose of bortezomib at the onset of peripheral neuropathy was 16.3 mg/m², the median cumulative dose at onset of peripheral neuropathy ≥ grade 2 was 19.5 mg/m², and the median cumultative dose at onset of ≥ grade 3 peripheral neuropathy was 20.2 mg/m². Patients with peripheral neuropathy received a total median cumulative dose of bortezomib of 38.0 mg/m². The complete response rate did not vary based on treatment-emergent peripheral neuropathy; of those who developed treatment-emergent peripheral neuropathy (85%), the complete response rate was 30% compared to the 29% complete response rate among patients who did not develop peripheral neuropathy. Expressed another way, 53% of patients with complete response developed peripheral neuropathy.

3.5.3.8   Rituximab with and without Bortezomib

In a phase III trial of 676 rituximab-naïve or rituximab-sensitive patients with relapsed grade 1 or 2 follicular lymphoma, patients were randomized to receive five 35-day cycles of 375 mg/m² intravenous rituximab on days 1, 8, 15, and 22 of cycle 1, and starting on day 1 of the second through fifth cycles, the rituximab would be administered alone or with 1.6 mg/m² bortezomib on days 1, 8, 15, and 22 of all cycles (Coiffier et al., 2011). Overall adverse event rates ≥ grade 3 were 21% in the rituximab-only group versus 46% in the rituximab-bortezomib group, the most common of which was neutropenia. In the rituximab-bortezomib group, 17% of patients suffered peripheral neuropathy (3% of which was ≥ grade 3), compared to 1% of patients in the rituximab-only group, none of which had grade 3 or higher neuropathy.

3.5.4 DOSING FREQUENCY OF BORTEZOMIB

There is growing evidence that suggests the incidence of peripheral neuropathy may be exacerbated by higher frequency of bortezomib treatment, for example, when chemotherapy is delivered twice weekly rather than once a week. In a study of 372 multiple myeloma patients receiving once-weekly or twice-weekly bortezomib, long-term outcomes were similar (3-year progression-free survival rates were 50% in the once-weekly group versus 47% in the twice-weekly group, NS), with an overall 3-year survival of 88% versus 89%, respectively (Bringhen et al., 2010). There was no statistically significant difference in complete response rate (30% for once weekly and 35% for twice weekly). Peripheral neuropathy ≥ grade 3 occurred in 8% of the once-weekly group compared to 28% of the twice-weekly group ($p < 0.001$), and 5% of patients in the once-weekly group versus 15% in the twice-weekly group discontinued bortezomib treatment on account of peripheral neuropathy ($p < 0.001$). In this study, the improved safety profile with respect to peripheral neuropathy of once-weekly bortezomib administration did not appear to affect the agent's efficacy rates.

The dosing frequency of bortezomib combined with rituximab was investigated in a study of 81 patients with relapsed or refractory follicular or marginal zone B-cell lymphoma. Patients were randomized to receive 1.3 mg/m² bortezomib twice a week on days 1, 4, 8, and 11 of a 21-day cycle for five cycles or 1.6 mg/m² bortezomib weekly on days 1, 8, 15, and 22 of a 35-day cycle for three cycles. Both groups received 375 mg/m² rituximab weekly for 4 weeks (de Vos et al., 2009). Although dose intensity was greater in the twice-weekly group, the mean total dose of bortezomib was similar in both twice-weekly and once-weekly groups (18.5 and 17.1 mg/m², respectively). Results appear in Table 3.3. It should be noted that no grade 4 toxicities of any kind occurred in the weekly regimen. This study suggests that dosing regimen may play a greater role than cumulative dose in avoiding bortezomib-induced peripheral neuropathy.

TABLE 3.3
Results Showing Bortezomib and Rituximab Dosing Schedules and Rates of Treatment-Emergent Peripheral Neuropathy

Dosing	Overall Response Rate	Complete Response Rate	Median Time to Progression (Duration of Response)	Overall Adverse Events ≥ Grade 3 (Peripheral Neuropathy ≥ Grade 3)
Twice weekly	49%	14%	7.0 months (not reached)	54% (10%)
Once weekly	43%	10%	10.0 months (9.3 months)	35% (5%)

Source: Data from de Vos, S. et al., *J Clin Oncol* 27(30):5023–5030, 2009.

3.5.5 Subcutaneous Bortezomib

Bortezomib is typically administered intravenously, but new studies are evaluating subcutaneous drug delivery as an alternative. In a phase III multicenter study ($n = 222$), subcutaneous bortezomib was shown to be noninferior to intravenous bortezomib but with significantly lower rates of peripheral neuropathy (Moreau et al., 2011). In this study, peripheral neuropathy (any grade) occurred in 38% of subcutaneous versus 53% of intravenous patients ($p = 0.044$), while peripheral neuropathy ≥ grade 2 occurred in 24% versus 41% of patients, respectively ($p = 0.012$) and peripheral neuropathy ≥ grade 3 was observed in 6% versus 16%, respectively ($p = 0.026$).

3.5.6 Bortezomib in Special Populations

In a study of 55 treatment-naïve and treatment-experienced multiple myeloma patients receiving bortezomib for the first time to treat relapsed or refractory multiple myeloma, age was identified as a risk factor for peripheral neuropathy as an adverse event during bortezomib therapy, with every year increasing the risk by about 6% (Corso et al., 2010). This finding is disputed, in that other investigators have not found age as a risk factor in bortezomib-induced peripheral neuropathy (Kanbayashi et al., 2010).

In a study of 117 multiple myeloma patients with some degree of renal impairment (14 of whom required dialysis), bortezomib was administered with at least a partial response documented in 73% of evaluable patients (19% complete response) (Morabito et al., 2010). Response rates were similar across subgroups based on degree of severity of renal dysfunction. The rate of discontinuation on account of adverse events was 11% in patients with severe renal impairment, compared to 5% in those with moderate and no mild renal impairment. This same trend occurred in cases of peripheral neuropathy, which occurred in five patients with severe renal impairment and four patients with moderate renal impairment, but no patients with mild renal impairment. Another study investigating this same population of newly diagnosed multiple myeloma patients with renal impairment ($n = 18$) found that treatment with a median of four cycles of bortezomib and dexamethasone resulted in an overall response rate of 83.3% (33.3% complete response) and a reversal of renal impairment in 38.9% of patients, which occurred at a median of 16 days (Li et al., 2009). Three patients (17%) in that latter study developed a grade 3 or 4 peripheral neuropathy.

Preexisting peripheral neuropathy has been implicated as a risk factor for many types of chemotherapy-induced peripheral neuropathy. Peripheral neuropathy may be secondary to the patient's malignancy or an adverse effect of previous treatment. In a murine model, the presence of severe neuropathy prior to treatment with bortezomib resulted in a more marked neuropathy with greater involvement of peripheral nerves (Bruna et al., 2011). In a subanalysis of the phase III VISTA trial, investigators found through multivariate analysis that the only consistent risk factor for chemotherapy-induced peripheral neuropathy in newly diagnosed multiple myeloma patients treated with bortezomib-melphalan-prednisone was preexisting neuropathy (hazard ratio, 1.786; $p = 0.0065$). In this study, factors such as age, preexisting diabetes, obesity, and creatinine clearance were not significant risk factors for peripheral neuropathy in multiple myeloma patients treated with the aforementioned combination therapy (Dimopoulos et al., 2011).

3.6 THALIDOMIDE

Thalidomide was first sold as a sedative and antiemetic agent in the 1950s but was taken off the market in 1961 because of its teratogenic effects (Lenz, 1985). In 1994, preclinical studies showed that thalidomide had antiangiogenic effects, so the drug's potential use in treating diseases associated with angiogenesis, such as malignant tumors, was explored (D'Amato et al., 1994). Thalidomide has been shown to be effective in many chemotherapeutic regimens, particularly in the treatment of multiple myeloma. However, thalidomide is associated with a number of treatment-emergent adverse events, including peripheral neuropathy. The underlying mechanisms of thalidomide-induced peripheral neuropathy remain unclear. The drug causes a downregulation of tumor necrosis factor alpha (TNF-α) synthesis that could, in theory at least, affect the process of Wallerian degeneration of nerve fibers. It is also possible that this might explain thalidomide's beneficial activity in response to neuropathic pain (George et al., 2000).

Peripheral neuropathy is a frequently reported adverse effect of thalidomide chemotherapy and may be treatment limiting. The incidence of thalidomide-induced peripheral neuropathy in the treatment of cancer varies widely and may be as high as 70%. The correlation, if any, between thalidomide dosage, duration of treatment, and the rate, onset, and severity of thalidomide-induced neuropathy remains unclear (Bastuji-Garin et al., 2002; Chaudhry et al., 2002; Plasmati et al., 2007; Hattori et al., 2008). Older patients may be more susceptible to thalidomide-induced neuropathy than younger ones (Molloy et al., 2001). Thalidomide has been shown to induce dose-dependent peripheral neuropathy in pediatric patients (53.8%) (Priolo et al., 2008).

3.6.1 MONOTHERAPIES

Thalidomide is considered an effective monotherapeutic regimen for first-line treatment of multiple myeloma. In a study of 31 patients with newly diagnosed multiple myeloma, patients were administered 200 mg/day thalidomide aimed at debulking multiple myeloma in advance of autologous transplantation. Posttransplantation, patients took 200 mg/day thalidomide for 3 more months. The overall response rate was 100%. At the conclusion of the study, 83% of patients had clinical and electrophysiological evidence of mild sensory neuropathy (not motor, axonal, or length-dependent polyneuropathy).

In a regulatory phase II trial for the Ministry of Health, Labor, and Welfare of Japan, the safety, efficacy, pharmacokinetics, and pharmacodynamics of thalidomide in 34 multiple myeloma patients was assessed. Patients were given 100 mg/day oral thalidomide for the first 4 weeks, then 200 mg/day for weeks 5 to 8, 300 mg/day for weeks 9 through 12, and finally 400 mg/day (maximum dose) for the 13th week of the study, providing toxicity was acceptable (Murakami et al., 2009). The overall response rate was 35.3%. Peripheral neuropathy ≤ grade 2 occurred in about a quarter of patients; no peripheral neuropathy ≥ grade 3 occurred. This rate of peripheral neuropathy was reported to be similar to rates observed in American and European studies.

Thalidomide for maintenance therapy in multiple myeloma patients was evaluated in 100 patients in five dose-escalating groups of equal size ($n = 20$). The target doses for the groups were 50, 100, 200, 250, and 300 mg/day (Feyler et al., 2007). All patients started at 50 mg/day and were escalated to target doses. The 3-year overall survival rate was 76% (95% confidence interval, 63 to 85%). Median progression-free survival was 34 months for the entire group. At a median follow-up period of 32.3 months (range, 9 to 48), 77% had discontinued thalidomide therapy (53% because of adverse events, 23% owing to disease progression, and 1% out of financial concerns). Patients took thalidomide for a median of 14 months (range, 0.5 to 37), and those who chose to discontinue thalidomide because of adverse effects took the drug an average of 10 months before stopping (range, 0.5 to 26). The most common side effect was peripheral neuropathy, occurring in 72% of all patients. Thirty-four patients discontinued thalidomide maintenance therapy because of peripheral neuropathy. Doses of 200 mg or greater were associated with major toxicity and could not be tolerated long term.

A 2002 study of thalidomide for the treatment of refractory multiple myeloma (Kakimoto et al., 2002) was extended to a single-center phase II study with a larger patient population and longer study duration (Hattori et al., 2008). Patients ($n = 61$) were administered 200 mg oral thalidomide at night and observed; if this dose was tolerated, it was increased to 400 mg/day and continued as maintenance therapy. During thalidomide therapy, patients had no other chemotherapy or radiotherapy. If disease progression was observed, combination therapy of dexamethasone with thalidomide was considered. The median duration of therapy was 14 weeks and the overall response rate was 39%. Twenty-two of the patients could be considered responders, and of them, 15 achieved a partial response and 3 achieved a near-complete response. There was no apparent association between thalidomide dose and responders, suggesting that dose intensity may not be an important factor in patient response to thalidomide monotherapy for multiple myeloma. Two-year progression-free survival was 10.7 weeks. The 2-year survival rate was 41.3%. Mean daily dose did not have an association with progression-free survival or overall survival. In this study, 100% of patients experienced at least one adverse event. Fifty-six percent had peripheral neuropathy (all grades), while 79% experienced somnolence (all grades) and 57% had constipation (all grades). While in this study, peripheral neuropathy could be correlated significantly with the total dose of thalidomide and with the duration of thalidomide therapy, it could not be correlated with the daily dose of thalidomide or its plasma concentration. Most cases of peripheral neuropathy were mild; only 2% of patients reported peripheral neuropathy ≥ grade 3. While some adverse events, such as somnolence, fever, and neutropenia, emerged in the first weeks of treatment initiation, peripheral neuropathy (like dry mouth and constipation) was more likely to emerge later in treatment and, in fact, increased in frequency as the study continued. At 6 months, peripheral neuropathy was observed in roughly half of the patients in this study, and by 1 year, all patients (100%) had some degree of peripheral neuropathy.

Peripheral neuropathy caused a dose reduction of thalidomide in 18% of patients; one patient discontinued therapy because of peripheral neuropathy.

Double autologous peripheral blood stem cell transplant (APBSCT) has been shown to be effective in treating multiple myeloma patients by extending progression-free and overall survival durations, but the disease often recurs. Thalidomide was evaluated in 17 multiple myeloma patients as maintenance therapy (Martino et al., 2007). Patients were administered 100 mg/day oral thalidomide beginning 3 to 5 months after the second transplantation and continuing until toxicity or disease progression occurred. Median administration was 13 months (range, 3 to 26) and 76.5% of patients discontinued treatment. Two patients (2/17) discontinued treatment because of peripheral neuropathy. The most common side effects were constipation, dizziness, somnolence, and peripheral neuropathy, with constipation and peripheral neuropathy also the most persistent side effects. After the first transplant, 17.6% of patients were in complete remission and 82.4% were in partial remission. After the second transplant but before thalidomide therapy commenced, 11.8% were in complete remission and 35.3% were in near complete remission, while 52.9% were in partial remission. Four-year estimated progression-free survival was 38.1% ± 14.2%. While thalidomide is effective in this population, toxicity is high and may limit its potential application.

Smoldering or indolent multiple myeloma is a slow-growing, asymptomatic form of multiple myeloma, which puts the patient at risk for the development of active or overt multiple myeloma. A phase II clinical study of 29 patients initiated therapy with 200 mg/day thalidomide and then adjusted the dose as tolerated (Detweiler-Short et al., 2010). Median follow-up for the patients was 10.2 years (range, 7.5 to 11.0 years). The partial response rate was 34% and the minimal response rate was 31%, with a median time to progression to a symptomatic form of the disease observed to be 35 months. Median overall survival from diagnosis was 86 months, and median survival from onset of symptomatic myeloma was 49 months. Peripheral neuropathy ≤ grade 2 occurred in 83% of patients. Peripheral neuropathy ≥ grade 3 occurred in 14% of patients.

In a multicenter study of 64 patients with advanced relapsed or refractory multiple myeloma treated with thalidomide (initiated at 100 mg/day; increased in increments of 200 mg/day every other week; maximum dose, 800 mg/day; median dose, 400 mg/day), peripheral neuropathy ≥ grade 3 occurred in 14% of patients (Tosi et al., 2002). In this study, 28.3% showed ≥50% reduction in serum or urinary M protein concentration.

In a study of 41 patients with myelofibrosis with myeloid metaplasia, patients were administered 200 mg/day thalidomide with a weekly 200 mg/day dose escalation until the best-tolerated dose or 800 mg/day was achieved (Thomas et al., 2006). Five patients started therapy at a reduced dose of 50 or 100 mg/day because of their age. Forty-one percent of patients who were treated for at least 15 days exhibited a response: 10% complete response, 10% partial response, and hematologic improvements in 21%. The median tolerated dose of thalidomide was 400 mg (range, 100 to 800). Peripheral neuropathy was a common drug-related toxicity; grade 1 or 2 peripheral neuropathy occurred in 20% and grade 3 or 4 peripheral neuropathy in 2% of patients.

The optimal treatment of metastatic carcinoid and islet cell tumors remains unclear. These types of tumors are highly vascular, so it was hypothesized that because of its antiangiogenic activity, thalidomide might be effective in treating these neuroendocrine metastases. In a study of 18 patients, patients were treated with 200 mg/day oral thalidomide and were escalated to 400 mg/day after 2 weeks (Varker et al., 2008). No partial or complete responses occurred, although 69% of patients achieved stable disease state. Peripheral neuropathy ≤ grade 2 occurred in 28% of patients ($n = 5$). Grade 3 sensory neuropathy occurred in 11% of patients ($n = 2$). In this study, thalidomide therapy was not effective (no objective responses occurred) but was reasonably well tolerated.

The antiangiogenic properties of thalidomide also led to the hypothesis that it might be effective in treating the growth of malignant gliomas in glioblastoma. In a study of 17 patients with recurrent glioblastoma that had been previously treated with surgery and radiotherapy, patients were treated with thalidomide (Morabito et al., 2004). One patient had a minimal response and eight patients were noted to have disease stabilization, with an overall 52.9% rate of clinical benefit. Median time to progression and median overall survival for responders were 25 weeks (range, 12 to 40) and 36 weeks (range, 16 to 64), respectively. The most common side effects were constipation (76.5%), somnolence (47%), and peripheral neuropathy (11.8%). These side effects were considered to be mild to moderate by investigators.

In a phase II trial of 18 patients with recurrent gliomas who had failed radiotherapy and chemotherapy, 100 mg/day oral thalidomide was administered and responses evaluated every 4 weeks (Short et al., 2001). Median treatment duration was 42 days (range, 7 to 244 days), and treatment had to be discontinued in one patient (5.5%) because of peripheral sensory neuropathy. Median survival from the start of the study was 2.5 months. Twelve patients could be considered responders and continued treatment for more than 4 weeks. Of these 12 patients, 1 had clinical and radiological response, 2 had stable disease for 2 and 4 months, respectively, and 9 patients experienced disease progression. Thus, the partial response rate was low at about 6% and there was one case of treatment-limiting peripheral neuropathy.

Thalidomide was also studied in an open-label phase II trial of 20 men with androgen-independent prostate cancer (Drake et al., 2003). Patients were treated with 100 mg oral thalidomide once daily for up to 6 months (mean time of study, 109 days; median, 107 days; range, 4 to 184 days). A decline in serum prostate-specific antigen (PSA) of at least 50% sustained over the entire course of the study was observed in 15% of the patient population. Of the patients treated for a minimum of 2 months ($n = 16$), 37% showed a fall in absolute PSA of 48% (median). Three patients withdrew from the study because of adverse events, which included constipation, drowsiness, dizziness, and rash. Seven patients completed the entire 6-month course of treatment and all of them (100%) had peripheral neuropathy. Of these patients, four had subclinical evidence of neuropathy prior to thalidomide therapy.

Twenty patients (ages, 6 to 41 years; mean age, 17.5 years) with plexiform neurofibroma inneurofibromatosis I were treated with escalating doses of thalidomide (1, 2, 3, and 4 mg/kg/day) for 12 months (Gupta et al., 2003). Doses up to 200 mg/day were well tolerated. Twelve patients completed the full year of treatment, of which eight showed no change in the size of the plexiform neurofibroma while four had a minor response, defined as a tumor size reduction of 26% to 50%. Two patients developed reversible peripheral neuropathy, and the investigators found no association between higher doses of thalidomide and the frequency of peripheral neuropathy or any other adverse events.

In a pilot study of 19 patients with progressive metastatic renal cell carcinoma, patients were treated with oral thalidomide starting at doses of 200 mg/day and increasing by increments of 100 to 200 mg/day weekly until a target daily dose of 1,200 mg was achieved (Daliani et al., 2002). Eighteen of the 19 patients achieved the target dose. Nine patients in the study had stable disease for a median of 14 months (range, 3 to 17) and median time to progression was 4.7 months (range, 0.7 to 31.3). Median survival was 4.7 months. Peripheral neuropathy occurred in 15/19 patients after a prolonged duration of treatment and was treatment limiting. Most peripheral neuropathy was grade 1, but one patient, who had preexisting neuropathy and diabetes, developed grade 3 peripheral neuropathy. This patient discontinued thalidomide with significant improvement in his symptoms.

In another study of renal cell cancer, 25 adult male patients were treated with oral thalidomide, escalated to the target dose of 600 mg/day (Stebbing et al., 2001). Treatment continued until disease progression or intolerable levels of toxicity occurred. Two patients (9%) showed a partial response (95% confidence interval, 1 to 29%) and 32% had stable disease for more than 6 months (95% confidence interval, 14 to 55%). No cases of grade 1 or grade 4 peripheral neuropathy occurred. Patients who developed grade 2 or 3 neuropathy (16 and 4%, respectively) required a dose reduction but were able to continue treatment.

There are few studies reported in the literature to guide the optimal therapy for Langerhans cell histiocytosis (LCH). Since TNF-α is present in LCH lesions, it appeared an important therapeutic target for chemotherapy. Thalidomide is known to inhibit the production of TNF-α, so it was hypothesized that thalidomide might be effective in such patients. In this study, 16 pediatric and adult LCH patients who had failed primary and at least one secondary therapeutic regimen were enrolled (McClain and Kozinetz, 2007). Patients ranged in age from 19 months to 45 years. Of these patients, six were considered high risk because of the involvement of the spleen, lung, liver, or bone marrow. Thalidomide dose was based on patient weight, with doses typically starting at 50 mg/day for children and 100 mg/day for adults. If there was no toxicity in the first month, the dose was increased in increments of 50 mg/day until efficacy or the first signs of toxicity were noted. Of the six high-risk patients, no response was observed. In contrast, four of the low-risk patients (25%) had complete response and three had a partial response (19%). The responses to thalidomide therapy were significantly better for the low-risk than high-risk patients ($p < 0.05$). The study reported three cases of grade 2 and one case of grade 3 paresthesia, but investigators commented that paresthesia rates in children may be underreported, because some children were not able to clearly verbalize their symptoms.

The long-term toxicity of thalidomide was studied in 40 patients (median age, 61.5 years) who had received salvage thalidomide therapy (with or without dexamethasone) for more than 12 months (Tosi et al., 2005). All patients had stable disease upon commencement of 200 to 400 mg/day thalidomide monotherapy ($n = 20$) or 200 mg/day thalidomide and 40 mg/day dexamethasone for 4 days in a 28-day cycle ($n = 20$). The incidence of any form of neurotoxicity in both groups averaged about 75% with long-term treatment, with grades 1, 2, and 3 occurring in 15, 32.5, and 27.5%, respectively. Electromyographic evaluations were conducted in patients with any neurotoxicity ≥ grade 2 and revealed a symmetrical type of mostly sensory peripheral neuropathy with minor motor involvement. The severity of peripheral neuropathy was associated with the duration of disease prior to thalidomide treatment and was not significantly associated with the cumulative or daily dose of thalidomide. Investigators speculate that multiple myeloma might cause subclinical neurological alterations that set the stage for subsequent thalidomide-induced peripheral neuropathy.

Dose-dependent thalidomide-induced peripheral neuropathy was reported in a study of 59 multiple myeloma patients who were treated with 100 mg/day thalidomide, increasing weekly by 100 mg/day increments, until a maximum dose of 400 mg/day was achieved (Offidani et al., 2004). A subset of these patients ($n = 27$) was also treated with 0.20 mg/kg/day oral melphalan for four out of every 28 days. Peripheral neuropathy occurred in 39% of patients and could be significantly associated with a median daily dose of thalidomide 150 mg. That dose was associated with a higher frequency and greater actuarial risk of peripheral neuropathy, but not an improved overall response rate. Other thalidomide-associated side effects, such as nausea, constipation, and somnolence, were not dose dependent, at least up to a daily dose of 400 mg. Furthermore, therapeutic response and patient survival did not depend on the dose, leading investigators to suggest that daily doses of thalidomide <150 mg may be effective and reduce the risk of peripheral neuropathy.

3.6.2 COMBINATION THERAPIES

3.6.2.1 Thalidomide and Dexamethasone

In a phase II study of 66 patients with refractory multiple myeloma, the safety and efficacy of low-dose thalidomide combined with low-dose dexamethasone was tested (Murakami et al., 2007). Patients were treated with 100 mg/day oral thalidomide for the first week and dexamethasone was administered at 4 mg/day for the first 4 weeks, then decreased by 1 mg each week until a dose of 1 mg/day was achieved and then maintained. The thalidomide dose was increased, if tolerated, to 200 mg/day for the second week and then maintained. The maintenance dose of thalidomide to responding patients was 50 mg/day for five patients, 100 mg/day for 23 patients, and 200 mg/day for 26 patients. Patients were treated for a median of 4.0 months. The overall response rate was 63.6%, and progression-free and overall survival times were 6.2 and 25.4 months, respectively. Peripheral neuropathy (any grade) occurred in 27% of patients and was grade 1 in 20%. This study was conducted in Japan, and investigators noted that the rates of adverse events differed somewhat from studies conducted in the United States or Europe; namely, the rates of peripheral neuropathy and deep vein thrombosis were lower in this Japanese study, while leukopenia rates are higher in Japanese than American or European studies.

In a study of 29 pretreated patients with multiple myeloma with a median number of three relapses per patient (range, 1 to 7), patients underwent therapy with

400 mg/day oral thalidomide and 20 mg/m^2 oral dexamethasone daily for four consecutive days on a 21-day cycle (Schutt et al., 2005). Thalidomide therapy continued but dexamethasone cycles were given until maximal decline of myeloma protein was observed. A response occurred in 62% of the patients, including 17% having complete responses. The median event-free survival time was 7.2 months, and the median overall survival was 26.1 months. Peripheral neuropathy was observed in 55% of patients. Thalidomide dose reductions were made in several patients, 17% of whom had polyneuropathy.

3.6.2.2 Thalidomide and Dexamethasone and Cyclophosphamide

In an open-label phase II study, 68 patients with newly diagnosed multiple myeloma were treated with pulse cyclophosphamide, thalidomide, and dexamethasone chemotherapy for induction therapy (Yang et al., 2010). The overall response was 79.4% (42.6% complete or very good partial response) after a median of 28 months of follow-up. Peripheral sensory neuropathy occurred in 14.3% of patients.

3.6.2.3 Thalidomide and Bortezomib

In a study of 27 patients with newly diagnosed multiple myeloma, patients were given 1.3 mg/m^2 bortezomib on days 1, 4, 8, and 11 of a 21-day cycle and 150 mg/day oral thalidomide every day for a maximum of eight cycles (Ghosh et al., 2011). The overall response rate was 81.5%, with 25.8% achieving a complete or near-complete response. Several grade 3 toxicities occurred, with a 22% incidence of peripheral neuropathy, 15% pneumonia, 7% fatigue, and 7% anemia. Upon conclusion of the therapy, peripheral neuropathy completely resolved in 80% of the patients. The 3-year overall survival rate is 74%. This regimen was steroid-free and treatment-emergent peripheral neuropathy was often reversible.

In a phase II trial conducted in China, 34 patients with newly diagnosed multiple myeloma received 1.3 mg/m^2 bortezomib on days 1, 4, 8, and 11 and 100 mg/day oral thalidomide on a 21-day cycle (Chen, Jiang et al., 2010). Twenty-six patients completed eight cycles of treatment with a 100% overall response rate (31% complete response). The responses were rapid; the best response occurred within the first four cycles in 96% of patients. Peripheral neuropathy (all grades) occurred in 38% of patients. Overall, 12% of patients had to have a dose reduction of thalidomide (from 100 to 50 mg/day) because of peripheral neuropathy; no dose reductions of bortezomib were required. One patient (3%) developed grade 3 peripheral neuropathy and motor neuropathy that improved with dose reduction.

3.6.2.4 THALIDOMIDE AND MELPHALAN AND DEXAMETHASONE

In this study of 50 patients of ≥75 years of age with multiple myeloma, patients were treated with 8 mg/m^2 melphalan on days 1 through 4, 12 mg/m^2 dexamethasone on days 1 through 4 and again on days 17 through 20, and 300 mg/day oral thalidomide on days 1 through 4 and 17 through 20 on a 35-day cycle (Dimopoulos et al., 2006). If there was no evidence of disease progression, patients continued with up to nine more cycles of melphalan, dexamethasone, and thalidomide but without the dexamethasone and thalidomide doses on days 17 through 20. A partial response was achieved in 62% and a complete response in 10% of patients. Median time to response was 2 months, and median time to progression was 21.2 months. Peripheral neuropathy occurred in 9% of patients and was, in all instances, ≤ grade 2. Among patients who received four or more courses of therapy, the incidence of peripheral neuropathy was 11%.

3.6.2.5 Thalidomide and Melphalan and Lenalidomide and Prednisone

In an open-label multicenter trial of thalidomide, melphalan, lenalidomide, and prednisone (RMPT) combination therapy in 44 relapsed or refractory multiple myeloma patients, 10 mg/day oral lenalidomide was administered on days 1 through 21, 0.81 mg/kg oral melphalan and 2 mg/kg oral prednisone on days 1 through 4, and 60 or 100 mg/day oral thalidomide on days 1 through 28 of a 28-day cycle (Palumbo et al., 2010b). Patients underwent six cycles and then went on to maintenance therapy (10 mg/day lenalidomide on days 1 through 21 of a 28-day cycle). Patients continued until disease progression or adverse events warranted treatment cessation. Seventy-five percent of patients achieved at least a partial response (2% complete response) and 1-year progression-free survival was 51%. In this study, 36% of patients experienced grade 1 or 2 neurological symptoms, deemed manageable with routine support, and no cases of grade 3 or 4 peripheral neuropathy were reported. This particular study suggests that RMPT salvage therapy holds promise and is associated with manageable adverse effects, including only mild to moderate levels of peripheral neuropathy.

3.6.2.6 Thalidomide and Bortezomib with Chemotherapy (Cisplatin, Cyclophosphamide, Etoposide, and Dexamethasone)

A phase I clinical trial investigated the use of bortezomib and thalidomide along with combination chemotherapy to treat newly diagnosed multiple myeloma patients (Badros et al., 2006). Patients received escalating doses of bortezomib (0.7, 1.0, and 1.3 mg/m^2 on days 1, 4, and 8) and 10 mg/m^2 cisplatin, 10 mg/m^2 doxorubicin, 400 mg/m^2 cyclophosphamide, and 40 mg/m^2 etoposide per day on days 1 through 4 by continuous infusion. Patients were also administered 40 mg oral dexamethasone on days 1 through 4 and 200 mg/day oral thalidomide on days 1 through 8. Peripheral blood stem cells were collected after the first cycle. A total of 12 patients completed the study and all went on to autologous stem cell transplantation. After two cycles, 83% of patients exhibited a partial response or better. Peripheral neuropathy ≥ grade 3 occurred in 25% of patients. While this phase I trial does not provide any data on how this treatment might impact survival, it suggests that this combination therapy may allow for adequate collection of peripheral blood stem cells and early autologous stem cell transplant in multiple myeloma patients.

3.6.2.7 Thalidomide and Bortezomib with Epirubicin and Dexamethasone

Bortezomib combined with epirubicin, dexamethasone, and thalidomide (BADT) has been proposed as a combination therapy for treating multiple myeloma. Twelve patients with multiple myeloma (four were treatment naïve and eight were pretreated with at least one cycle of systemic chemotherapy) were enrolled. Patients received 1.0 mg/m^2 intravenous bortezomiub and 12 mg/m^2 intravenous epirubicin on days 1, 4, 8, and 11 of a 28-day cycle and 20 mg dexamethasone on days 1, 2, 4, 5, 8,

9, 11, and 12 and 100 mg/day oral thalidomide on days 1 through 28 (Lu et al., 2009). On average, patients underwent five cycles (minimum of two). The complete response rate was 83.3% and the disease stabilization rate was 16.7%. The average number of cycles required to achieve complete response in this single-center study was 1.9 (range, 1 to 6). One-third of patients (33%) developed peripheral neuropathy ≥ grade 3. Other adverse effects included thrombocytopenia (25%), neutropenia (42%), infection (33%), weakness (42%), and constipation (25%). Investigators in this study suggested that predictive factors for developing peripheral neuropathy might be preexisting neuropathy, prior thalidomide use, and type 2 diabetes mellitus. The rapid achievement of high rates of complete response along with acceptable toxicity make this drug appear promising as a treatment for multiple myeloma.

3.6.2.8 Thalidomide and a Combination of Bortezomib, Melphalan, and Dexamethasone

In a phase II trial, 62 pretreated patients with refractory or relapse multiple myeloma were administered combination chemotherapy consisting of 1.0 mg/m^2 intravenous bortezomib on days 1, 4, 8, and 11 of a 28-day cycle with 0.15 mg/kg oral melphalan administered on days 1 through 4 (Terpos et al., 2008). Thalidomide was administered intermittently at a dose of 100 mg/day on days 1 through 4 and again on days 17 to 20. In patients who developed grade 2 peripheral neuropathy, bortezomib was reduced to a dose of 0.7 mg/m^2 on the same schedule. The overall response rate was 66% and the complete response rate was 13%. The median time to response was 35 days (range, 10 to 150 days) and median time to progression was 9.3 months. Peripheral neuropathy was frequent and developed (all grades) in 66% of patients. Broken down by grade, grades 1, 2, and 3 peripheral neuropathy occurred in 30.6, 22.6, and 9.7% of patients, respectively. Of the six patients who developed grade 3 peripheral neuropathy, five of them had preexisting peripheral neuropathy. No patients developed grade 4 peripheral neuropathy. While toxicities were described in this study to be manageable, 22% of patients discontinued therapy on account of adverse events.

A multicenter trial ($n = 30$) evaluated the addition of thalidomide and bortezomib to the standard treatment of oral melphalan and prednisone in relapsed multiple myeloma patients (Palumbo et al., 2007). In this study, bortezomib was administered in three dose levels: 1.0, 1.3, and 1.6 mg/m^2 on days 1, 4, 15, and 22 of a 35-day cycle. On days 1 through 5, patients were administered 6 mg/m^2 melphalan and 60 mg/m^2 prednisone. Patients received 50 mg oral thalidomide every day. The maximum tolerated dose of bortezomib was 1.3 mg/m^2. Twenty patients (67%) had a partial response or better; 43% achieved a very good partial response. One-year progression-free survival was 61% and 1-year overall survival was 84%. The rate of peripheral neuropathy ≥ grade 3 was 7%, and both cases were grade 3 ($n = 2$). There were no grade 4 toxicities of any kind. Investigators described the rate of treatment-related peripheral neuropathy as "unexpectedly low."

3.6.2.9 Thalidomide and Capecitabine

In a phase II study, 12 patients with progressive, measurable metastatic renal cell carcinoma were treated with 200 mg/day oral thalidomide and capecitabine 1,250 mg/m^2

twice daily for 14 days of a 21-day cycle (Harshman et al., 2008). Nine patients in the study had had a prior nephrectomy. Patients received a median number of four cycles (range, 2 to 10) and 42% achieved stable disease. There were no cases of radiographic responses, and 58% of the patients experienced disease progression with a median overall survival rate of 10.2 months. Peripheral neuropathy occurred in 25% of patients and was considered mild to moderate (grade 1 or 2). Hand-foot syndrome likewise occurred in 25% of patients.

3.6.2.10   Thalidomide and Cyclophosphamide

In a phase I clinical trial of 16 pretreated patients with hormone refractory prostate cancer, oral thalidomide at two doses (100 and 200 mg/day) was evaluated (Di Lorenzo et al., 2007). Patients were assigned to 100 mg/day or 200 mg/day of thalidomide, started on day 1 and continued for a 28-day cycle. All patients also received 50 mg/day oral cyclophosphamide. Two patients (15%) had a decrease in prostate-specific antigen (PSA) levels of >50%, and one patient (8%) had a decrease in PSA of <50%. The overall decrease in PSA levels was 23%. Rates of peripheral neuropathy ≤ grade 2 were similar in both dose groups (30% and 33% for 100 and 200 mg/day, respectively). Peripheral neuropathy ≥ grade 3 occurred in none and one patient (1/16) of the 100 and 200 mg/day groups, respectively. The maximum tolerated dose of thalidomide in this trial was 100 mg/day. Overall, the incidence of peripheral neuropathy in this study (all grades) was 31.25%. All adverse events in this study resolved with cessation of treatment.

A trial of thalidomide and cyclophosphamide enrolled 27 patients with a variety of recurrent or refractory pediatric malignancies, including central nervous system (CNS) tumors, Ewing sarcoma, neuroblastoma, fibrosarcoma, and other non-CNS solid tumors, such as germ cell tumors, osteosarcomas, and so on (Gilheeney et al., 2007). Patients ranged from one to 54 years of age and had exhausted all other therapeutic options. The median number of prior treatment regimens per patient was four. Patients began this treatment with oral thalidomide (starting at 6 mg/kg/day, divided into four equal doses, with maximum daily dose of 800 mg, and maximum single dose of 200 mg) and 1,200 mg/m^2/day cyclophosphamide administered over 60 minutes on day 1 of a 28-day cycle. Thalidomide and cyclophosphamide were initiated on the same day. Patients continued taking thalidomide daily unless there was unacceptable toxicity or disease progression. After therapy commenced, some patients were allowed to take thalidomide as one single daily dose at bedtime. Therapy was administered in repeated cycles, as tolerated. Twenty-one patients were evaluable for response, of which one had a partial response (Hodgkin's disease), one had stable disease (neuroendocrine tumor), and 19 had progressive disease. Although this study screened patients for treatment-emergent peripheral neuropathy as part of the protocol, there were no cases of peripheral neuropathy of any grade observed. The study was stopped early because patient accrual waned and results were not encouraging.

3.6.2.11   Thalidomide, Cyclophosphamide, and Dexamethasone

In a study of 53 pretreated multiple myeloma patients, patients were administered an oral regimen of 150 mg/m^2 cyclophosphamide every 12 hours before meals on days 1 through 5, 400 mg thalidomide in the evenings on days 1 through 5 and 14 through 18, and 20 mg/m^2 dexamethasone in the mornings after breakfast on days 1 through 5 and 14 through 18 (Dimopoulos et al., 2004). Treatment was scheduled on a 28-day cycle. Patients were to receive three cycles and responders would receive maintenance therapy of cyclophosphamide, thalidomide, and dexamethasone but only on the first five days of the 28-day cycle. Based on an intent-to-treat analysis, 60% of patients achieved a partial response with a median time to response of 1.5 months. Of the thalidomide-naïve patients in the study, 67% were responders. Peripheral neuropathy occurred in 2% of patients, an unexpectedly low rate.

3.6.2.12 Thalidomide and Dacarbazine

An open-label phase II study of 13 patients with histologically confirmed measurable metastatic melanoma without brain metastases received 1,000 mg/m^2 intravenous dacarbazine every 3 weeks and oral thalidomide daily (Ott et al., 2009). Patients were started at 200 mg/day of thalidomide and escalated every 3 weeks as tolerated up to a maximum of 800 mg/day. Nine of the patients in the study had not had any prior adjuvant therapy. Patients received a median of five cycles of chemotherapy (range, 1 to 18), and the median daily dose of thalidomide was 200 mg/day. The maximum tolerated dose of thalidomide in this study was 400 mg/day ($n = 1$); no patient tolerated the intended maximum dose of 800 mg/day. One patient (1/13) had a partial response, three had stable disease, and nine had progressive disease. Several toxicities ≥ grade 3 occurred, including constipation, fatigue, edema, neutropenia, thrombocytopenia, nausea, and peripheral neuropathy. In this study, the rates of peripheral neuropathy for grades 2, 3, and 4 were 15, 8, and 0%, respectively. Peripheral neuropathy occurred in all patients taking >200 mg/day thalidomide and the single patient who developed grade 3 peripheral neuropathy was taking a daily dose of 400 mg. Thus, thalidomide did not contribute to the efficacy of this treatment regimen, but did increase the toxicity.

3.6.2.13 Thalidomide and Fludarabine

Fludarabine is a purine analog that inhibits DNA synthesis; it is used in a variety of hematological malignancies. In a trial of patients with chronic lymphocytic leukemia ($n = 13$), patients received continuous daily doses of oral thalidomide at levels of 100, 200, and 300 mg/day (Chanan-Khan et al., 2005). Overall response rates were 100%, with 55% of patients achieving a complete remission. At median follow-up of 15 months, no patient had had a relapse and median time to disease progression could not be assessed. Grade 1 or 2 peripheral neuropathy occurred in 61.5% of patients, but no cases of more severe neuropathy were observed. All cases of peripheral neuropathy resolved completely when treatment stopped.

3.6.2.14 Thalidomide and Granulocyte Macrophage-Colony Stimulating Factor (GM-CSF)

Rising levels of prostate specific antigen (PSA) in advanced prostate cancer patients is an indicator of biochemical relapse and may indicate residual cancer or active cancer before overt clinical signs appear. Prognosis in such patients often relies on parameters such as time to PSA nadir, time to PSA recurrence, and the pattern of PSA recurrence. Granulocyte macrophage-colony stimulating factor (GM-CSF) has been studied in patients with androgen-independent prostate cancer and was evaluated in a phase II clinical trial in combination with thalidomide in hormone-naïve prostate carcinoma patients ($n = 20$) (Amato et al., 2009). Patients were administered $250\,\mu g/m^2$ (maximum $500\,\mu g/m^2$) GM-CSF subcutaneously three times a week with injections a minimum of 24 hours apart. Thalidomide was administered concurrently with an initial dose of 100 mg/day. After 7 days, during weeks 2 through 4, the thalidomide dose was escalated by increments of 100 mg every week until the maximum tolerated dose was determined or the patient reached 400 mg/day. The maximum tolerated dose of thalidomide or 400 mg/day was continued daily without interruption over the course of the study. PSA levels and other laboratory parameters were assessed every 6 weeks. At baseline, PSA levels ranged from 1.3 to 61.0 ng/ml. Of the 18 responders in the study, the median PSA level reduction was 59% (range, 26 to 89) and the median duration of response was 11 months (range, 4.5 to 36). The maximum tolerated doses of thalidomide in this study ranged from 50 mg/day to 400 mg/day, with 60% of patients receiving a dose of ≤100 mg/day. Nineteen patients left the study at points from 3.0 to 33.3 months, because of disease progression, development of a second primary tumor, or toxicity. Peripheral neuropathy ≤ grade 2 occurred in 18 patients, two of which had grade 2. No more severe cases of peripheral neuropathy were observed.

3.6.2.15 Thalidomide and Interleukin-2 Plus Granulocyte Macrophage-Colony Stimulating Factor (GM-CSF)

Many patients with primary renal tumors develop metastatic disease, and there has yet to emerge a standard of care. Front-line treatment is generally interleukin-2 (IL-2) or cytokine therapy. Granulocyte macrophage-colony stimulating factor (GM-CSF) is cytokine tested as both monotherapy and combined with IL-2 in the treatment of metastatic renal cell carcinoma. A phase II study was designed to test the hypothesis that thalidomide's antiangiogenic and immunomodulary activities would be effective to add to this therapy (Amato et al., 2008). Thirty-one patients were enrolled, of whom 94% had undergone a prior nephrectomy. Median time from diagnosis of metastatic disease to enrollment was 3 months. Patients were given one 200 mg dose of oral thalidomide before starting IL-2 and GM-CSF therapy. Patients were administered IL-2 and GM-CSF, subcutaneously, fixed at $7\,mIU/m^2$ and $250\,\mu g/m^2$, respectively, on days 1 through 5 of weeks 2 to 5. At 48 hours after chemotherapy commenced, patients were increased to a daily dose of 400 mg oral thalidomide. In the first course, patients were not treated during weeks 6 and 7; in subsequent courses, weeks 5 and 6 were the weeks off. After six courses of combination therapy (slightly over 9 months), patients then continued on thalidomide alone. Patients with complete response continued on oral thalidomide for 6 months, while other patients continued thalidomide until disease progression or intolerable toxicity occurred. Twenty-eight patients completed the first 13 weeks of treatment, and of those, 10% had complete response, 26% partial response, and 19% stabilized disease. Three of the patients who achieved complete response continued taking maintenance doses of thalidomide for 15 months, with responses lasting 15, 17, and 24 months, respectively. Median time to progression for all 31 patients was 5 months (range, 1 to 24) and median overall survival was 18 months (range, 1 to 31). In this study, 29% developed paresthesia and 13% experienced numbness, in all cases ≤ grade 2. Four patients (13%) required dose reductions from 400 mg/day thalidomide to 200 mg/day.

3.6.2.16 Thalidomide and Rituximab

Waldenström macroglobulinemia (WM), also known as lymphoplasmacytic lymphoma, is a relatively rare cancer and is a type of non-Hodgkin's lymphoma, which involves the liver and spleen. In a phase II clinical trial ($n = 25$), symptomatic WM patients were treated with 200 mg/day oral thalidomide for 2 weeks, increased to 400 mg/day for 50 weeks, and 375 mg/m^2 rituximab per week on weeks 2 to 5 and again on weeks 13 to 16 (Treon et al., 2008). None of the patients had been previously treated with either thalidomide or rituximab. When evaluated on an intent-to-treat basis, the overall response rate was 72%, with a 64% major response rate. Median time to progression for responders was 38 months. Patients did not tolerate the high dose of thalidomide; a dose reduction of thalidomide was made in all patients and led to 14/25 (56%) patients discontinuing thalidomide treatment. Discontinuation of treatment occurred at a median of 4.1 months (range, 1.2 to 10.4). Peripheral neuropathy ≥ grade 2 occurred in 44% of patients and was the most commonly reported adverse event in this study. Broken down by grades, grade 1, 2, and 3 peripheral neuropathy occurred in 16, 16, and 28% of patients, respectively; no patient developed grade 4 peripheral neuropathy. Among patients who had peripheral neuropathy ≥ grade 2 ($n = 11$), the neuropathy was first reported at a median of 6.3 months (range, 0.64 to 11.8) after starting thalidomide. Peripheral neuropathy was frequently reversible. Resolution to peripheral neuropathy ≤ grade 1 occurred in 91% of patients at a median time of 5.3 months (range, 1 to 22.5), and 63.6% reported peripheral neuropathy completely resolved at a median of 8.8 months (range, 2.3 to 43.7).

3.6.2.17 Thalidomide and Semaxanib

Semaxanib is a small molecule tyrosine kinase inhibitor of vascular endothelial growth factor (VEGF) receptor-2. Combining semaxanib with thalidomide offers dual antiangiogenetic activities. In a phase II pharmacokinetic study, 12 patients with metastatic melanoma who had failed at least one prior course of treatment (biologic or chemotherapy) were treated with fixed-dose (145 mg/m^2) intravenous semaxanib twice weekly, combined with oral daily thalidomide, commencing with a dose of 200 mg/day and escalated as tolerated (Mita et al., 2007). In the first course, patients were treated with semaxanib 1 day in advance of starting thalidomide therapy in order to allow pharmacokinetics of semaxanib with and without thalidomide to be evaluated. Only 2 of the 12 patients tolerated dose escalation of thalidomide from 200 mg/day to 300 and 400 mg/day, respectively. Peripheral neuropathy (any grade) was reported in 42% of patients ($n = 5$). There was no grade 3 and one case of grade 4 peripheral neuropathy reported, the latter occurring in the first course of treatment.

3.6.2.18 Thalidomide and Vincristine with Pegylated Doxorubicin and Dexamethasone

Combination therapy of vincristine and doxorubicin, both administered as a continuous 96-hour infusion via a central line, and intermittent high-dose dexamethasone as a front-line treatment for newly diagnosed multiple myeloma has resulted in high response rates (55 to 85%). However, these high response rates did not translate into a survival advantage when compared to melphalan and prednisone therapy (Hussein, 2003; Durie et al., 2004). Adults with newly diagnosed or relapsed/refractory multiple myeloma were evaluated in a study of pegylated liposomal doxorubicin, vincristine, and decreased-frequency dexamethasone (DVd) combined with thalidomide (n = 102) (Hussein et al., 2006). Patients were treated with DVd therapy and received 50 mg/day oral thalidomide, increased slowly to a maximum daily dose of 400 mg. At the time of best response, patients were administered oral prednisone 50 mg every other day. The overall response rate was 87% for newly diagnosed and 90% for previously treated multiple myeloma. Complete response rates were 49% for newly diagnosed patients and 45% for pretreated patients. Peripheral neuropathy (all grades) occurred frequently and was observed in 84% of patients. Grade 3 or 4 peripheral neuropathy occurred in 22% of patients and was the most frequent grade 3 or 4 adverse event. In patients with grade 3 or 4 peripheral neuropathy, dose modification of both thalidomide and vincristine resulted in improved symptoms.

In a similar study, 39 patients with multiple myeloma were treated with 2 mg/m^2 intravenous vincristine and 40 mg/m^2 intravenous liposomal doxorubicin, administered as a single dose on day 1, and 40 mg oral dexamethasone for 4 days and, in the first cycle of treatment only, repeated again on days 15 through 18 (Zervas et al., 2004). Oral thalidomide (200 mg/day) was administered at bedtime every day. Response was 74% (10% achieved complete response), evaluated after four cycles. After completion of four cycles, patients could advance to high-dose chemotherapy or continue this regimen for another two cycles. Eighteen percent of patients could be classified as nonresponders. Peripheral neuropathy ≥ grade 3 occurred in 5% of patients. Grade 1 or 2 peripheral neuropathy was more frequent and occurred in 46% of patients.

3.6.3 COMPARATIVE STUDIES

3.6.3.1 Carboplatin with and without Thalidomide

Forty patients with stage Ic/IV ovarian cancer were randomized to be treated with intravenous carboplatin (area under the curve = 7) every 4 weeks for a maximum of six cycles or carboplatin at the same dosing schedule plus 100 mg/day oral thalidomide (Muthuramalingam et al., 2011). Median follow-up was 1.95 years and overall response rates were similar (90% for carboplatin only versus 75% for carboplatin-thalidomide, p = 0.41). Several adverse events, including peripheral neuropathy, occurred significantly more often in the carboplatin-thalidomide group. Thus, thalidomide conferred no efficacy benefit to patients in this study, but was associated with an increased incidence of adverse events.

3.6.3.2 Carboplatin and Gemcitabine with and without Thalidomide

In a study of 722 patients with advanced non-small-cell lung cancer, all patients were treated with gemcitabine (1,200 mg/m^2 on days 1 and 8) and carboplatin (area under the curve = 5 or 6) chemotherapy on a 21-day cycle for a maximum of four cycles (Lee et al., 2009a). Patients were randomized to receive daily oral thalidomide (starting at 100 mg and increasing, as tolerated, to a maximum of 200 mg) or placebo for up to 2 years. Overall survival rates were similar between groups (8.5 months thalidomide versus 8.9 months placebo) with a hazard ratio of 1.13 (95% confidence interval, 0.97 to 1.32, $p = 0.12$). The 2-year survival rates were 12 and 16% for thalidomide and placebo, respectively. Thalidomide patients had a 74% increased risk of a thrombotic events compared to placebo patients. Peripheral neuropathy rates were similar with 4% of thalidomide and 2% of placebo patients reporting peripheral neuropathy ≥ grade 3.

3.6.3.3   Carboplatin and Epotoside with and without Thalidomide

In a study of 724 patients with various stages of small-cell lung cancer (51% with limited and 49% with extensive disease), patients all received etoposide and carboplatin chemotherapy on a 21-day cycle for a maximum of six cycles (Lee et al., 2009b). Patients were randomized to receive 100 mg/day oral thalidomide (increased, as tolerated, to a maximum of 200 mg/day) or placebo for 2 years. Overall survival rates were similar (10.1 months for thalidomide versus 10.5 months for placebo) with a hazard ratio for mortality of 1.09 (95% confidence interval, 0.93 to 1.27, $p = 0.28$). For patients with limited disease, there was no survival difference between thalidomide and placebo (hazard ratio, 0.91; 95% confidence interval, 0.73 to 1.15), but thalidomide was associated with a worse survival rate in patients with extensive disease (hazard ratio, 1.36; 95% confidence interval, 1.10 to 1.68). Peripheral neuropathy ≥ grade 3 occurred in 6% of thalidomide versus 2% of placebo patients.

3.6.3.4   Dexamethasone with and without Thalidomide

Patients with newly diagnosed multiple myeloma ($n = 207$) were randomized in a phase III clinical trial to receive thalidomide with or without dexamethasone (Rajkumar et al., 2006). Patients in arm A received 200 mg/day oral thalidomide for 4 weeks and 40 mg/day oral dexamethasone on days 1 through 4, 9 through 12, and 17 to 20 on a 28-day cycle. Patients in arm B of the study received only the dexamethasone on the same schedule. The response rate was significantly higher in arm A than arm B (63% versus 41%, respectively; $p = 0.0017$). However, the incidence of adverse events ≥ grade 3 was significantly higher in arm B (21% versus 45%, respectively; $p < 0.001$). The incidence of peripheral neuropathy ≥ grade 3 was 4% in group A compared to 7% in group B, a difference that did not achieve statistical significance.

3.6.3.5   Thalidomide and Dexamethasone with and without Bortezomib

A standard induction therapy for multiple myeloma is thalidomide combined with dexamethasone. In a study of treatment-naïve newly diagnosed multiple myeloma patients, patients were randomized to receive three 21-day cycles of 100 mg of oral thalidomide for the first 14 days (and 200 mg/day thereafter) plus 40 mg/day dexamethasone on 8 of the first 12 days but not consecutively, with or without 1.3 mg/m^2 bortezomib on days 1, 4, 8, and 11 of the 21-day cycle (Cavo et al., 2010). After double autologous stem cell transplantation, patients received two 35-day cycles of their assigned drug regimen. Patients on the thalidomide-dexamethasone regimen had significantly better response than patients taking thalidomide-dexamathesone-bortezomib.

Of the 474 evaluable patients, those with complete or near-complete response were 31% (95% confidence interval, 25.0 to 36.8%) in the thalidomide-dexamethasone group versus 11% (range, 7.3 to 15.4) in the thalidomide-dexamethasone-bortezomib group ($p < 0.0001$). Adverse events $\geq$ grade 3 occurred significantly more often in the thalidomide-dexamethasone-bortezomib group (56% versus 33%, respectively; $p < 0.0001$), including peripheral neuropathy (10% versus 2%, respectively; $p = 0.0004$). At the conclusion of treatment, 78% of patients with peripheral neuropathy in the thalidomide-dexamethasone-bortezomib group saw improvement or resolution of symptoms compared to 60% in the thalidomide-dexamethasone group.

3.6.3.6 Thalidomide with and without Interferon

In a dose-escalating study of thalidomide with and without interferon, 75 patients with relapsed or refractory multiple myeloma were enrolled (Mileshkin et al., 2006). Patients underwent nerve electrophysiological studies (NES) at baseline, and 39% had some degree of NES abnormality upon enrollment. Patients received thalidomide at a median dose intensity of 373 mg/day. During the therapy, 41% developed peripheral neuropathy and 15% discontinued treatment specifically because of peripheral neuropathy. Delayed neuropathy was observed. At 6 months, the actuarial incidence of peripheral neuropathy in this study population was 38%, but by 12 months it was 73%. NES evaluations could not reliably predict which patients would or would not develop peripheral neuropathy. In general, patients who developed peripheral neuropathy had a significantly longer duration of thalidomide exposure than patients who did not develop peripheral neuropathy (median, 268 days versus 89 days; $p = 0.0001$). However, cumulative thalidomide dose and dose intensity was not shown to have predictive power.

3.6.3.7 Thalidomide and Dexamethasone versus Interferon-Alpha and Dexamethasone as Maintenance Therapy

Multiple myeloma patients pretreated with conventional thalidomide, dexamethasone, and pegylated liposomal doxorubicin with at least a minor response after six courses were randomized in a clinical study to receive 3 MU interferon-alpha three times weekly or 100 mg/day oral thalidomide until relapse ($n = 103$) (Offidani et al., 2009). All patients received 20 mg pulsed dexamethasone 4 days per month. Two-year progression-free survival times were significantly better in the thalidomide than interferon-alpha patients (63% versus 32%, respectively; $p = 0.024$); overall survival was likewise significantly better for thalidomide maintenance patients (84% versus 68%, respectively; $p = 0.030$). Peripheral neuropathy occurred more often in thalidomide than interferon patients (31% versus 12%, respectively) and was more severe in thalidomide patients (6% of thalidomide patients had peripheral neuropathy $\geq$ grade 3 compared to no such cases in the interferon group). However, many side effects were more common in the interferon-alpha group, including fever, anorexia, fatigue, liver and heart abnormalities, and hematological toxicities. Interferon-alpha patients discontinued the regimen significantly more often than thalidomide patients because of treatment-emergent side effects (26% versus 8%, $p = 0.017$). The estimated 3-year risk of discontinuing treatment because of treatment-emergent side effects was 44% for interferon-alpha patients compared to 21% for thalidomide patients ($p = 0.014$).

3.6.3.8 Melphalan and Prednisone with and without Thalidomide

Multiple myeloma frequently occurs in geriatric patients, for whom the standard of care has been chemotherapy with melphalan and prednisone. A phase III clinical trial of 229 newly diagnosed multiple myeloma patients age ≥ 75 years administered to all patients 0.2 mg/kg/day melphalan and 2 mg/kg/day prednisone on days 1 through 4 on a 6-week cycle (Hulin et al., 2009). Patients were randomized to receive, in addition, either 100 mg/day oral thalidomide or placebo for the entire 12 courses of treatment (72 weeks). Overall survival was significantly longer in patients who received thalidomide than in those who received placebo (median, 44.0 months versus 29.1 months, respectively; $p = 0.028$). Progression-free survival was also significantly improved (24.1 months versus 18.5 months, respectively; $p = 0.001$). However, thalidomide patients also experienced significantly higher rates of peripheral neuropathy ≥ grade 2 (20% versus 5%, respectively; $p < 0.001$). Most cases of peripheral neuropathy were mild and could be managed. In comparing the control to the thalidomide groups, rates of peripheral neuropathy were 17% versus 18% for grade 1, 3% versus 19% for grade 2, 2% versus 2% for grade 3, and no cases of grade 4. Thalidomide patients in this study were significantly more likely than control patients to develop peripheral neuropathy ($p = 0.003$). Thus, thalidomide in combination with melphalan and prednisone was seen as conferring a survival benefit to elderly patients but with added toxicity.

3.6.3.9 Vincristine, Liposomal Doxorubicin, and Dexamethasone with and without Thalidomide

Vincristine, liposomal doxorubicin, and dexamethasone (VAD-doxil) have been demonstrated as effective in treating newly diagnosed multiple myeloma (Hussein et al., 2002, 2006). A multicenter trial evaluated the feasibility and results of adding thalidomide to this regimen in treatment-naïve multiple myeloma patients of <75 years old (Zervas et al., 2007). Patients ($n = 232$) were randomized to VAD-doxil treatment (arm A) or VAD-doxil plus thalidomide (arm B). Patients in arm A received 2 mg intravenous vincristine and 40 mg/m^2 liposomal doxorubicin on day 1 and 40 mg oral dexamethasone on days 1 through 4, 9 through 12, and 17 through 20 for the first 28-day cycle and on days 1 through 4 only on the next three cycles. Patients in arm B received the same therapy with the addition of 200 mg oral thalidomide daily at bedtime. Based on an intent-to-treat analysis, the addition of thalidomide significantly increased the response rate; partial response or better occurred in 62.6% of arm A versus 81.2% of arm B patients ($p = 0.003$). Progression-free survival and overall survival were also significantly improved with thalidomide (44.8% versus 58.9%, respectively; $p = 0.013$; and 64.6% versus 77%, respectively; $p = 0.037$). Overall, toxicities grade 3 or 4 were not significantly different between arms. However, peripheral neuropathy (any grade) occurred in 13 and 45.3% of patients in arms A and B, respectively ($p < 0.01$). Peripheral neuropathy ≥ grade 3 occurred in 1.7% versus 7.7% of arms A and B, respectively (NS). Treatment was discontinued on account of adverse events in 6.1% of arm A and 9.4% of arm B patients (NS). Peripheral neuropathy was the reason that one patient in arm A and seven patients in arm B discontinued treatment. Thus, treatment discontinuation occurred at a relatively low rate (<10%) in both arms, and side effects were described by investigators as manageable. It should be noted that the rate of peripheral neuropathy ≥ grade 3 in the thalidomide group (arm B) was much lower in this study (7.7%) than in a similar study by Hussein and colleagues of the same agents (22%) (Hussein et al., 2006). This discrepancy might be explained by the fact that thalidomide-induced peripheral neuropathy may be delayed, and that this study was of shorter duration than the Hussein study. It is not known if more prolonged observation of these patients would have resulted in higher rates of peripheral neuropathy ≥ grade 3.

3.6.4 SINGLE NUCLEOTIDE POLYMORPHISMS AND THALIDOMIDE-INDUCED PERIPHERAL NEUROPATHY

In a study of 28 patients with relapsed or refractory multiple myeloma treated with thalidomide monotherapy, single nucleotide polymorphisms (SNPs) were identified. SNPs in 12 genes involving multidrug resistance, drug metabolic pathways, DNA repair systems, and cytokines were identified and results correlated with chemotherapeutic response, toxicity, and overall survival rates (Cibeira et al., 2011). Patients with SNPs in ERCC1 (rs735482), ERCC5 (rs17655), or XRCC5 (rs1051685) had significantly better responses to thalidomide monotherapy than other patients. Significantly longer overall survival times were associated with the SNPs in ERCC1 (rs735482) and XRCC5 (rs1051685). SNPs in GSTT1 (rs4630) could be associated with a significantly lower rate of thalidomide-induced peripheral neuropathy ($p = 0.04$). Further research is warranted.

3.7 LENALIDOMIDE

Lenalidomide, first approved for U.S. market release in 2004, is a derivative of thalidomide developed for the treatment of multiple myeloma. Lenalidomide is an immunomodulator that has been demonstrated to be effective in the treatment of other hematological disorders as well. Lenalidomide has a direct antitumor effect and induces apoptosis of tumor cells both directly and indirectly by inhibiting stromal cell activity in the bone marrow. Like thalidomide, lenalidomide is antiangiogenic. It is not known if lenalidomide shares the teratogenic effects of thalidomide, but it should not be prescribed to women who are pregnant or may become pregnant.

An open-label randomized phase II clinical trial examined two different dose regimens of lenalidomide in the setting of relapsed, refractory multiple myeloma (Richardson et al., 2006). For the first 21 days of a 28-day treatment cycle, 102 patients were randomized to receive either 30 mg lenalidomide once daily or 15 mg lenalidomide twice daily. The overall response rate to lenalidomide was 25% and was similar between groups. In the once-daily group, the response rate was 24% (95% confidence interval, 14 to 36%), with 6% achieving complete response. In this group, the median duration of response to lenalidomide was 19 months (range, 2 to 22). In the twice-daily group, the response rate was 29%

(95% confidence interval, 15 to 46%), with no patient achieving complete response. The median duration of response in the twice-daily group was 23 months (range, 2 to 25). Treatment-emergent peripheral neuropathy occurred more frequently in the twice-daily group: 23% versus 10%, respectively.

In a study of 102 newly diagnosed multiple myeloma patients between the ages of 65 and 75 years, patients received induction therapy in a 21-day cycle of 1.3 mg/m^2 bortezomib on days 1, 4, 8, and 11, 30 mg/m^2 pegylated liposomal doxorubicin on day 4, and 40 mg/day dexamethasone on days 1 to 4, 8 to 11, and 15 to 18 during the first cycle and for the next two cycles on days 1 through 4 only (Palumbo et al., 2010a). Patients underwent autologous transplantation with stem cell support and received consolidation therapy in the form of four 28-day cycles of 25 mg/day lenalidomide on days 1 through 21 plus 50 mg prednisone every other day, followed by maintenance therapy of 10 mg/day lenalidomide on days 1 through 21 until relapse. After induction chemotherapy, 58% of patients had a very good partial response or better and 13% had complete response. After lenalidomide maintenance therapy, 86% had a very good partial response or better and 66% had complete response. At a median 21-month follow-up time, 2-year progression-free survival was 69% and overall survival was 86%. During chemotherapy, 16% of patients developed peripheral neuropathy ≥ grade 3 (95% confidence interval, 9 to 24) and 1% developed peripheral neuropathy during lenalidomide maintenance therapy (95% confidence interval, 0 to 7).

3.8   SURAMIN

Suramin is a polysulfonated naphthylurea that had been previously used to treat acquired immune deficiency syndrome and other conditions, but has been hypothesized to be an effective anticancer agent because of its ability to bind cellular growth factors. Suramin has been associated with treatment-limiting adverse effects. Risk factors for surarmin-induced peripheral neuropathy have not been thoroughly studied, but may relate to peak serum concentrations of ≥350 µg/ml (Chaudhry et al., 1996). In some cases, suramin-induced peripheral neuropathy may resolve at least partially with cessation of treatment.

3.8.1   Monotherapy

In a study of 75 patients with hormone-refractory prostate cancer, patients were administered three different targeted plasma concentrations of suramin (275, 215, and 175 µg/ml, respectively) for different durations (2, 4, or 8 weeks). Suramin was administered by continuous intravenous infusion (Bowden et al., 1996). Toxicity was observed to be most severe at the highest target plasma concentration (275 µg/ml) for the longest duration (8 weeks), with the most frequent toxicities in these patients observed to be paresthesias and motor nerve neuropathy. Overall, grade 3 or 4 neuromotor toxicity occurred in 9.4% of patients, typically manifested as symmetric paresthesias and weaknesses in the lower extremities. The overall response rate of evaluable patients was 17%.

3.8.2 COMBINATION THERAPY

3.8.2.1 Suramin and Epirubicin

In a study of patients ($n = 26$) with hormone-independent advanced prostate carcinoma with progressive refractory disease, including antiandrogen withdrawal, patients were administered intravenous suramin in a 6-day continuous infusion every week through a central line with an initial daily dose of 350 mg/m² (first 6 days) (Falcone et al., 1999). After that, the dose for the weekly infusion was determined based on pharmacokinetic parameters in order to maintain a suramin plasma concentration of approximately 200 to 250 µg/ml. Patients were administered 25 mg/m² epirubicin as a weekly intravenous bolus at the start of suramin infusion for a maximum of 6 months. Thereafter, this regimen was repeated every 4 weeks for a maximum of 6 months. There was an objective response in 27% of patients and 33% of patients evaluated for prostate-specific antigen (PSA) levels had a decrease of ≥50%, which lasted a median of 32 weeks (range, 8 to 52). Peripheral neuropathy was common but usually mild, with 23% of patients reporting grade 1 peripheral neuropathy and 4% reporting grade 3 peripheral neuropathy (no other cases were observed).

3.8.2.2 Suramin and Mitomycin C

Thirty-two hormone-resistant prostate cancer patients were treated with 350 mg/m² suramin daily for 5 days followed by 350 mg/m² weekly starting on day 14 of a 35-day cycle (Rapoport et al., 1993). Mitomycin C 12 mg/m² was administered to patients every 5 weeks starting on day 14. There was one complete and six partial responses and 15 patients achieved disease stabilization. The median time to treatment failure was 103 days and median survival was 209 days. Ten patients (31%) exhibited some form of neurotoxicity, including temporary sensory peripheral neuropathy ($n = 8$), upper limb motor neuropathy ($n = 1$), and restless leg syndrome ($n = 1$).

3.9 EPOTHILONES

Epothilones are a new class of anticancer agent thought to work by interfering with tubulin, and thus preventing the division of cancer cells. In that way, epothilones may be considered similar to taxanes, but they hold promise in that they may be more efficacious and less toxic. Epothilones are more water soluble than taxanes and thus do not need a solubizing agent (such as cremophor) like that used with paclitaxel. A variety of epothilone agents (including ixabepilone, patupilone, sagopilone, and so on) exist and were developed with names epothilone A through epithilone F (these older names sometimes still appear in the literature). The epothilones will be discussed here together rather than separated by individual agent.

3.9.1 MONOTHERAPIES

In a phase I drug interaction study, 10 mg/m² patupilone was administered intravenously to patients on days 8 and 29 of a 29-day cycle with 20 mg oral warfarin (days 1 through 29) (Tsimberidou et al., 2011b). The purpose of this study was to evaluate the pharmacokinetics and pharmacodynamics of warfarin coadministered with patupilone. Seventeen patients were enrolled, and the study found that the pharmacokinetics and pharmacodynamics of warfarin were not affected by patupilone, suggesting that patupilone has no clinically important effect on CYP2C9 metabolism. In patients who participated in two cycles of treatment ($n = 17$), peripheral neuropathy of any grade occurred in 23.4% and peripheral neuropathy ≥ grade 3 did not occur at all. Some patients ($n = 9$) continued to receive three cycles or more and received 10 mg/m^2 patupilone once every 3 weeks. In those patients, peripheral neuropathy of any grade occurred in 33.3%, but no cases were more severe than grade 2.

In a phase I dose escalation study of patupilone in 45 patients with advanced ovarian, primary fallopian, or primary peritoneal cancer, patients were administered 6.5 to 11.0 mg/m^2 patupilone every 3 weeks in a 20-minute infusion (Ten Bokkel Huinink et al., 2009). The maximum tolerated dose was not reached and 4% of patients developed peripheral neuropathy ≥ grade 3. The overall response rate was 19.5% and median duration of disease stabilization (complete and partial responses plus stable disease) was 15.8 months.

Ixabepilone monotherapy was evaluated in 24 patients with histologically confirmed stage IV melanoma (Ott et al., 2010). Patients received 20 mg/m^2 intravenous ixabepilone on days 1, 8, and 15 of a 28-day cycle. Patients were grouped in two arms: previously untreated and previously treated. There were no confirmed cases of complete or partial responses in either group. Median time to progression was similar in both groups: 1.7 and 1.5 months in the previously untreated and previously treated arms, respectively. Peripheral neuropathy occurred among previously untreated patients at rates of 27, 18, 9, and 0% for grades 1, 2, 3, and 4, respectively. In previously treated patients, peripheral neuropathy rates were 31, 0, 8, and 0%, respectively. This study suggests that ixabepilone has no clinical role in the treatment of melanoma.

On the other hand, another study found safety and efficacy of ixabepilone treatment of taxane- and platinum-resistant primary ovarian or peritoneal carcinoma (De Geest et al., 2010). Forty-nine such patients received 20 mg/m^2 intravenous ixabepilone administered over 1 hour on days 1, 8, and 15 of a 28-day cycle in a phase II clinical study. The objective response rate was 14.3% (95% confidence interval, 5.9 to 27.2%) with a 6% rate of complete response ($n = 3$). The median time to progression was 4.4 months (95% confidence interval, 0.8 to 32.6 months) and median survival time was 14.8 months (95% confidence interval, 0.8 to 50.0 months). The median number of treatment cycles per patient was two (range, 1 to 29) and 18.4% of patients received six or more cycles. Peripheral neuropathy ≥ grade 3 occurred in 6.1% of patients, although lower-grade neuropathy was more common than higher grade. Peripheral neuropathy grade 1 occurred in 24.5% of patients and grade 2 in 28.6% of patients. Fourteen percent of patients discontinued treatment and 6% required a dose reduction because of peripheral neuropathy.

In a phase II genomics study of ixabepilone as neoadjuvant therapy for invasive breast cancer not amenable to breast conservation surgery, patients ($n = 161$) were administered 40 mg/m^2 ixabepilone as a 3-hour infusion on day 1 of a 21-day cycle for four or fewer cycles (Baselga et al., 2009). The overall complete pathologic response rate was 18% in breast and 29% in estrogen-receptor-negative (ER–)

patients. Ixabepilone-induced peripheral neuropathy $\geq$ grade 3 was observed in 3% of patients and was reversible in 6 to 12 weeks after cessation of treatment. Mild peripheral neuropathy (grades 1 and 2) occurred in 40% of patients (26 and 14% for grades 1 and 2, respectively).

In a phase I study of sagopilone, 52 patients with advanced solid tumors received a 30-minute intravenous infusion of escalating doses of sagopilone ranging from 0.6 to 29.4 mg/m^2 every 21 days (Schmid et al., 2010). Nine more patients were recruited to this study to a 3-hour infusion arm (16.53 to 22.0 mg/m^2) specifically to evaluate the rate of sagopilone-induced peripheral neuropathy. The maximum tolerated dose established by this study was 22.0 mg/m^2. Peripheral sensory neuropathy was the most commonly observed grade 3 adverse effect and was more prevalent in the 3-hour group. Peripheral neuropathy (all grades) developed in 40.4% of 30-minute and 88.9% of 3-hour patients, and peripheral neuropathy $\geq$ grade 3 developed in 15.4% of the 30-minute and 55.6% of the 3-hour group. Investigators describe sagopilone-induced peripheral neuropathy as being similar to taxane-induced peripheral neuropathy, in that it includes paresthesia, anesthesia, and the "glove-and-stocking" pattern.

In another study to determine the maximum tolerated dose of sagopilone in patients with refactory or resistant tumors ($n = 23$), the maximum weekly dose was established to be 5.3 mg/m^2 with an 8.7% incidence of peripheral neuropathy $\geq$ grade 3 (Arnold et al., 2009). Peripheral neuropathy (any grade) occurred in 35% of patients and was the most frequent adverse effect. The rates of hematological and nonhematological adverse events were low, with the other highest rates of adverse effects being decreased hemoglobin (22%) and nausea (22%).

3.9.2 COMBINATION THERAPIES

The safety and efficacy of ixabepilone combined with capecitabine was evaluated in a study of 21 patients with metastatic breast cancer pretreated with or resistant to anthracyclines and taxanes (Wang et al., 2010). Patients received intravenous 40 mg/m^2 ixabepilone on day 1 of a 21-day cycle plus 2,000 mg/m^2 oral capcitabine on days 1 through 14. Patients received a total of 146 cycles of treatment (range, 1 to 13) with a median of five cycles per patient. Rates of partial response, stable disease, and progressive disease were 66.7, 23.8, and 9.5%, respectively. Two-thirds of patients (66.7%) discontinued therapy because of adverse events and 38.1% required a dose reduction. A third of patients (33.3%) had peripheral neuropathy $\geq$ grade 3, which was observed to be reversible after a median duration of 6 weeks.

In a phase I/II dose-escalating study of ixabepilone and capecitabine, 106 patients were treated on a 21-day cycle with schedule A (40 mg/m^2 ixabepilone on day 1 plus 1,640 to 2,000 mg/m^2 capecitabine on days 1 through 14) or schedule B (8 to 10 mg/m^2 ixabepilone on days 1 through 3 plus 1,650 mg/m^2 capectiabine on days 1 through 14) (Bunnell et al., 2008). Patients had either anthracycline-pretreated, anthracycline-resistant, or taxane-resistant metastatic breast cancer. The maximum tolerated doses were determined in this study to be 40/2,000 mg/m^2 for schedule A patients. The objective response rate was 30%, the median time to response was 6 weeks, and the median duration of response was 6.9 months. The median progression-free survival time was 3.8 months. Peripheral neuropathy $\geq$ grade 3 occurred in 19 and 13% of patients (schedules A and B, respectively). Ixabepilone-induced peripheral neuropathy in this study was described as sensory, cumulative, and reversible. Eleven percent of patients discontinued treatment because of peripheral neuropathy. Treatment-emergent neuropathy in schedule A patients resolved to baseline or grade 1 in 94% of patients with a median time to resolution of 2.6 weeks (95% confidence interval, 1.1 to 6.9 weeks).

3.10   CONCLUSION

The literature provides considerable evidence of the prevalence of chemotherapy-induced peripheral neuropathy in a wide variety of regimens for treating a variety of malignancies. Chemotherapy-induced peripheral neuropathy occurs frequently and may sometimes be severe enough to limit treatment. Efforts to determine risk factors for chemotherapy-induced peripheral neuropathy suggest that it varies with different agents; for certain drugs, cumulative dose may be important, while dosing schedule may be more crucial for other agents. Although geriatric patients are generally considered to be at higher risk for treatment-emergent peripheral neuropathy, studies on this subject are equivocal. In some cases, peripheral neuropathy may be entirely or partially reversible upon cessation of therapy. The development of new chemotherapeutic agents and changes in combination therapies, routes of administration, or dosing schedules may produce in the future more effective and less toxic forms of chemotherapy.

REFERENCES

Adams R, Meade A, et al. (2011). Intermittent versus continuous oxaliplatin and fluoropyrimidine combination chemotherapy for first-line treatment of advanced colorectal cancer: Results of the randomised phase 3 MRC COIN trial. *Lancet Oncol* 12(7):642–53.

Amato RJ, Hernandez-McClain J, et al. (2009). Phase 2 study of granulocyte-macrophage colony-stimulating factor plus thalidomide in patients with hormone-naive adenocarcinoma of the prostate. *Urol Oncol* 27(1):8–13.

Amato RJ, Malya R, et al. (2008). Phase II study of combination thalidomide/interleukin-2 therapy plus granulocyte macrophage-colony stimulating factor in patients with metastatic renal cell carcinoma. *Am J Clin Oncol* 31(3):237–43.

Andre T, Boni C, et al. (2004). Oxaliplatin, fluorouracil, and leucovorin as adjuvant treatment for colon cancer. *N Engl J Med* 350(23):2343–51.

Andre T, Boni C, et al. (2009). Improved overall survival with oxaliplatin, fluorouracil, and leucovorin as adjuvant treatment in stage II or III colon cancer in the MOSAIC trial. *J Clin Oncol* 27(19):3109–16.

Arnold D, Voigt W, et al. (2009). Weekly administration of sagopilone (ZK-EPO), a fully synthetic epothilone, in patients with refractory solid tumours: Results of a phase I trial. *Br J Cancer* 101(8):1241–47.

Badros A, Goloubeva O, et al. (2006). Phase I trial of first-line bortezomib/thalidomide plus chemotherapy for induction and stem cell mobilization in patients with multiple myeloma. *Clin Lymphoma Myeloma* 7(3):210–16.

Baselga J, Zambetti M, et al. (2009). Phase II genomics study of ixabepilone as neoadjuvant treatment for breast cancer. *J Clin Oncol* 27(4):526–34.

Bastuji-Garin S, Ochonisky S, et al. (2002). Incidence and risk factors for thalidomide neuropathy: A prospective study of 135 dermatologic patients. *J Invest Dermatol* 119(5):1020–26.

Bensinger W, Jagannath S, et al. (2010). Phase 2 study of two sequential three-drug combinations containing bortezomib, cyclophosphamide and dexamethasone, followed by bortezomib, thalidomide and dexamethasone as frontline therapy for multiple myeloma. *Br J Haematol* 148(4):562–68.

Berenson J, Yellin O, et al. (2011). A modified regimen of pegylated liposomal doxorubicin, bortezomib and dexamethasone (DVD) is effective and well tolerated for previously untreated multiple myeloma patients. *Br J Haematol* 155(5):580–87.

Blum JL, Savin MA, et al. (2007). Phase II study of weekly albumin-bound paclitaxel for patients with metastatic breast cancer heavily pretreated with taxanes. *Clin Breast Cancer* 7(11):850–56.

Boccardo F, Amadori D, et al. (2010). Epirubicin followed by cyclophosphamide, methotrexate and 5-fluorouracil versus paclitaxel followed by epirubicin and vinorelbine in patients with high-risk operable breast cancer. *Oncology* 78(3–4):274–81.

Bowden CJ, Figg WD, et al. (1996). A phase I/II study of continuous infusion suramin in patients with hormone-refractory prostate cancer: Toxicity and response. *Cancer Chemother Pharmacol* 39(1–2):1–8.

Boyette-Davis J, Cata J, et al. (2011). Follow-up psychophysical studies in bortezomib-related chemoneuropathy patients. *J Pain* 12(9):1017–24.

Bringhen S, Larocca A, et al. (2010). Efficacy and safety of once-weekly bortezomib in multiple myeloma patients. *Blood* 116(23):4745–53.

Brouwers EE, Huitema AD, et al. (2009). Persistent neuropathy after treatment with cisplatin and oxaliplatin. *Acta Oncol* 48(6):832–41.

Bruna J, Alé A, et al. (2011). Evaluation of pre-existing neuropathy and bortezomib retreatment as risk factors to develop severe neuropathy in a mouse model. *J Periph Nerv Syst* 16(3):199–212.

Bunnell C, Vahdat L, et al. (2008). Phase I/II study of ixabepilone plus capecitabine in anthracycline-pretreated/resistant and taxane-resistant metastatic breast cancer. *Clin Breast Cancer* 8(3):234–41.

Carlomagno C, Farella A, et al. (2009). Neo-adjuvant treatment of rectal cancer with capecitabine and oxaliplatin in combination with radiotherapy: A phase II study. *Ann Oncol* 20(5):906–12.

Cavaletti G, Jakubowiak A. (2010). Peripheral neuropathy during bortezomib treatment of multiple myeloma: A review of recent studies. *Leuk Lymphoma* 51(7):1178–87.

Cavo M, Tacchetti P, et al. (2010). Bortezomib with thalidomide plus dexamethasone compared with thalidomide plus dexamethasone as induction therapy before, and consolidation therapy after, double autologous stem-cell transplantation in newly diagnosed multiple myeloma: A randomised phase 3 study. *Lancet* 376(9758):2075–85.

Cella D, Huang H, et al. (2010). Patient-reported peripheral neuropathy of doxorubicin and cisplatin with and without paclitaxel in the treatment of advanced endometrial cancer: Results from GOG 184. *Gynecol Oncol* 119(3):538–42.

Chanan-Khan A, Miller KC, et al. (2005). Results of a phase 1 clinical trial of thalidomide in combination with fludarabine as initial therapy for patients with treatment-requiring chronic lymphocytic leukemia (CLL). *Blood* 106(10):3348–52.

Ch'ang HJ, Huang CL, et al. (2009). Phase II study of biweekly gemcitabine followed by oxaliplatin and simplified 48-h infusion of 5-fluorouracil/leucovorin (GOFL) in advanced pancreatic cancer. *Cancer Chemother Pharmacol* 64(6):1173–79.

Chang MH, Kim KH, et al. (2009). Irinotecan and oxaliplatin combination as the first-line treatment for patients with advanced non-small cell lung cancer. *Cancer Chemother Pharmacol* 64(5):917–24.

Chaudhry V, Cornblath DR, et al. (2002). Thalidomide-induced neuropathy. *Neurology* 59(12):1872–75.

Chaudhry V, Eisenberger MA, et al. (1996). A prospective study of suramin-induced peripheral neuropathy. *Brain* 119(Pt 6):2039–52.

Chen S, Jiang B, et al. (2010). Bortezomib plus thalidomide for newly diagnosed multiple myeloma in China. *Anat Rec (Hoboken)* 293(10):1679–84.

Chen S, Qiu L, et al. (2011). The efficacy and safety of bortezomib plus thalidomide in treatment of newly diagnosed multiple myeloma. *Zhonghua Nei Ke Za Zhi* 50(4):291–94.

Chen XS, Nie XQ, et al. (2010). Weekly paclitaxel plus carboplatin is an effective nonanthracycline-containing regimen as neoadjuvant chemotherapy for breast cancer. *Ann Oncol* 21(5):961–67.

Chen YM, Reury Perng P, Shih JF, Tsai CM, Whang-Peng, J. (2005). A randomized phase II study of vinorelbine plus gemcitabine with/without cisplatin against inoperable, non-small-lung cancer previously untreated. *Lung Cancer* 47(3):373–80.

Chen YM, Perng RP, et al. (2006). A phase II randomized study of paclitaxel plus carboplatin or cisplatin against chemo-naive inoperable non-small cell lung cancer in the elderly. *J Thorac Oncol* 1(2):141–45.

Chin SN, Pinto V, et al. (2009). Evaluation of an intraperitoneal chemotherapy program implemented at the Princess Margaret Hospital for patients with epithelial ovarian carcinoma. *Gynecol Oncol* 112(3):450–54.

Cibeira MT, de Larrea CF, et al. (2011). Impact on response and survival of DNA repair single nucleotide polymorphisms in relapsed or refractory multiple myeloma patients treated with thalidomide. *Leuk Res* 35(9):1178–83.

Coiffier B, Osmanov E, et al. (2011). Bortezomib plus rituximab versus rituximab alone in patients with relapsed, rituximab-naive or rituximab-sensitive, follicular lymphoma: A randomised phase 3 trial. *Lancet Oncol* 12(8):773–84.

Comella P, Chiuri VE, et al. (2010). Gemcitabine combined with either pemetrexed or paclitaxel in the treatment of advanced non-small cell lung cancer: A randomized phase II SICOG trial. *Lung Cancer* 68(1):94–98.

Conlin AK, Seidman AD, et al. (2010). Phase II trial of weekly nanoparticle albumin-bound paclitaxel with carboplatin and trastuzumab as first-line therapy for women with HER2-overexpressing metastatic breast cancer. *Clin Breast Cancer* 10(4):281–87.

Corso A, Mangiacavalli S, et al. (2010). Bortezomib-induced peripheral neuropathy in multiple myeloma: A comparison between previously treated and untreated patients. *Leuk Res* 34(4):471–74.

Daliani DD, Papandreou CN, et al. (2002). A pilot study of thalidomide in patients with progressive metastatic renal cell carcinoma. *Cancer* 95(4):758–65.

D'Amato R, Loughnan M, et al. (1994). Thalidomide is an inhibitor of angiogenesis. *Proc Natl Acad Sci USA* 91:4082–85.

De Geest K, Blessing JA, et al. (2010). Phase II clinical trial of ixabepilone in patients with recurrent or persistent platinum- and taxane-resistant ovarian or primary peritoneal cancer: A Gynecologic Oncology Group study. *J Clin Oncol* 28(1):149–53.

Delforge M, Bladé J, et al. (2010). Treatment-related peripheral neuropathy in multiple myeloma: The challenge continues. *Lancet Oncol* 11(11):1086–95.

de Vos S, Goy A, et al. (2009). Multicenter randomized phase II study of weekly or twice-weekly bortezomib plus rituximab in patients with relapsed or refractory follicular or marginal-zone B-cell lymphoma. *J Clin Oncol* 27(30):5023–30.

Detweiler-Short K, Hayman S, et al. (2010). Long-term results of single-agent thalidomide as initial therapy for asymptomatic (smoldering or indolent) myeloma. *Am J Hematol* 85(10):737–40.

Di Lorenzo G, Autorino R, et al. (2007). Thalidomide in combination with oral daily cyclophosphamide in patients with pretreated hormone refractory prostate cancer: A phase I clinical trial. *Cancer Biol Ther* 6(3):313–17.

Di Lorenzo G, Buonerba C, et al. (2011). Phase II study of docetaxel re-treatment in docetaxel-pretreated castration-resistant prostate cancer. *BJU Int* 107(2):234–39.

Dimopoulos M, Mateos M, et al. (2011). Risk factors for, and reversibility of, peripheral neuropathy associated with bortezomib-melphalan-prednisone in newly diagnosed patients with multiple myeloma: Subanalysis of the phase 3 VISTA study. *Eur J Haematol* 86(1):23–31.

Dimopoulos MA, Anagnostopoulos A, et al. (2006). Primary treatment with pulsed melphalan, dexamethasone and thalidomide for elderly symptomatic patients with multiple myeloma. *Haematologica* 91(2):252–54.

Dimopoulos MA, Hamilos G, et al. (2004). Pulsed cyclophosphamide, thalidomide and dexamethasone: An oral regimen for previously treated patients with multiple myeloma. *Hematol J* 5(2):112–17.

Dong NN, Wang MY, et al. (2009). Oxaliplatin combined with capecitabine as first-line chemotherapy for patients with advanced gastric cancer. *Ai Zheng* 28(4):412–15.

Drake MJ, Robson W, et al. (2003). An open-label phase II study of low-dose thalidomide in androgen-independent prostate cancer. *Br J Cancer* 88(6):822–27.

Durie B, Jacobson J, et al. (2004). Magnitude of response with myeloma frontline therapy does not predict outcome: Importance of time to progression in Southwest Oncology Group chemotherapy trials. *J Clin Oncol* 15(22):1857–63.

Eigentler TK, Radny P, et al. (2008). Adjuvant treatment with vindesine in comparison to observation alone in patients with metastasized melanoma after complete metastasectomy: A randomized multicenter trial of the German Dermatologic Cooperative Oncology Group. *Melanoma Res* 18(5):353–58.

Ejlertsen B, Mouridsen HT, et al. (2004). Phase III study of intravenous vinorelbine in combination with epirubicin versus epirubicin alone in patients with advanced breast cancer: A Scandinavian Breast Group Trial (SBG9403). *J Clin Oncol* 22(12):2313–20.

Falcone A, Antonuzzo A, et al. (1999). Suramin in combination with weekly epirubicin for patients with advanced hormone-refractory prostate carcinoma. *Cancer* 86(3):470–76.

Feliu J, Martin G, et al. (2006). Docetaxel and mitomycin as second-line treatment in advanced non-small cell lung cancer. *Cancer Chemother Pharmacol* 58(4):527–31.

Ferrari D, Fiore J, et al. (2009). A phase II study of carboplatin and paclitaxel for recurrent or metastatic head and neck cancer. *Anticancer Drugs* 20(3):185–90.

Feyler S, Rawstron A, et al. (2007). Thalidomide maintenance following high-dose therapy in multiple myeloma: A UK myeloma forum phase 2 study. *Br J Haematol* 139(3):429–33.

Gasparetto C, Gockerman J, et al. (2010). "Short course" bortezomib plus melphalan and prednisone as induction prior to transplant or as frontline therapy for nontransplant candidates in patients with previously untreated multiple myeloma. *Biol Blood Marrow Transplant* 16(1):70–77.

Gebbia V, Caruso M, et al. (2002). Vinorelbine and cisplatin for the treatment of recurrent and/or metastatic carcinoma of the uterine cervix. *Oncology* 63(1):31–37.

George A, Marziniak M, et al. (2000). Thalidomide treatment in chronic constrictive neuropathy decreases endoneurial tumor necrosis factor-alpha, increases interleukin-10 and has long-term effects on spinal cord dorsal horn met-enkephalin. *Pain* 88(3):267–75.

Ghobrial I, Hong F, et al. (2010). Phase II trial of weekly bortezomib in combination with rituximab in relapsed or relapsed and refractory Waldenstrom macroglobulinemia. *J Clin Oncol* 28(8):1422–28.

Ghobrial I, Weller E, et al. (2011). Weekly bortezomib in combination with temsirolimus in relapsed or relapsed and refractory multiple myeloma: A multicentre, phase 1/2, open-label, dose-escalation study. *Lancet Oncol* 12(3):263–72.

Ghosh N, Ye X, et al. (2011). Bortezomib and thalidomide, a steroid free regimen in newly diagnosed patients with multiple myeloma. *Br J Haematol* 152(5):593–99.

Gilheeney SW, Lyden DC, et al. (2007). A phase II trial of thalidomide and cyclophosphamide in patients with recurrent or refractory pediatric malignancies. *Pediatr Blood Cancer* 49(3):261–65.

Ginopoulos P, Kontomanolis E, et al. (2002). A phase II study of non-platinum based chemotherapy with paclitaxel and vinorelbine in non-small cell lung cancer. *Lung Cancer* 38(2):199–203.

Goedhals L, Falkson G, et al. (2005). Vinorelbine and cisplatin in advanced squamous cell carcinoma of the cervix: The South African experience. *Anticancer Res* 25(3c):2489–92.

Gradishar WJ, Krasnojon D, et al. (2009). Significantly longer progression-free survival with nab-paclitaxel compared with docetaxel as first-line therapy for metastatic breast cancer. *J Clin Oncol* 27(22):3611–19.

Gruenberger B, Schueller J, et al. (2010). Cetuximab, gemcitabine, and oxaliplatin in patients with unresectable advanced or metastatic biliary tract cancer: A phase 2 study. *Lancet Oncol* 11(12):1142–48.

Gu Y, Shu Y, et al. (2009). A study of weekly paclitaxel plus 5-fluorouracil and cisplatin for patients with advanced or recurrent inoperable gastric cancer. *Biomed Pharmacother* 63(4):293–96.

Gupta A, Cohen BH, et al. (2003). Phase I study of thalidomide for the treatment of plexiform neurofibroma in neurofibromatosis 1. *Neurology* 60(1):130–32.

Harousseau J, Attal M, et al. (2010). Bortezomib plus dexamethasone is superior to vincristine plus doxorubicin plus dexamethasone as induction treatment prior to autologous stem-cell transplantation in newly diagnosed multiple myeloma: Results of the IFM 2005-01 phase III trial. *J Clin Oncol* 28(30):4621–29.

Harrison S, Quach H, et al. (2011). A high rate of durable responses with romidepsin, bortezomib, and dexamethasone in relapsed or refractory multiple myeloma. *Blood* 118(24):6274–83.

Harshman LC, Li M, et al. (2008). The combination of thalidomide and capecitabine in metastatic renal cell carcinoma—is not the answer. *Am J Clin Oncol* 31(5):417–23.

Hattori Y, Okamoto S, et al. (2008). Single-institute phase 2 study of thalidomide treatment for refractory or relapsed multiple myeloma: Prognostic factors and unique toxicity profile. *Cancer Sci* 99(6):1243–50.

Hideshima T, Richardson P, et al. (2001). The proteasome inhibitor PS-341 inhibits growth, induces apoptosis, and overcomes drug resistance in human multiple myeloma cells. *Cancer Res* 61(7):3071–76.

Horn L, Bernardo P, et al. (2009). A phase II study of paclitaxel + etoposide + cisplatin + concurrent radiation therapy for previously untreated limited stage small cell lung cancer (E2596): A trial of the Eastern Cooperative Oncology Group. *J Thorac Oncol* 4(4):527–33.

Hulin C, Facon T, et al. (2009). Efficacy of melphalan and prednisone plus thalidomide in patients older than 75 years with newly diagnosed multiple myeloma: IFM 01/01 trial. *J Clin Oncol* 27(22):3664–70.

Hussein M. (2003). Modifications to therapy for multiple myeloma: Pegylated liposomal doxorubicin in combination with vincristine, reduced-dose dexamethasone, and thalidomide. *Oncologist* 8(Suppl):39–45.

Hussein M, Wood L, et al. (2002). A phase II trial of pegylated liposomal doxorubicin, vincristine, and reduced-dose dexamethasone combination therapy in newly diagnosed multiple myeloma patients. *Cancer* 95(10):2160–68.

Hussein MA, Baz R, et al. (2006). Phase 2 study of pegylated liposomal doxorubicin, vincristine, decreased-frequency dexamethasone, and thalidomide in newly diagnosed and relapsed-refractory multiple myeloma. *Mayo Clin Proc* 81(7):889–95.

Hwang J, Cho SH, et al. (2008). Phase II study of paclitaxel, cisplatin, and 5-fluorouracil combination chemotherapy in patients with advanced gastric cancer. *J Korean Med Sci* 23(4):586–91.

Isayama H, Nakai Y, et al. (2011). Gemcitabine and oxaliplatin combination chemotherapy for patients with refractory pancreatic cancer. *Oncology* 80(1–2):97–101.

Iwamoto T, Ishibashi M, et al. (2010). Drug interaction between itraconazole and bortezomib: Exacerbation of peripheral neuropathy and thrombocytopenia induced by bortezomib. *Pharmacotherapy* 30(7):661–64.

Jagiello-Gruszfeld A, Tjulandin S, et al. (2010). A single-arm phase II trial of first-line paclitaxel in combination with lapatinib in HER2-overexpressing metastatic breast cancer. *Oncology* 79(1–2):129–35.

Jones S, Erban J, et al. (2005). Randomized phase III study of docetaxel compared with paclitaxel in metastatic breast cancer. *J Clin Oncol* 23(24): 5542–51.

Kakimoto T, Hattori Y, et al. (2002). Thalidomide for the treatment of refractory multiple myeloma: Association of plasma concentrations of thalidomide and angiogenic growth factors with clinical outcome. *Jpn J Cancer Res* 93(9):1029–36.

Kanbayashi Y, Hosokawa T, et al. (2010). Statistical identification of predictors for peripheral neuropathy associated with administration of bortezomib, taxanes, oxaliplatin or vincristine using ordered logistic regression analysis. *Anticancer Drugs* 21(9):877–81.

Kato K, Inaba Y, et al. (2011). A multicenter phase-II study of 5-FU, leucovorin and oxaliplatin (FOLFOX6) in patients with pretreated metastatic colorectal cancer. *Jpn J Clin Oncol* 41(1):63–68.

Kim Y, Sohn S, et al. (2010). Clinical efficacy of a bortezomib, cylcophosphamide, thalidomide, and dexamethsaone (Vel-CTD) regimen in patients with relapsed or refractory multiple myeloma: A phase II study. *Ann Hematol* 89(5):475–82.

Koizumi W, Akiya T, et al. (2009). Second-line chemotherapy with biweekly paclitaxel after failure of fluoropyrimidine-based treatment in patients with advanced or recurrent gastric cancer: A report from the gastrointestinal oncology group of the Tokyo Cooperative Oncology Group, TCOG GC-0501 trial. *Jpn J Clin Oncol* 39(11):713–19.

Krzakowski M, Ramlau R, et al. (2010). Phase III trial comparing vinflunine with docetaxel in second-line advanced non-small-cell lung cancer previously treated with platinum-containing chemotherapy. *J Clin Oncol* 28(13):2167–73.

Lamm W, Kaufmann H, et al. (2011). Bortezomib combined with rituximab and dexamethasone is an active regimen for patients with relapsed and chemotherapy-refractory mantle cell lymphoma. *Haematologica* 96(7):1008–14.

Lancet J, Duong V, et al. (2011). A phase I clinical-pharmacodynamic study of the farnesyltransferase inhibitor tipifarnib in combination with the proteasome inhibitor bortezomib in advanced acute leukemias. *Clin Cancer Res* 17(5):1140–46.

Lassen U, Molife LR, et al. (2010). A phase I study of the safety and pharmacokinetics of the histone deacetylase inhibitor belinostat administered in combination with carboplatin and/or paclitaxel in patients with solid tumours. *Br J Cancer* 103(1):12–17.

Lee JL, MH Ryu, et al. (2008). A phase II study of docetaxel as salvage chemotherapy in advanced gastric cancer after failure of fluoropyrimidine and platinum combination chemotherapy. *Cancer Chemother Pharmacol* 61(4):631–37.

Lee SM, Rudd R, et al. (2009a). Randomized double-blind placebo-controlled trial of thalidomide in combination with gemcitabine and carboplatin in advanced non-small-cell lung cancer. *J Clin Oncol* 27(31):5248–54.

Lee SM, Woll PJ, et al. (2009b). Anti-angiogenic therapy using thalidomide combined with chemotherapy in small cell lung cancer: A randomized, double-blind, placebo-controlled trial. *J Natl Cancer Inst* 101(15):1049–57.

Lee Y, Nassikas N, et al. (2011). The role of the central nervous system in the generation and maintenance of chronic pain in rheumatoid arthritis, osteoarthritis and fibromyalgia. *Arth Res Ther* 13:211–21.

Lenz W. (1985). Thalidomide embryopathy in Germany, 1959–1961. *Prog Clin Biol* Res 163C:77–83.

Li J, Zeng L, et al. (2009a). Combination of bortezomib and dexamethasone for newly diagnosed multiple myeloma. *Zhonghua Xue Ye Xue Za Zhi* 30(8):543–47.

Li J, Zhou D, et al. (2009b). Bortezomib and dexamethasone therapy for newly diagnosed patients with multiple myeloma complicated by renal impairment. *Clin Lymphoma Myeloma* 9(5):394–98.

Lilenbaum RC, Chen CS, et al. (2005). Phase II randomized trial of vinorelbine and gemcitabine versus carboplatin and paclitaxel in advanced non-small-cell lung cancer. *Ann Oncol* 16(1):97–101.

Lincoln S, Blessing J, et al. (2003). Activity of paclitaxel as second-line chemotherapy in endometrial carcinoma: A Gynecologic Oncology Group study. *Gynceol Oncol* 88:277–81.

Lobo C, Lopes G, et al. (2010). Final results of a phase II study of nab-paclitaxel, bevacizumab, and gemcitabine as first-line therapy for patients with HER2-negative metastatic breast cancer. *Breast Cancer Res Treat* 123(2):427–35.

Loprinzi CL, Reeves BN, et al. (2011). Natural history of paclitaxel-associated acute pain syndrome: Prospective cohort study NCCTG N08C1. *J Clin Oncol* 29(11):1472–1478.

Lou F, Zhu YH, et al. (2009). Oxaliplatin combined with ELF regimen in the treatment of patients with advanced gastric cancer. *Zhonghua Zhong Liu Za Zhi* 31(1):75–78.

Loven D, Levavi H, et al. (2009). Long-term glutamate supplementation failed to protect against peripheral neurotoxicity of paclitaxel. *Eur J Cancer Care (Engl)* 18(1):78–83.

Lu S, Wang J, et al. (2009). Bortezomib in combination with epirubicin, dexamethasone and thalidomide is a highly effective regimen in the treatment of multiple myeloma: A single-center experience. *Int J Hematol* 89(1):34–38.

Machover D, Delmas-Marsalet B, et al. (2010). Treatment with rituximab, dexamethasone, high-dose cytarabine, and oxaliplatin (R-DHAOx) produces a strong long-term anti-tumor effect in previously treated patients with follicular non-Hodgkin's lymphoma. *Biomed Pharmacother* 64(2):83–87.

Mannel R, Brady M, et al. (2011). A randomized phase III trial of IV carboplatin and paclitaxel × 3 courses followed by observation versus weekly maintenance low-dose paclitaxel in patients with early-stage ovarian carcinoma: A Gynecologic Oncology Group study. *Gynecol Oncol* 122(1):89–94.

Martino M, Console G, et al. (2007). Low tolerance and high toxicity of thalidomide as maintenance therapy after double autologous stem cell transplant in multiple myeloma patients. *Eur J Haematol* 78(1):35–40.

Mateos M, Oriol A, et al. (2010). Bortezomib, melphalan, and prednisone versus bortezomib, thalidomide, and prednisone as induction therapy followed by maintenance treatment with bortezomib and thalidomide versus bortezomib and prednisone in elderly patients with untreated multiple myeloma: A randomised trial. *Lancet Oncol* 11(10):934–41.

McClain KL, Kozinetz CA (2007). A phase II trial using thalidomide for Langerhans cell histiocytosis. *Pediatr Blood Cancer* 48(1):44–49.

Messinger Y, Gaynon P, et al. (2010). Phase I study of bortezomib combined with chemotherapy in children with relapsed childhood acute lymphoblastic leukemia (ALL): A report from the therapeutic advances in childhood leukemia (TACL) consortium. *Pediatr Blood Cancer* 55(2):254–59.

Mielke S, Sparreboom A, et al. (2006). Peripheral neuropathy: A persisting challenge in paclitaxel-based regimens. *Eur J Cancer* 42(1):24–30.

Mileshkin L, Stark R, et al. (2006). Development of neuropathy in patients with myeloma treated with thalidomide: Patterns of occurrence and the role of electrophysiologic monitoring. *J Clin Oncol* 24(27):4507–14.

Milla P, Airoldi M, et al. (2009). Administration of reduced glutathione in FOLFOX4 adjuvant treatment for colorectal cancer: Effect on oxaliplatin pharmacokinetics, Pt-DNA adduct formation, and neurotoxicity. *Anticancer Drugs* 20(5):396–402.

Mir O, Alexandre J, et al. (2009). Vinorelbine and oxaliplatin in stage IV nonsmall cell lung cancer patients unfit for cisplatin: A single-center experience. *Anticancer Drugs* 20(2):105–8.

Mita MM, Rowinsky EK, et al. (2007). A phase II, pharmacokinetic, and biologic study of semaxanib and thalidomide in patients with metastatic melanoma. *Cancer Chemother Pharmacol* 59(2):165–74.

Mitsiades N, Mitsiades C, et al. (2003). The proteasome inhibitor PS-341 potentiates sensitivity of multiple myeloma cells to conventional chemotherapeutic agents: Therapeutic applications. *Blood* 101(6):2377–380.

Molloy FM, Floeter MK, et al. (2001). Thalidomide neuropathy in patients treated for metastatic prostate cancer. *Muscle Nerve* 24(8):1050–57.

Morabito A, Fanelli M, et al. (2004). Thalidomide prolongs disease stabilization after conventional therapy in patients with recurrent glioblastoma. *Oncol Rep* 11(1):93–95.

Morabito F, Gentile M, et al. (2010). Safety and efficacy of bortezomib-based regiments for multiple myeloma patients with renal impairment: A retrospective study of Italian Myeloma Network GIMEMA. *Eur J Haematol* 84:223–28.

Moreau P, Avet-Loiseau H, et al. (2011a). Bortezomib plus dexamethasone versus reduced-dose bortezomib, thalidomide plus dexamethasone as induction treatment prior to autologous stem cell transplantation in newly diagnosed multiple myeloma. *Blood* 118(22):5752–58.

Moreau P, Pylypenko H, et al. (2011b). Subcutaneous versus intravenous administration of bortezomib in patients with relapsed multiple myeloma: A randomised, phase 3, non-inferiority study. *Lacent Oncol* 12(5):431–40.

Murakami H, Handa H, et al. (2007). Low-dose thalidomide plus low-dose dexamethasone therapy in patients with refractory multiple myeloma. *Eur J Haematol* 79(3):234–39.

Murakami H, Shimizu K, et al. (2009). Phase II and pharmacokinetic study of thalidomide in Japanese patients with relapsed/refractory multiple myeloma. *Int J Hematol* 89(5):636–41.

Muthuramalingam S, Braybrooke J, et al. (2011). A prospective randomised phase II trial of thalidomide with carboplatin compared with carboplatin alone as a first-line therapy in women with ovarian cancer, with evaluation of potential surrogate markers of angiogenesis. *Eur J Gynaecol Oncol* 32(3):253–58.

Nabhan C, Villines D, et al. (2011). Bortezomib (Velcade), rituximab, cyclophosphamide, and dexamethasone combination regimen is active as front-line therapy of low-grade non-Hodgkin lymphoma. *Clin Lymphoma Myeloma Leuk* 12(1):26–31.

Nakano A, Abe M, et al. (2011). Delayed treatment with vitamin C and N-acetyl-L-cysteine protects Schwann cells without compromising the anti-myeloma activity of bortezomib. *Int J Hematol* 93(6):727–34.

Offidani M, Corvatta L, et al. (2004). Common and rare side-effects of low-dose thalidomide in multiple myeloma: Focus on the dose-minimizing peripheral neuropathy. *Eur J Haematol* 72(6):403–9.

Offidani M, Corvatta L, et al. (2009). Thalidomide-dexamethasone versus interferon-alpha-dexamethasone as maintenance treatment after ThaDD induction for multiple myeloma: A prospective, multicentre, randomised study. *Br J Haematol* 144(5):653–59.

Ott PA, Chang JL, et al. (2009). Phase II trial of dacarbazine and thalidomide for the treatment of metastatic melanoma. *Chemotherapy* 55(4):221–27.

Ott PA, Hamilton A, et al. (2010). A phase II trial of the epothilone B analog ixabepilone (BMS-247550) in patients with metastatic melanoma. *PLoS ONE* 5(1):e8714.

Overman MJ, Varadhachary GR, et al. (2009). Phase II study of capecitabine and oxaliplatin for advanced adenocarcinoma of the small bowel and ampulla of Vater. *J Clin Oncol* 27(16):2598–603.

Pace A, Giannarelli D, et al. (2010). Vitamin E neuroprotection for cisplatin neuropathy: A randomized, placebo-controlled trial. *Neurology* 74(9):762–66.

Palumbo A, Ambrosini MT, et al. (2007). Bortezomib, melphalan, prednisone, and thalidomide for relapsed multiple myeloma. *Blood* 109(7):2767–72.

Palumbo A, Gay F. (2009). How to treat elderly patients with multiple myeloma: Combination of therapy or sequencing. *Hematol Am Soc Hematol Educ Program* 566–77.

Palumbo A, Gay F, et al. (2010a). Bortezomib as induction before autologous transplantation, followed by lenalidomide as consolidation-maintenance in untreated multiple myeloma patients. *J Clin Oncol* 28(5):800–7.

Palumbo A, Larocca A, et al. (2010b). Lenalidomide, melphalan, prednisone, and thalidomide (RMPT) for relapsed/refractory multiple myeloma. *Leukemia* 24(5):1037–42.

Palumbo A, Mateos M, et al. (2011). Practical management of adverse events in multiple myeloma: Can therapy be attenuated in older patients? *Blood Rev* 25(4):181–91.

Pereira JR, Martins SJ, et al. (2004). Chemotherapy with cisplatin and vinorelbine for elderly patients with locally advanced or metastatic non-small-cell lung cancer (NSCLC). *BMC Cancer* 4:69.

Plasmati R, Pastorelli F, et al. (2007). Neuropathy in multiple myeloma treated with thalidomide: A prospective study. *Neurology* 69(6):573–81.

Priolo T, Lamba LD, et al. (2008). Childhood thalidomide neuropathy: A clinical and neurophysiologic study. *Pediatr Neurol* 38(3):196–99.

Pujade-Lauraine E, Wagner U, et al. (2010). Pegylated liposomal doxorubicin and carboplatin compared with paclitaxel and carboplatin for patients with platinum-sensitive ovarian cancer in late relapse. *J Clin Oncol* 28(20):3323–29.

Rajkumar SV, Blood E, et al. (2006). Phase III clinical trial of thalidomide plus dexamethasone compared with dexamethasone alone in newly diagnosed multiple myeloma: A clinical trial coordinated by the Eastern Cooperative Oncology Group. *J Clin Oncol* 24(3):431–36.

Rapoport BL, Falkson G, et al. (1993). Suramin in combination with mitomycin C in hormone-resistant prostate cancer. A phase II clinical study. *Ann Oncol* 4(7):567–73.

Richardson P, Chanan-Khan A, et al. (2011). Tanespimycin and bortezomib combination treatment in patients with relapsed or relapsed and refractory multiple myeloma: Results of a phase 1/2 study. *Br J Haematol* 153(6):729–40.

Richardson P, Badros A, et al. (2010a). Tanespimycin with bortezomib: Activity in relapsed/refractory patients with multiple myeloma. *Br J Haematol* 150(4):428–37.

Richardson P, Laubach J, et al. (2010b). Complications of multiple myeloma therapy, part 1: Risk reduction and management of peripheral neuropathy and asthenia. *J Natl Compr Canc Netw* 8(Suppl 1):S4–12.

Richardson PG, Blood E, et al. (2006). A randomized phase 2 study of lenalidomide therapy for patients with relapsed or relapsed and refractory multiple myeloma. *Blood* 108(10):3458–64.

Rifkin R, Greenspan A, et al. (2010). A phase II open-label trial of bortezomib in patients with multiple myeloma who have undergone an autologous peripheral blood stem cell transplant and failed to achieve a complete response. *Invest New Drugs* 30(2):714–22.

Rixe O, Gatineau M, et al. (2005). Sequential administration of docetaxel followed by cisplatin-vindesine: A pilot study in patients with locally advanced or metastatic non-small cell lung cancer (NSCLC). *Bull Cancer* 92(1):E1–6.

Rose A, Smith B, et al. (2002). Glucocorticoids and rituximab *in vitro*: Synergistic direct antiproliferative and apoptotic effects. *Blood* 100(5):1765–73.

Roussel M, Moreau P, et al. (2009). Bortezomib and high-dose melphalan as conditioning regimen before autologous stem cell transplantation in patients with *de novo* multiple myeloma: A phase 2 study of the Intergroupe Francophone due Myélome (IFM). *Blood* 115(1):32–37.

Sakakibara T, Inoue A, et al. (2010). Randomized phase II trial of weekly paclitaxel combined with carboplatin versus standard paclitaxel combined with carboplatin for elderly patients with advanced non-small-cell lung cancer. *Ann Oncol* 21(4):795–99.

San Miguel J, Schlag R, et al. (2008). Bortezomib plus melphalan and prednisone for initial treatment of multiple myeloma. *N Engl J Med* 359(9):906–17.

Sarosy GA, Hussain MM, et al. (2010). Ten-year follow-up of a phase 2 study of dose-intense paclitaxel with cisplatin and cyclophosphamide as initial therapy for poor-prognosis, advanced-stage epithelial ovarian cancer. *Cancer* 116(6):1476–84.

Schmid P, Heilmann V, et al. (2005). Gemcitabine as prolonged infusion and vinorelbine in anthracycline and/or taxane pretreated metastatic breast cancer: A phase II study. *J Cancer Res Clin Oncol* 131(9):568–74.

Schmid P, Kiewe P, et al. (2010). Phase I study of the novel, fully synthetic epothilone sagopilone (ZK-EPO) in patients with solid tumors. *Ann Oncol* 21(3):633–39.

Schmitt S, Goldschmidt H, et al. (2011). Inflammatory autoimmune neuropathy, presumably induced by bortezomib, in a patient suffering from multiple myeloma. *Int J Hematol* 93(6):791–94.

Schonnemann KR, Jensen HA, et al. (2008). Phase II study of short-time oxaliplatin, capecitabine and epirubicin (EXE) as first-line therapy in patients with non-resectable gastric cancer. *Br J Cancer* 99(6):858–61.

Schutt P, Ebeling P, et al. (2005). Thalidomide in combination with dexamethasone for pre-treated patients with multiple myeloma: Serum level of soluble interleukin-2 receptor as a predictive factor for response rate and for survival. *Ann Hematol* 84(9):594–600.

Seo HY, Lee HJ, et al. (2011). Phase II study of vinorelbine monotherapy in anthracycline and taxane pre-treated metastatic breast cancer. *Invest New Drugs* 29(2):360–65.

Shim HJ, Cho SH, et al. (2010). Phase II study of docetaxel and cisplatin chemotherapy in 5-fluorouracil/cisplatin pretreated esophageal cancer. *Am J Clin Oncol* 33(6):624–28.

Short SC, Traish D, et al. (2001). Thalidomide as an anti-angiogenic agent in relapsed gliomas. *J Neurooncol* 51(1):41–45.

Sikov WM, Dizon DS, et al. (2009). Frequent pathologic complete responses in aggressive stages II to III breast cancers with every-4-week carboplatin and weekly paclitaxel with or without trastuzumab: A Brown University Oncology Group Study. *J Clin Oncol* 27(28):4693–700.

Spicka I, Mateos M, et al. (2011). An overview of the VISTA trial: Newly diagnosed, untreated patients with multiple myeloma ineligible for stem cell transplantation. *Immunotherapy* 3(9):1033–40.

Stathopoulos GP, Antoniou D, et al. (2010). Liposomal cisplatin combined with paclitaxel versus cisplatin and paclitaxel in non-small-cell lung cancer: A randomized phase III multicenter trial. *Ann Oncol* 21(11):2227–32.

Stebbing J, Benson C, et al. (2001). The treatment of advanced renal cell cancer with high-dose oral thalidomide. *Br J Cancer* 85(7):953–58.

Sugimoto S, Katano K, et al. (2009). Multicenter safety study of mFOLFOX6 for unresectable advanced/recurrent colorectal cancer in elderly patients. *J Exp Clin Cancer Res* 28:109.

Sun Q, Liu C, et al. (2009). Multi-center phase II trial of weekly paclitaxel plus cisplatin combination chemotherapy in patients with advanced gastric and gastro-esophageal cancer. *Jpn J Clin Oncol* 39(4):237–43.

Syrigos KN, Dannos I, et al. (2005). Bi-weekly administration of docetaxel and gemcitabine as first-line therapy for non-small cell lung cancer: A phase II study. *Anticancer Res* 25(5):3489–93.

Tabata T, Tanida K, et al. (2008). Weekly low-dose paclitaxel and carboplatin therapy in gynecological cancer patients with venous thrombosis. *Anticancer Res* 28(6B):3971–75.

Tahara M, Minami H, et al. (2011). Weekly paclitaxel in patients with recurrent or metastatic head and neck cancer. *Cancer Chemother Pharmacol* 68(3):769–76.

Ten Bokkel Huinink WW, Sufliarsky J, et al. (2009). Safety and efficacy of patupilone in patients with advanced ovarian, primary fallopian, or primary peritoneal cancer: A phase I, open-label, dose-escalation study. *J Clin Oncol* 27(19):3097–103.

Terpos E, Kastritis E, et al. (2008). The combination of bortezomib, melphalan, dexamethasone and intermittent thalidomide is an effective regimen for relapsed/refractory myeloma and is associated with improvement of abnormal bone metabolism and angiogenesis. *Leukemia* 22(12):2247–56.

Thomas DA, Giles FJ, et al. (2006). Thalidomide therapy for myelofibrosis with myeloid metaplasia. *Cancer* 106(9):1974–84.

Thomas DA, Kantarjian HM, et al. (2009). Phase 1 multicenter study of vincristine sulfate liposomes injection and dexamethasone in adults with relapsed or refractory acute lymphoblastic leukemia. *Cancer* 115(23):5490–98.

Tiersten AD, Sill MW, et al. (2010). A phase I trial of dose-dense (biweekly) carboplatin combined with paclitaxel and pegfilgrastim: A feasibility study in patients with untreated stage III and IV ovarian, tubal or primary peritoneal cancer: A Gynecologic Oncology Group study. *Gynecol Oncol* 118(3):303–7.

Tosi P, Zamagni E, et al. (2002). Salvage therapy with thalidomide in patients with advanced relapsed/refractory multiple myeloma. *Haematologica* 87(4):408–14.

Tosi P, Zamagni E, et al. (2005). Neurological toxicity of long-term (>1 yr) thalidomide therapy in patients with multiple myeloma. *Eur J Haematol* 74(3):212–16.

Treon SP, Soumerai JD, et al. (2008). Thalidomide and rituximab in Waldenstrom macroglobulinemia. *Blood* 112(12):4452–57.

Tsimberidou AM, Letourneau K, et al. (2011a). Phase I clinical trial of hepatic arterial infusion of paclitaxel in patients with advanced cancer and dominant liver involvement. *Cancer Chemother Pharmacol* 68(1):247–53.

Tsimberidou AM, Takimoto CH, et al. (2011b). Effects of patupilone on the pharmacokinetics and pharmacodynamics of warfarin in patients with advanced malignancies: A phase I clinical trial. *Mol Cancer Ther* 10(1):209–17.

Uhm JE, Park JO, et al. (2009). A phase II study of oxaliplatin in combination with doxorubicin as first-line systemic chemotherapy in patients with inoperable hepatocellular carcinoma. *Cancer Chemother Pharmacol* 63(5):929–35.

Valero V, Forbes J, et al. (2011). Multicenter phase III randomized trial comparing docetaxel and trastuzumab with docetaxel, carboplatin, and trastuzumab as first-line chemotherapy for patients with HER2-gene-amplified metastatic breast cancer (BCIRG 007 study): Two highly active therapeutic regimens. *J Clin Oncol* 29(2):149–56.

van Herpen CM, Eskens FA, et al. (2010). A Phase Ib dose-escalation study to evaluate safety and tolerability of the addition of the aminopeptidase inhibitor tosedostat (CHR-2797) to paclitaxel in patients with advanced solid tumours. *Br J Cancer* 103(9):1362–68.

Varker KA, Campbell J, et al. (2008). Phase II study of thalidomide in patients with metastatic carcinoid and islet cell tumors. *Cancer Chemother Pharmacol* 61(4):661–68.

Verstappen CC, Koeppen S, et al. (2005). Dose-related vincristine-induced peripheral neuropathy with unexpected off-therapy worsening. *Neurology* 64(6):1076–77.

Wainberg Z, Lin L, et al. (2011). Phase II trial of modified FOLFOX6 and erlotinib in patients with metastatic or advanced adenocarcinoma of the oesophagus and gastro-oesophageal junction. *Br J Cancer* 105(6):760–65.

Wang J, Fan Y, et al. (2010). Ixabepilone plus capecitabine for Chinese patients with metastatic breast cancer progressing after anthracycline and taxane treatment. *Cancer Chemother Pharmacol* 66(3):597–603.

Wang M, Han X, et al. (2008). Bortezomib is synergistic with rituximab and cyclophosphamide in inducing apoptosis of mantle cell lymphoma cells *in vitro* and *in vivo*. *Leukemia* 22(1):179–85.

Waterman G, Yellin O, et al. (2011). A modified regimen of pegylated liposomal doxorubicin, bortezomib, and dexamethasone is effective and well tolerated in the treatment of relapsed or refractory multiple myeloma. *Ann Hematol* 90(2):193–200.

Winer E, Berry D, et al. (2004). Failure of higher-dose paclitaxel to improve outcome in patients with metastatic breast cancer: Cancer and Leukemia Group B Trial 9342. *J Clin Oncol* 22:2061–68.

Yang DH, Kim YK, et al. (2010). Induction treatment with cyclophosphamide, thalidomide, and dexamethasone in newly diagnosed multiple myeloma: A phase II study. *Clin Lymphoma Myeloma Leuk* 10(1):62–67.

Zervas K, Dimopoulos MA, et al. (2004). Primary treatment of multiple myeloma with thalidomide, vincristine, liposomal doxorubicin and dexamethasone (T-VAD doxil): A phase II multicenter study. *Ann Oncol* 15(1):134–38.

Zervas K, Mihou D, et al. (2007). VAD-doxil versus VAD-doxil plus thalidomide as initial treatment for multiple myeloma: Results of a multicenter randomized trial of the Greek Myeloma Study Group. *Ann Oncol* 18(8):1369–75.

Zhang X, Shi H, et al. (2011). Prospective, randomized trial comparing 5-FU/LV with or without oxaliplatin as adjuvant treatment following curative resection of gastric adenocarcinoma. *Eur J Surg Oncol* 37(6):466–72.

Zhao JG, Qiu F, et al. (2009). A phase II study of modified FOLFOX as first-line chemotherapy in elderly patients with advanced gastric cancer. *Anticancer Drugs* 20(4):281–86.

Zhu AX, Meyerhardt JA, et al. (2010). Efficacy and safety of gemcitabine, oxaliplatin, and bevacizumab in advanced biliary-tract cancers and correlation of changes in 18-fluorodeoxyglucose PET with clinical outcome: A phase 2 study. *Lancet Oncol* 11(1):48–54.

4 Orofacial Neuropathy and Pain in Cancer Patients

Yehuda Zadik, Noam Yarom, and Sharon Elad

CONTENTS

4.1 Introduction 95
4.2 Cancer-Related Orofacial Pain 96
    4.2.1 Orofacial Pain in Head and Neck Malignancies 96
    4.2.2 Other Malignancies 97
4.3 Cancer-Related Orofacial Neuropathy 98
    4.3.1 Mental Nerve Neuropathy 98
    4.3.2 Trigeminal Neuralgia 99
    4.3.3 Facial Palsy 99
4.4 Radiotherapy- and Surgery-Related Neuropathies 100
    4.4.1 Taste Dysfunction 100
    4.4.2 Postoperative Neuropathies 101
    4.4.3 Auriculotemporal Syndrome 101
4.5 Chemotherapy-Related Orofacial Neuropathy 102
    4.5.1 Chemotherapy-Related Neurotoxicity 102
    4.5.2 Neuralgia-Inducing Cavitational Osteonecrosis of Jaws 103
    4.5.3 Neuropathies Secondary to Oral Complications of Chemotherapy 104
        4.5.3.1 Drug-Induced Osteonecrosis of Jaws 104
        4.5.3.2 Recurrent Orofacial Viral Infections 104
4.6 Chemotherapy-Related Odontalgia 104
    4.6.1 Dental Hypersensitivity 105
    4.6.2 Dental Pain 105
4.7 Other Types of Orofacial Pain 108
4.8 Conclusion 108
References 108

4.1 INTRODUCTION

The orofacial region, which includes the lower half of the face and the oral cavity, commonly causes oncologic patients to seek medical attention for pain. Orofacial pain is unique because its potential influence is much wider than pain in other regions of the body. Orofacial pain impairs: (1) orofacial functions such as eating, drinking, speaking, and facial expression; (2) quality of life; and (3) the ability to maintain adequate oral hygiene, which might result in the deterioration of oral health (teeth and gums) and halitosis. These difficulties may have a significant medical, nutritional, functional, or social-psychological impact in the cancer patient, especially during periods of cytotoxic chemotherapy-related neutropenia. The debilitating effects of orofacial pain may limit the administration of anticancer chemotherapy or cause other treatment modifications (e.g., percutaneous endoscopic gastrostomy for feeding). Furthermore, orofacial neuropathies manifesting as parasthesia may cause aspiration of oral intakes, with adverse consequences.

In this chapter, orofacial neuropathy—both as a result of the cancer or as an adverse effect of anticancer therapy—will be described, with a focus on chemotherapy-related neuropathic pain.

It should be noted that orofacial pain in the oncology patient may be coincidental and unrelated to cancer. The reader should also note that despite the high prevalence of the phenomenon, the data regarding cancer-related orofacial pain and neuropathy are incomplete, and rely largely on case reports and expert opinion.

4.2   CANCER-RELATED OROFACIAL PAIN

Orofacial pain affects up to 70% of oncology patients (Benoliel et al., 2007). In these patients, pain may be due to the cancer, the surgical interventions, the radiotherapy, the chemotherapy, or the other cancer interventions, such as stem cell transplantation or immunobiologic treatments. Table 4.1 lists the possible causes of orofacial pain in oncology patients according to treatment modality.

There is a bidirectional relationship between emotional stress/anxiety and orofacial pain in oncology patients; some orofacial pain may not be directly related to cancer, or anticancer treatment may be exacerbated by the stress and anxiety typically experienced during the period of cancer diagnosis or anticancer treatments. Furthermore, orofacial pain occurring in cancer patients is likely to be associated with heightened anxiety, which affects the presentation and associated behavior of pain and patient (Epstein et al., 2007).

4.2.1   Orofacial Pain in Head and Neck Malignancies

Pain is the first clinical symptom in one-fifth of oral cancer patients (Cuffari et al., 2006). The pain is usually unilateral and nonspecific, and therefore an unreliable predictor of orofacial malignancy. More than one-third of patients described the pain as a sore throat, pain when swallowing, and regional pain (tongue, intraoral, tooth, and ear) (Cuffari et al., 2006). Nevertheless, the combination of pain, parasthesia, and swelling may predict malignancy, especially when other systemic signs, such as weight loss, fatigue, or anemia, are present (Elad et al., 2008).

Approximately 50 to 85% of head and neck cancer patients suffer from pain prior to cancer therapy, usually of low-grade intensity (Epstein and Van Der Waal, 2008), 80% during therapy, and 70 to 78% at the end of therapy. Approximately one-third of patients suffer from pain at and beyond 6 months after treatment, and this late pain is typically more severe than initial (pretreatment) pain, but less severe than the immediate posttreatment period (Epstein et al., 2010). Among head and neck cancer patients, increased pain intensity was reported by individuals treated with bimodal

TABLE 4.1

Possible Causes of Orofacial Pain in the Oncology Patient

Etiology	Pathophysiology
Cancer related	Mass effect (direct pressure, invasion)
	Chemical neurosensitization
	Ulceration (exposure of nerves)
	Secondary anemia
	Infection (tumor necrosis or impaired granulocytes)
Surgery related	Postoperative pain[a]
	Postoperative infection
	Neuropathy[b]
Radiotherapy related	Oral mucositis[a]
	Tissue atrophy, necrosis, and fibrosis[b]
	Oral dysesthesia secondary to dry mouth[a,b] and candidiasis[a]
	Neuropathy[b]
	Radiation dental caries[b]
	Osteoradionecrosis[b]
Chemotherapy related	Infection[a]
	Oral mucositis[a]
	Postherpetic neuralgia[b]
	Neuropathy[b]
	Targeted therapy related to oral ulcers (e.g., mTOR inhibitors[a])
	Drug-related osteonecrosis of jaw[b]
Allogeneic HSCT related	Acute GVHD[a]
	Chronic GVHD[b]
	Thalidomide-induced neuropathy
Other	Orofacial pain unrelated to cancer (or anticancer therapy)
	Burning mouth syndrome

Notes: mTOR, mammalian target of rapamycin; GVHD, graft versus host disease; HSCT, hematopoietic stem cell transplantation.

[a] Highly prevalent.

[b] May be chronic.

therapy (i.e., radiotherapy combined with chemotherapy) (Epstein et al., 2010). Despite ongoing pain management measures, these patients experience nociceptive and neuropathic pain, which impact considerably on quality of life, even when the levels of pain are low to moderate (Epstein et al., 2009).

4.2.2 OTHER MALIGNANCIES

Orofacial pain has also been reported in patients with either distant metastasized or nonmetastasized malignant lung tumors (Capobianco, 1995; Sarlani et al., 2003). Several mechanisms have been proposed to explain orofacial pain induced by non-metastasized (lung) cancer, including activation of nociceptive pathways in the mediastinum and head and neck structures, invasion or compression of the vagus nerve, referred pain from the phrenic nerve, and production of inflammatory mediators (i.e., a paraneoplastic process) (Elad et al., 2008). Typically, pain presents as a dull unilateral ache located in the periotic jaw or temporal area ipsilateral to the lung lesion (Sarlani et al., 2003).

Pain has also been reported in nonsolid cancers. The common mechanisms in hematologic malignancies include pressure from a leukemic infiltrate, penetration of closed anatomical compartments (i.e., attached gingiva), and infiltration of malignant cells in proximity to peripheral nerves or the central nervous system (Chamberlain, 2005). Cancer-related intracranial hemorrhage is another possible etiology for orofacial neuropathy (Chamberlain, 2005). Unique to cancer patients undergoing hematopoietic stem cell transplantation, oral pain may be associated with graft versus host disease (GVHD), particularly the erosive or ulcerative type (Meier et al., 2011).

4.3 CANCER-RELATED OROFACIAL NEUROPATHY

One in six cancer patients suffers from cancer-related orofacial neuropathy (Epstein, 2001). One in nine head and neck cancer patients suffers from treatment-related neuropathic pain (Grond et al., 1996). The entities related directly to cancer include mental nerve neuropathy and trigeminal neuralgia. Radiotherapy may cause taste disorders and surgery may cause postoperative neuropathic or auriculotemporal nerve dysfunction (*Frey syndrome*). Coincidently, burning mouth syndrome may be aggravated by anxiety associated with cancer. These entities are further described below.

4.3.1 MENTAL NERVE NEUROPATHY

Although the discussion is focused on neuropathy of the mental (chin) region, neuropathies occasionally involve other orofacial regions. Mental nerve neuropathy, also called *numb chin syndrome*, is characterized by numbness or paresthesia, and rarely with pain. This condition is associated with malignant lesions in one-fifth of cases (Kalladka et al., 2008). Similarly, space-occupying lesions, such as nasopharyngeal or sinus carcinoma, may cause facial neuralgia, often with physical signs (sensory or motor impairment) (Scully, 2008b). A malignant lesion may cause neuropathy by three mechanisms:

1. Peripheral inflammation induced by early malignant encroachment on peripheral neural tissue and production of perineural inflammation and neuritis. This inflammation primarily affects the large myelinated Aβ fibers reducing the detection threshold (hypersensitivity).
2. Compression of a peripheral nerve by the malignancy (Figure 4.1) or infiltration of the nerve (Figure 4.2). This type of nerve injury affects all sensory nerve fibers (large myelinated Aβ, thin myelinated Aδ, and unmyelinated C fibers) elevating the detection threshold (hyposensitivity) (Eliav et al., 2004; Eliav and Gracely, 2008).
3. Central nervous system involvement of a primary or, more often, a secondary neoplasm, or infiltration of a hematologic malignancy (Scully, 2008b).

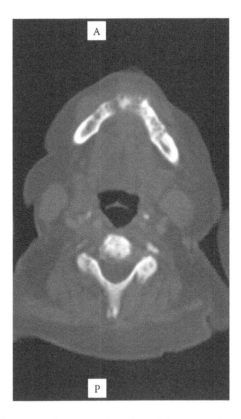

FIGURE 4.1 Axial computed tomography view of breast carcinoma metastasis to the mandible causing extensive regional neuropathy. Despite the extensive bilateral mandibular lesions, only the right side was symptomatic. A: anterior; P: posterior.

When the positive symptom (pain) is combined with the negative symptom (anesthesia), the condition is called *anesthesia dolorosa* or *painful trigeminal neuropathy*, and suggests complete denervation (Benoliel et al., 2008).

4.3.2 Trigeminal Neuralgia

About 10% of patients diagnosed with trigeminal neuralgia (TN) have symptomatic TN, caused by intracranial neoplasms. These tumors are often metastases (Scully, 2008a), posterior fossa tumors, and meningiomas (Benoliel et al., 2008). Symptomatic TN is more prevalent in young (<29 years old) TN patients (Benoliel et al., 2008).

4.3.3 Facial Palsy

In patients undergoing iodine radioablation for thyroid cancer, facial palsy may develop (Levenson et al., 1994). This could be a consequence of inflammation in the adjacent parotid gland (Mandel and Mandel, 2003). Upon remission of the acute parotitis the paralysis usually resolves.

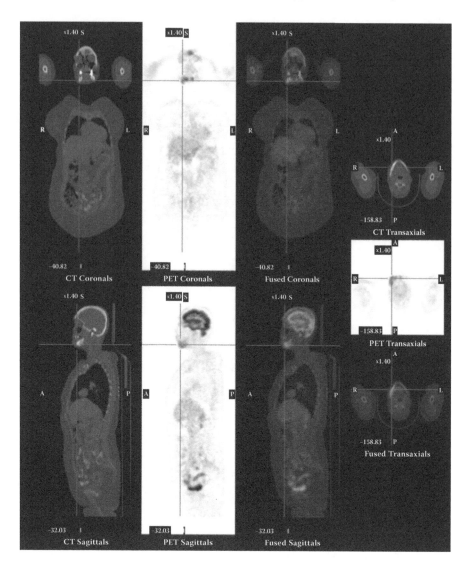

FIGURE 4.2   F-18 fluorodeoxyglucose (FDG) positron emission tomography with computed tomography (PET-CT) of a patient diagnosed with primary diffuse large B cell lymphoma of the mandible. Mandibular pain and mental neuropathy were the first manifestations of the malignant lesion. Plain mandibular radiographs were not contributory.

4.4   RADIOTHERAPY- AND SURGERY-RELATED NEUROPATHIES

4.4.1   TASTE DYSFUNCTION

Taste dysfunctions (dysgeusia, ageusia, hypogeusia, hypergeusia) are common adverse effects of anticancer therapy (radiotherapy, chemotherapy), affecting 56 to 76% of patients (Hovan et al., 2010). Greater changes in taste are reported by female patients (Epstein et al., 2002). This phenomenon is caused by damage to the neuroepithelial taste receptors, specifically their microvilli, or to the innervating fibers. During a course of head and neck radiation therapy, taste impairments are an early complication, appearing within the first week, and a bitter flavor dominates. Loss of taste begins with a cumulative radiation dose of 20 Gy, and at 30 Gy all taste qualities are affected. Almost all patients experience a complete taste loss at 60 Gy of cumulative radiation (Fischer et al., 2008). The adverse taste sensation may be exacerbated by concomitant hyposalivation (Epstein et al., 2002), and nausea and vomiting. In addition, the diffusion of chemotherapy drugs into the oral cavity may also aggravate the sensation, inducing a bitter taste, as well as unpleasant odor (halitosis) and aversions to certain foods (Little et al., 2008; Lalla et al., 2011).

Radioactive iodine (^{131}I) targets differentiated papillary and follicular cancers of the thyroid gland, is concentrated in the salivary gland, and is secreted into the saliva. Therefore one of the oral complications of this treatment is altered taste (Mandel and Mandel, 2003).

Due to the fact that the taste receptors have a 10-day turnover, the taste dysfunction usually recovers within weeks or months of the cessation of treatment. Most patients return to normal or near-normal taste sensation within 1 year (Fischer et al., 2008); however, in some patients it takes as long as 5 years, and in others the hypogeusia is permanent.

4.4.2 Postoperative Neuropathies

Surgical procedures may cause inflammatory and neuropathic pain. Neuropathic pain is the result of stretching or transecting the nerve during surgery (Clark and Ram, 2008), may be acute (short-term) or chronic in nature, and is aggravated by adjuvant therapies (e.g., irradiation) and dysfunction (e.g., lack or impaired function due to motor, sensory, or behavioral factors) (Elad et al., 2008). Acute pain following surgery is universal (Epstein and Van Der Waal, 2008); chronic pain may affect 50% of patients after mandibular resection (Chow and Teh, 2000) and up to 90% of postmaxillectomy patients (Rogers et al., 2003).

In about 50% of cases of repaired traumatic trigeminal neuropathies, patients recover full sensory function by about 7 months postop (Benoliel et al., 2008), and at 54 to 60 months, only about 15% of patients suffer from pain (Gellrich et al., 2002). Considering that the surgical intervention itself may exacerbate the symptoms, painful traumatic neuropathies are best managed medically.

4.4.3 Auriculotemporal Syndrome

Nearly half of the patients diagnosed with auriculotemporal syndrome (also called Frey syndrome) underwent parotid surgery, most commonly the excision of a salivary gland neoplasm. The syndrome is due to abnormal reinnervation (Scully, 2008a), and in the affected patients the severed parasympathetic fibers of the auriculotemporal nerve regenerated along the sympathetic fibers. Therefore a gustatory stimulus causes sympathetic activation of sweat glands and blood vessels, instead of (parasympathetic) salivation (Gonzales, 2009). Clinical manifestations include paroxysmal mild burning pain, parasthesia (hypo- or hyperesthesia) in the temporal area or the posterior cheek, with eating-related flushing and sweating of the cheek.

4.5 CHEMOTHERAPY-RELATED OROFACIAL NEUROPATHY

Chemotherapy may directly affect the nervous system (i.e., chemotherapy-related neurotoxicity, neuralgia inducing cavitational osteonecrosis of the jaws) or may cause oral complications that indirectly result in neuropathy (drug-induced osteonecrosis of the jaws and neutropenia-induced viral infections).

4.5.1 CHEMOTHERAPY-RELATED NEUROTOXICITY

Peripheral neurotoxicity and neuropathic pain, including thermal (cold or heat) allodynia and hyperalgesia, are well-known complications of several cytotoxic chemotherapeutic agents, including vinca plant alkaloids (vincristine, vinblastine, and vindesine), taxanes such as paclitaxel and docetaxel, bortezomib (a proteasome inhibitor), suramin (a growth factor antagonist), and platinum derivatives, such as cisplatin and oxaliplatin (Binder et al., 2007; Clark and Ram, 2008; Fischer and Epstein, 2008; Lalla et al., 2011). The platinum derivatives may also cause masticatory muscle spasms, which typically resolve within days, but may recur and intensify with repeated administration (Leonard et al., 2005). Orofacial cold sensitivity was the most common reported transient neuropathic symptom among oxaliplatin-treated (metastatic) colorectal cancer patients, experienced while eating and drinking (Leonard et al., 2005). This sensitivity, however, was of short duration, and only rarely made the patients avoid cold stimuli (Leonard et al., 2005). Vinca alkaloids, taxanes, and platinum-derived agents preferentially affect the large myelinated Aβ nerve fibers, although small myelinated Aδ and unmyelinated C fibers are also affected (Fischer et al., 2008). In addition, other medications used in management of cancer patients, such as thalidomide (and its derivative lenalidomide), interferons, or amphotericin-B, may cause peripheral neuropathy in the face and jawbones (Elad et al., 1997; Benoliel et al., 2007). Cetuximab, a monoclonal antibody targeting the epidermal growth factor receptor, commonly used in head and neck and colorectal cancers, may also cause polyneuropathy (Beydoun and Shatzmiller, 2010). Facial sensory loss may be caused by methotrexate (Scully, 2008b).

Thus, most neuropathy patients present with combined signs and symptoms that indicate involvement of the sensory and motor systems, with positive as well as negative sensory symptoms, and muscle weakness and atrophy, respectively (Fischer et al., 2008). Various sites along the trigeminal and glossopharyngeal nerves can be affected, primarily the temporomandibular joint, the mandible, mandibular teeth, and the ears (whereas the tongue, lips, maxilla, and edentulous ridges are rarely affected) (Benoliel et al., 2007). The neurotoxicity in the orofacial structures is mainly described as constant deep-seated, diffuse, throbbing jaw pain or numbness.

Factors affecting the prevalence of this phenomenon include the agent used, dose and cumulative dose, age, preexisting nerve damage (e.g., diabetes mellitus, alcoholism, inherited neuropathy, neurologic paraneoplastic syndrome) (Fischer et al., 2008), and concomitant treatments (i.e., combination of chemotherapeutics, radiation, and surgery) (Fischer and Epstein, 2008). The dysfunction of the nervous tissue may be exacerbated by the long-term inflammatory pain caused by radiation or surgery (Fischer et al., 2008).

In one study, up to 65% of chemically treated breast cancer patients suffered from orofacial neurotoxicity during a 7-week course; of these patients, 86% suffered from orofacial pain (i.e., 56% of the cohort) (McCarthy and Skillings, 1992a). In another study the prevalence of orofacial pain in breast cancer patients during chemotherapy was found to be 45% (Macquart-Moulin et al., 2000).

This neuropathic pain usually resolves with discontinuation of the drugs (American Academy on Pediatric Dentistry, 2008–2009); therefore no treatment is needed, and neurosurgery is rarely considered. Recovery from neuropathy induced by oxaliplatin may be slow owing to residual platinum traces in peripheral nerves and dorsal root ganglia (Benoliel et al., 2007). In some patients, however, the pain evolves into a chronic phase, which may result in sensory and motor changes (Fischer and Epstein, 2008). Medications to consider in chronic cases, or when the pain is intense, include opioid analgesics, anticonvulsants, antidepressants, and other adjunctive medications and analgesics (Epstein, 2001; Clark and Ram, 2008). In addition, hypnosis, relaxation therapy, imagery, biofeedback, support groups, healing touch, acupuncture, and transcutaneous nerve stimulation may be beneficial (Clark and Ram, 2008; Epstein and Van Der Waal, 2008). Invasive interventions may be useful in unresponsive cases such as cranial nerve neurolysis by diathermic coagulation of the Gasserian ganglion or glycerol injection, peripheral neurolysis by epidural phenol injection, or continuous nerve blockade with a local anesthetic agent (Datta and Pai, 2006). These interventions have potential complications, such as unintentional intravascular injection (which may cause seizures and cardiovascular collapse), hematoma, inadvertent blockade of other cranial nerves, and risk of aspiration.

Since there is no evidence-based treatment protocol, authors have adopted a management protocol for cancer pain from non-head-and-neck settings (Clark and Ram, 2008). For example, Swarm et al. (2007) formulated a guideline that recommends the administration of escalating doses of short-acting opioids for opioid-naïve cancer patients with the concomitant administration of other analgesics, such as nonsteroidal anti-inflammatory drugs or acetaminophen (paracetamol), that provide a synergistic effect plus the concurrent administration of an anticonstipation agent.

4.5.2 Neuralgia-Inducing Cavitational Osteonecrosis of Jaws

The controversial neuralgia-inducing cavitational osteonecrosis (NICO) of jaws may be the result of multiple systemic conditions, including chemotherapy (Gonzales, 2009; Sciubba, 2009). It is defined as a nonsuppurative osteomyelitis secondary to bone marrow ischemia. Currently there is no consensus regarding definition, clinical features, pathophysiology, or even the existence of the entity. Most reports describe the phenomenon in adult women, in the posterior body of the mandible. Pain features (intensity, deepness, nature) are not specific, pain localization is often difficult, and radiology is commonly noncontributory. Additional possible conditions that may be associated with NICO are coagulopathies, alcoholism, trauma, sickle cell disease, and use of prednisone (Gonzales, 2009; Sciubba, 2009).

4.5.3 Neuropathies Secondary to Oral Complications of Chemotherapy

4.5.3.1 Drug-Induced Osteonecrosis of Jaws

Bisphosphonate-related osteonecrosis of jaws (BRONJ) is defined as the presence of necrotic bone for more than 8 weeks anywhere in the oral cavity of an individual on bisphosphonate therapy with no history of radiation of the head and neck (Ruggiero et al., 2009). Although the most common indication for bisphosphonate therapy is osteoporosis, the prevalence of BRONJ in patients taking oral bisphosphonates for osteoporosis is much lower than the prevalence of BRONJ in patients receiving intravenous bisphosphonates for the management of multiple myeloma, bone metastasis, and cancer-related hypercalcemia or bone pain. The prevalence of BRONJ in these patients may be up to 13.3% (Migliorati et al., 2010).

Pain may be a major symptom of BRONJ, reported in 47% of oncologic BRONJ patients (range, 10 to 90%; Migliorati et al., 2010), and is among the staging criteria of BRONJ (Ruggiero et al., 2009). Consequently, pain control is an important treatment goal in the BRONJ patient (Ruggiero et al., 2009). However, pain in BRONJ is mostly due to secondary infection of the lesion and adjunct tissue inflammation (Ruggiero and Woo, 2008). Other factors contributing to the pain include altered alveolar bone metabolism (involving ischemia) (Assael, 2009). Neuropathy may also be a pain mechanism in oncology patients diagnosed with BRONJ patients (Otto et al., 2009; Elad et al., 2010a; Zadik et al., 2012). This neural damage may or may not be evident radiologically, for example, an impingement on the mandibular nerve canal (Figure 4.3) (Elad et al., 2010a; Zadik et al., 2012).

Contrary to the conservative treatment guidelines (Ruggiero et al., 2009), there are reports that patients with long-standing BRONJ-associated neuropathy may benefit from surgical intervention (Otto et al., 2009; Zadik et al., 2012). There is one report regarding the effectiveness of amitriptyline for the management of BRONJ-induced orofacial neuropathic pain (Zadik et al., 2012).

Osteonecrosis of the jaw has also been reported in cancer patients treated with bevacizumab (a monoclonal antibody targeting vascular endothelial growth factor A) or denosumab (a monoclonal antibody targeting receptor activator of nuclear factor-kappa B ligand) (Yarom et al., 2010).

4.5.3.2 Recurrent Orofacial Viral Infections

Recurrence of orofacial herpetic infections, such as herpes simplex (HSV) and varicella zoster (VZV) viruses, is quite common in cancer patients, especially during chemotherapy-induced periods of neutropenia (Elad et al., 2010b). These recurrences usually present as multiple acute painful mucocutaneous lesions. Both Herpesviridae infections may become complicated and cause chronic facial palsy, which, in the case of VZV, may be a part of Ramsay Hunt syndrome. VZV infection may also cause chronic postherpetic neuralgia.

4.6 CHEMOTHERAPY-RELATED ODONTALGIA

When discussing neuropathic odontalgia in cancer patients, a distinction needs to be made between dental hypersensitivity and pain.

4.6.1 DENTAL HYPERSENSITIVITY

Dental hypersensitivity is usually evoked in response to local thermal changes (e.g., cold drink intake), and it may be less intense than dental pain. In a study of 34 chemotherapy-treated breast cancer patients, 1 suffered from dental hypersensitivity (McCarthy and Skillings, 1992b).

Tooth hypersensitivity may also be related to decreased saliva flow following radiation therapy, a relative decrease in salivary pH (Rankin et al., 2008), and reduced salivary buffering and remineralizing capacity. These changes also significantly increase patient susceptibility to dental caries.

Patients may report dental hypersensitivity after hematopoietic stem cell transplantation (HSCT). This condition may be due to neurotoxicity caused by the conditioning regimen, or due to cyclosporine given to prevent graft versus host disease, or because of gingival recession (da Fonseca, 2000). Hyposalivation may also play a role in this condition.

4.6.2 DENTAL PAIN

In a cohort of vincristine-treated patients, 33 and 28% suffered from dental pain in their maxillary and mandibular teeth, respectively (McCarthy and Skillings, 1992b), although other authors stated that mandibular molars are more frequently affected (Rankin et al., 2008). An association between cyclophosphamide and dental neuropathy has also been reported (Zadik et al., 2010).

The characteristics of neuropathic dental pain are similar to those of atypical odontalgia, i.e., a severe throbbing pain localized to teeth or tooth supporting structures with no clinical or radiographic pathologic findings. Dental procedures (most commonly endodontic therapy, extraction, or apical surgery) might result in temporary relief, but the pain characteristically returns within days or weeks and can migrate after the dental procedure (including midline crossing and involving both jaws) (Benoliel et al., 2008; Blasberg et al., 2008; Zadik et al., 2010). The proposed mechanism of atypical odontalgia is pain due to nerve deafferentation from damage to peripheral nerves (Blasberg et al., 2008).

Dental and periodontal pathologies are highly prevalent in the general population; therefore it may be difficult to differentiate cancer-related dental neuropathy from ordinary odontogenic pain, and meticulous history taking and clinical, radiological, and even histological examinations are required (Zadik et al., 2010). Another rare cause of odontalgia, which may be of relevance in lymphoma patients, is the infiltration of the pulp or gingival tissues by lymphoma cells causing local pressure and pain (Biggs and Sabala, 1992; Payne and al-Damouk, 1993).

Dental pain and hypersensitivity are usually transient and subside shortly after dose reduction or cessation of chemotherapy (Rankin et al., 2008). Therefore, after neurotoxicity is diagnosed, management includes pain support for intense pain (with opioid-containing analgesics) (Lalla et al., 2011) and patient counseling. The patient may be advised to use a highly concentrated neutral fluoride gel, and desensitizing toothpaste, and to avoid oral intakes that trigger discomfort. The clinician should reassure the patient that this condition is transient (da Fonseca, 2000). However,

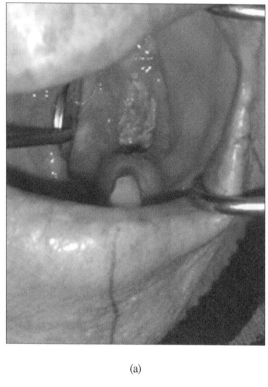

(a)

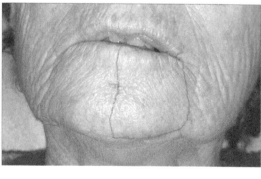

(b)

FIGURE 4.3 A patient diagnosed with mental neuropathy secondary to bisphosphonate-related osteonecrosis in the left body of the mandible. (a) Intraoral view of the inflamed osteonecrotic lesion. (b) Extraoral view of the lower lip and chin; the area of paresthesia is marked. (c) Cropped panoramic radiograph of the patient; the necrotic lesion is closely related to the mandibular nerve canal. (d) Coronal computer tomographic reconstruction demonstrating the relationship of the necrotic lesion (arrowheads) and the mandibular nerve canal (arrow).

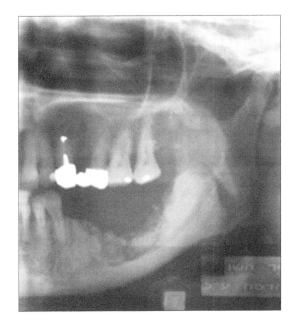

(c)

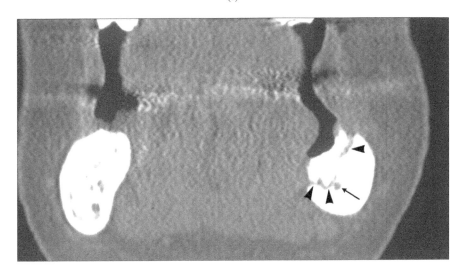

(d)

FIGURE 4.3 (continued)

resistant intense neuropathic dental pain that greatly compromises quality of life may be effectively relieved by pulpectomy (i.e., the removal of dental pulp tissue, including nerves) of the affected tooth (Zadik et al., 2010).

4.7   OTHER TYPES OF OROFACIAL PAIN

In the context of neuropathic pain and cancer, the common phenomenon of burning mouth syndrome (BMS), also called glossodynia, characteristically affecting postmenopausal women, must be mentioned. These patients suffer from persistent, annoying, burning neuropathic pain, mainly in the tongue. Currently, nerve dysfunction (e.g., of the chorda tympani nerve) is gaining acceptance as the underlying mechanism of BMS (Eliav et al., 2007; Nasri-Heir et al., 2011). Diagnosis is made by excluding other conditions that may cause similar symptoms, such as mucosal lesions, oral candidiasis, hyposalivation, anemia and other deficiencies, and diabetes mellitus; the former four conditions are not uncommon among cancer patients (Bensadoun et al., 2011). In BMS patients, the pain is mostly attributed to anxiety, stress, and cancer phobia, which may be aggravated in cancer patients (Lamey and Lamb, 1988; Lamey et al., 2005; Cavalcanti et al., 2007).

4.8   CONCLUSION

Orofacial neuropathy is one type of pain in cancer patients, who suffer from a heterogeneous group of pain disorders. It occurs frequently and has a significant impact on patient functioning, health, well-being, and quality of life. Therefore the importance of its treatment is clear. Orofacial neuropathy is often comorbidity in a compromised and complex oral environment. This complexity is due to possible hyposalivation, breakdown of the oral mucosal barrier, fibrosis of the masticatory muscles and perioral tissues, necrosis of the jaws, modified immunity, reduced healing capacity, and the inability to perform adequate oral hygiene procedures. The inclusion of an oral medicine practitioner in the oncologic supporting team is significant in this context, and ensures (1) dental preparation of the patient before anticancer therapy (such as cytotoxic chemotherapy, HSCT, bisphosphonate administration, and head and neck radiation); (2) oral and dental care during treatment, especially for oral mucositis, oral infections, and dental pain during nadir periods, and (3) lifelong postoperative follow-ups to help maintain oral health and function as well as relieve pain.

REFERENCES

American Academy on Pediatric Dentistry Clinical Affairs Committee; American Academy on Pediatric Dentistry Council on Clinical Affairs. (2008–2009). Guideline on dental management of pediatric patients receiving chemotherapy, hematopoietic cell transplantation, and/or radiation. *Pediatr Dent* 30S:219–25.

Assael LA. (2009). Oral bisphosphonates as a cause of bisphosphonate-related osteonecrosis of the jaws: Clinical findings, assessment of risks, and preventive strategies. *J Oral Maxillofac Surg* 67S:35–43.

Benoliel R, Zakik Y, Eliar E, Sharav Y. (2012). Peripheral painful traumatic trigeminal neuropathy: Clinical features in 91 cases and proposal of novel diagnostic criteria. *J Orofac Pain* 26:49–58.

Benoliel R, Epstein J, Eliav E, Jurevic R, Elad S. (2007). Orofacial pain in cancer: Part I—Mechanisms. *J Dent Res* 86:491–505.

Benoliel R, Heir GM, Eliav E. (2008). Neuropathic orofacial pain. In *Orofacial pain and headache*, ed. Sharav Y, Benoliel R, 255–94. Mosby Elsevier, Edinburgh.

Bensadoun RJ, Patton LL, Lalla RV, Epstein JB. (2011). Oropharyngeal candidiasis in head and neck cancer patients treated with radiation: Update 2011. *Support Care Cancer* 19:737–44.

Beydoun SR, Shatzmiller RA. (2010). Chronic immune-mediated demyelinating polyneuropathy in the setting of cetuximab treatment. *Clin Neurol Neurosurg* 112:900–2.

Biggs JT, Sabala C. (1992). Zebra XII. Part I. Large-cell lymphoma. *J Endod* 18:570–71.

Binder A, Stengel M, Maag R, Wasner G, Schoch R, Moosig F, Schommer B, Baron R. (2007). Pain in oxaliplatin-induced neuropathy—Sensitisation in the peripheral and central nociceptive system. *Eur J Cancer* 43:2658–63.

Blasberg B, Eliav E, Greenberg MS. (2008). Orofacial pain. In *Burket's oral medicine*, ed. Greenberg MS, Glick M, Ship JA, 257–88. 11th ed. BC Decker, Ontario.

Capobianco DJ. (1995). Facial pain as a symptom of nonmetastatic lung cancer. *Headache* 35:581–85.

Cavalcanti DR, Birman EG, Migliari DA, da Silveira FR. (2007). Burning mouth syndrome: Clinical profile of Brazilian patients and oral carriage of *Candida* species. *Braz Dent J* 18:341–45.

Chamberlain MC. (2005). Leukemia and the nervous system. *Curr Oncol Rep* 7:66–73.

Chow HT, Teh LY. (2000). Sensory impairment after resection of the mandible: A case report of 10 cases. *J Oral Maxillofac Surg* 58:629–35.

Clark GT, Ram S. (2008). Orofacial pain and neurosensory disorders and dysfunction in cancer patients. *Dent Clin North Am* 52:183–202.

Cuffari L, Tesseroli de Siqueira JT, Nemr K, Rapaport A. (2006). Pain complaint as the first symptom of oral cancer: A descriptive study. *Oral Surg Oral Med Oral Pathol Oral Radiol Endod* 102:56–61.

da Fonseca MA. (2000). Long-term oral and craniofacial complications following pediatric bone marrow transplantation. *Pediatr Dent* 22:57–62.

Datta S, Pai UT. (2006). Interventional approaches to management of pain of oral cancer. *Oral Maxillofac Surg Clin North Am* 18:627–41.

Elad S, Epstein J, Klasser G, Sroussi H. (2008). Orofacial pain in the medically complex patient. In *Orofacial pain and headache*, ed. Sharav Y, Benoliel R, 321–47. Mosby Elsevier, Edinburgh.

Elad S, Galili D, Garfunkel AA, Or R. (1997). Thalidomide-induced perioral neuropathy. *Oral Surg Oral Med Oral Pathol Oral Radiol Endod* 84:362–64.

Elad S, Gomori MJ, Ben-Ami N, Friedlander-Barenboim S, Regev E, Lazarovici TS, Yarom N. (2010a). Bisphosphonate-related osteonecrosis of the jaw: Clinical correlations with computerized tomography presentation. *Clin Oral Investig* 14:43–50.

Elad S, Zadik Y, Hewson I, Hovan A, Correa ME, Logan R, Elting LS, Spijkervet FK, Brennan MT; Viral Infections Section, Oral Care Study Group, Multinational Association of Supportive Care in Cancer/International Society of Oral Oncology. (2010b). A systematic review of viral infections associated with oral involvement in cancer patients: A spotlight on Herpesviridae. *Support Care Cancer* 18:993–1006.

Eliav E, Gracely RH. (2008). Measuring and assessing pain. In *Orofacial pain and headache*, ed. Sharav Y, Benoliel R, 45–56. Mosby Elsevier, Edinburgh.

Eliav E, Gracely RH, Nahlieli O, Benoliel R. (2004). Quantitative sensory testing in trigeminal nerve damage assessment. *J Orofac Pain* 18:339–44.

Eliav E, Kamran B, Schaham R, Czerninski R, Gracely RH, Benoliel R. (2007). Evidence of chorda tympani dysfunction in patients with burning mouth syndrome. *J Am Dent Assoc* 138:628–33.

Epstein JB. (2001). Orofacial pain in patients with cancer. In *Essentials of oral medicine*, ed. Silverman S Jr, Eversole LR, Truelove EL, 367–70. BC Decker, London.

Epstein JB, Elad S, Eliav E, Jurevic R, Benoliel R. (2007). Orofacial pain in cancer: Part II—Clinical perspectives and management. *J Dent Res* 86:506–518.

Epstein JB, Hong C, Logan RM, Barasch A, Gordon SM, Oberle-Edwards L, McGuire D, Napenas JJ, Elting LS, Spijkervet FK, Brennan MT. (2010). A systematic review of orofacial pain in patients receiving cancer therapy. *Support Care Cancer* 18:1023–31.

Epstein JB, Phillips N, Parry J, Epstein MS, Nevill T, Stevenson-Moore P. (2002). Quality of life, taste, olfactory and oral function following high-dose chemotherapy and allogeneic hematopoietic cell transplantation. *Bone Marrow Transplant* 30:785–92.

Epstein J, Van Der Waal I. (2008). Oral cancer. In *Burket's oral medicine*, ed. Greenberg MS, Glick M, Ship JA, 153–89. 11th ed. BC Decker, Ontario.

Epstein JB, Wilkie DJ, Fischer DJ, Kim YO, Villines D. (2009). Neuropathic and nociceptive pain in head and neck cancer patients receiving radiation therapy. *Head Neck Oncol* 1:26.

Fischer DJ, Epstein JB. (2008). Management of patients who have undergone head and neck cancer therapy. *Dent Clin North Am* 52:39–60.

Fischer DJ, Klasser GD, Epstein JB. (2008). Cancer and orofacial pain. *Oral Maxillofac Surg Clin North Am* 20:287–301.

Gellrich NC, Schramm A, Böckmann R, Kugler J. (2002). Follow-up in patients with oral cancer. *J Oral Maxillofac Surg* 60:380–86.

Gonzales TS. (2009). Facial pain and neuromuscular diseases. In *Oral and maxillofacial pathology*, ed. Neville BD, Damm DD, Allen CM, Bouquot JE, 859–86. 3rd ed. Saunders, Philadelphia.

Grond S, Zech D, Diefenbach C, Radbruch L, Lehmann KA. (1996). Assessment of cancer pain: A prospective evaluation in 2266 cancer patients referred to a pain service. *Pain* 64:107–14.

Hovan AJ, Williams PM, Stevenson-Moore P, Wahlin YB, Ohrn KE, Elting LS, Spijkervet FK, Brennan MT; Dysgeusia Section, Oral Care Study Group, Multinational Association of Supportive Care in Cancer/International Society of Oral Oncology. (2010). A systematic review of dysgeusia induced by cancer therapies. *Support Care Cancer* 18:1081–87.

Kalladka M, Proter N, Benoliel R, Czerninski R, Eliav E. (2008). Mental nerve neuropathy: Patient characteristics and neurosensory changes. *Oral Surg Oral Med Oral Pathol Oral Radiol Endod* 106:364–70.

Lalla RV, Brennan MT, Schubert MM. (2011). Oral complications of cancer therapy. In *Pharmacology and therapeutics for dentistry*, ed. Yagiela JA, Dowd FJ, Johnson BS, Mariotti AJ, Neidle EA, 782–98. 6th ed. Mosby Elsevier, St. Louis.

Lamey PJ, Freeman R, Eddie SA, Pankhurst C, Rees T. (2005). Vulnerability and presenting symptoms in burning mouth syndrome. *Oral Surg Oral Med Oral Pathol Oral Radiol Endod* 99:48–54.

Lamey PJ, Lamb AB. (1988). Prospective study of aetiological factors in burning mouth syndrome. *Br Med J* 296:1243–46.

Leonard GD, Wright MA, Quinn MG, Fioravanti S, Harold N, Schuler B, Thomas RR, Grem JL. (2005). Survey of oxaliplatin-associated neurotoxicity using an interview-based questionnaire in patients with metastatic colorectal cancer. *BMC Cancer* 5:116.

Levenson D, Coulec S, Sonneberg M, Lai E, Goldsmith SJ, Larson SM. (1994). Peripheral facial nerve palsy after high-dose radioiodine therapy in patients with papillary thyroid carcinoma. *Ann Int Med* 120:576–78.

Little JW, Falace DA, Miller CS, Rhodus NL. (2008). Cancer and oral care of the patient. In *Dental management of the medically compromised patient*, 433–61. 7th ed. Mosby Elsevier, St. Louis.

Macquart-Moulin G, Viens P, Palangie T, Bouscary ML, Delozier T, Roche H, Janvier M, Fabbro M, Moatti JP. (2000). High-dose sequential chemotherapy with recombinant granulocyte colony stimulating factor and repeated stem-cell support for inflammatory breast cancer patients: Does impact on quality of life jeopardize feasibility and acceptability of treatment? *J Clin Oncol* 18:754–64.

Mandel SJ, Mandel L. (2003). Radioactive iodine and the salivary glands. *Thyroid* 13:265–71.

McCarthy GM, Skillings JR. (1992a). Jaw and other orofacial pain in patients receiving vincristine for the treatment of cancer. *Oral Surg Oral Med Oral Pathol* 74:299–304.

McCarthy GM, Skillings JR. (1992b). Orofacial complications of chemotherapy for breast cancer. *Oral Surg Oral Med Oral Pathol* 74:172–78.

Meier JK, Wolff D, Pavletic S, Greinix H, Gosau M, Bertz H, Lee SJ, Lawitschka A, Elad S; International Consensus Conference on Clinical Practice in cGVHD. (2011). Oral chronic graft-versus-host disease: Report from the International Consensus Conference on clinical practice in cGVHD. *Clin Oral Investig* 15:127–39.

Migliorati CA, Woo SB, Hewson I, Barasch A, Elting LS, Spijkervet FK, Brennan MT; Bisphosphonate Osteonecrosis Section, Oral Care Study Group, Multinational Association of Supportive Care in Cancer/International Society of Oral Oncology. (2010). A systematic review of bisphosphonate osteonecrosis (BON) in cancer. *Support Care Cancer* 18:1099–106.

Nasri-Heir C, Gomes J, Heir GM, Ananthan S, Benoliel R, Teich S, Eliav E. (2011). The role of sensory input of the chorda tympani nerve and the number of fungiform papillae in burning mouth syndrome. *Oral Surg Oral Med Oral Pathol Oral Radiol Endod* 112:65–72.

Otto S, Hafner S, Grötz KA. (2009). The role of inferior alveolar nerve involvement in bisphosphonate-related osteonecrosis of the jaw. *J Oral Maxillofac Surg* 67:589–92.

Payne M, al-Damouk JD. (1993). Gingival swelling as a manifestation of non-Hodgkin's lymphoma. *Br Dent J* 175:293–94.

Rankin KV, Jones DL, Redding SW. (2008). *Oral health in cancer therapy—A guide for health care professionals*, 62–63. 3rd ed. Dental Oncology Education Program, Cancer Prevention and Research Institute of Texas, Baylor.

Rogers SN, Lowe D, McNally D, Brown JS, Vaughan ED. (2003). Health-related quality of life after maxillectomy: A comparison between prosthetic obturation and free flap. *J Oral Maxillofac Surg* 61:174–81.

Ruggiero SL, Dodson TB, Assael LA, Landesberg R, Marx RE, Mehrotra B; American Association of Oral and Maxillofacial Surgeons. (2009). American Association of Oral and Maxillofacial Surgeons position paper on bisphosphonate-related osteonecrosis of the jaws—2009 update. *J Oral Maxillofac Surg* 67S:2–12.

Ruggiero SL, Woo SB. (2008). Biophosphonate-related osteonecrosis of the jaws. *Dent Clin North Am* 52:111–28.

Sarlani E, Schwartz AH, Greenspan JD, Grace EG. (2003). Facial pain as first manifestation of lung cancer: A case of lung cancer-related cluster headache and a review of the literature. *J Orofac Pain* 17:262–67.

Sciubba JJ. (2009). Neuralgia-inducing cavitational osteonecrosis: A status report. *Oral Dis* 15:309–12.

Scully C. (2008a). Pain. In *Oral and maxillofacial medicine*, 97–108. 2nd ed. Elsevier, Edinburgh.

Scully C. (2008b). Sensory and motor changes and taste abnormalities. In *Oral and maxillofacial medicine*, 119–30. 2nd ed. Elsevier, Edinburgh.

Swarm R, Anghelescu DL, Benedetti C, Boston B, Cleeland C, Coyle N, Deleon-Casasola OA, Eidelman A, Eilers JG, Ferrell B, Grossman SA, Janjan NA, Levy MH, Lynch M, Montana GS, Nesbit S, Oakes L, Obbens EA, Paice J, Syrjala KL, Urba S, Weinstein SM; National Comprehensive Cancer Network. (2007). Adult cancer pain. *J Natl Compr Canc Netw* 5:726–51.

Yarom N, Elad S, Madrid C, Migliorati CA. (2010). Osteonecrosis of the jaws induced by drugs other than bisphosphonates—A call to update terminology in light of new data. *Oral Oncol* 46:e1.

Zadik Y, Benoliel R, Fleissig Y, Casap N. (2012). Painful trigeminal neuropathy induced by oral-bisphosphonate related osteonecrosis of jaw: A new etiology for the numb-chin syndrome. *Quintessence Int* 43:97–104.

Zadik Y, Vainstein V, Heling I, Neuman T, Drucker S, Elad S (2010). Cytotoxic chemotherapy-induced odontalgia: A differential diagnosis for dental pain. *J Endod* 36:1588–92.

5 Cancer Chemotherapy-Induced Neuropathic Pain
The Underlying Peripheral Neuropathy

Robert B. Raffa and Joseph V. Pergolizzi, Jr.

CONTENTS

5.1 Introduction 113
5.2 Peripheral Nervous System Vulnerability 115
5.3 Chemotherapeutic Drugs: Classes and Agents 116
    5.3.1 Platinum-Based Chemotherapeutic Agents 116
        5.3.1.1 Cisplatin 116
        5.3.1.2 Carboplatin 120
        5.3.1.3 Oxaliplatin 120
    5.3.2 Taxanes 122
        5.3.2.1 Paclitaxel 124
        5.3.2.2 Docetaxel 125
    5.3.3 Vinca Alkaloids 125
    5.3.4 Suramin 126
    5.3.5 Thalidomide 126
5.4 Some Major Unanswered Questions 127
5.5 Conclusion 128
Declarations and Acknowledgment 128
References 128

5.1 INTRODUCTION

The peripheral nervous system, in general, is vulnerable to chemotherapeutic agent toxicity, and chemotherapy-induced peripheral neuropathy (CIPN) underlies chemotherapy-induced neuropathic pain (CINP) during or following treatment with certain cancer chemotherapeutic drugs. The pain can persist long after cessation of drug administration, and is difficult to treat using currently available approaches. CIPN is characterized by distally predominant neuropathy, with lower limbs typically evidencing signs and symptoms before upper limbs. This chapter reviews CIPN; peripheral neuropathy associated with chemotherapeutic agents is well documented and there are putative mechanisms. Platinum-based drugs, taxanes, vinca alkaloids, suramin, and thalidomide, in particular, are associated with relatively high rates of CIPN. Platinum drugs are also known for coasting, a phenomenon in which symptoms persist or even worsen after the drug is discontinued. Taxanes are associated with rapid-onset cold-induced neuropathy, and thalidomide-induced CIPN is often irreversible. Different patterns of symptoms presumably reflect different mechanisms of toxicity, which include formation of DNA adducts, disruption of axonal transport, interference with ion channel function, and induction of apoptosis, among others. Greater understanding of the mechanisms involved in CIPN could better inform clinical practice regarding the optimal use of existing cancer chemotherapeutic drugs, individually or in combinations; stimulate the development of new antineoplastic agents with superior adverse effect profiles; and provide more optimal pain management in chemotherapy patients.

Neuropathy occurs relatively often in cancer patients either as a result of the paraneoplastic process (Malik and Stillman, 2008) or as an iatrogenic result of chemotherapy. For a variety of reasons, including imperfect assessment tools (Cavaletti et al., 2010) and differences among protocols, the prevalence of CIPN, although substantial (Zhou et al., 2009), can only be widely estimated to be between 10 and 80% (Authier et al., 2009). As one example, the rate of CIPN was found to be 64% for breast cancer patients during paclitaxel-based chemotherapy ($n = 430$) (Reyes-Gibby et al., 2009).

CIPN poses significant clinical challenges in that it can be dose limiting, adversely impact the patient's quality of life, and even result in chronic impairment in otherwise successfully treated patients (Cavaletti and Marmiroli, 2004). It can be acute or chronic. It can be permanent or reversible. But, even in cases where it can be reversed, resolution might be only partial. At present, there are no established treatments or approved drugs to treat CIPN.

CIPN resembles diabetic neuropathy insofar as it exhibits a "stocking glove" distribution pattern with similar pain, paresthesia, and dysesthesia (Wolf et al., 2008). However, treatments that are helpful for diabetic neuropathy are not always helpful for CIPN patients (Wolf et al., 2008), which suggests that distinct mechanisms are involved in the two.

This article addresses some well-known antineoplastic drugs: platinum-based compounds (cisplatin, carboplatin, and oxaliplatin, among others), taxanes (paclitaxel and docetaxel), vinca alkaloids, suramin, and thalidomide. All of these agents are associated with neurotoxicity and peripheral neuropathic pain (Gilbert, 1998; Plotkin and Wen, 2003). These antineoplastic agents were specifically designed to destroy rapidly replicating cells (Cavaletti and Marmiroli, 2004; Windebank and Grisold, 2008), so it might not be expected that such agents would damage neurons and glial cells, which have no or only a very low rate of replication (Cavaletti and Marmiroli, 2006). Nevertheless, peripheral nerve cells are quite vulnerable to chemotheraphy drugs.

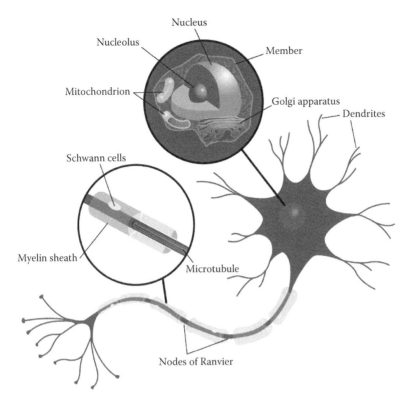

FIGURE 5.1 Access of chemotherapeutic drug molecules through fenestrated capillaries places peripheral neurons at greater risk than neurons within the central nervous system to neurotoxic adverse effects. All parts of the neuron are potential targets.

5.2 PERIPHERAL NERVOUS SYSTEM VULNERABILITY

The cells of the peripheral nervous system are supplied with blood through fenestrated capillaries that allow chemotherapeutic drug molecules to pass readily from the circulation into the extracellular fluid (Windebank and Grisold, 2008) (Figure 5.1). Since they are outside the blood-brain barrier, peripheral neurons can be affected by drugs that do not cause central nervous system toxicity.

Some of the mechanisms that chemotherapeutic agents use to attack fast-dividing cells can also affect the nervous system. Axonal transport within the neurons transmits material between the soma and axon terminals (Oztas, 2003) and relies on an infrastructure of microtubules. Axonal transport is essential to maintain neuronal health and proper function (Windebank and Grisold, 2008), and drugs that damage the axon or disrupt the microtubule assembly can result in neuropathy. Antineoplastic agents have these potential toxicities.

Sensory, motor, and autonomic fibers all have the potential to be affected by cancer chemotherapeutic agents, but if the cell body is spared, complete or partial functional recovery may be possible. Although autonomic nerves can be damaged by chemotherapeutic agents, autonomic symptoms are less commonly reported.

The most common forms of toxic neuropathies associated with chemotherapy have three presumed sites of cellular involvement: (1) axonopathy, which causes a "dying back" type of axonal degeneration and is characterized by distal predominance and centripetal progression; (2) ganglionopathy, which affects cell bodies in general and the dorsal root ganglion in particular; and (3) myelinopathy, a segmental demyelination of the nerve cell (Kimura, 2001). Since neurons are sensitive to DNA damage, if a chemotherapeutic agent can cause DNA damage to a neuron, it can induce programmed cell death (apoptosis) (Windebank and Grisold, 2008) (Figure 5.2).

The mechanisms of CIPN vary by agent. A frequently described neuropathy in chemotherapy patients is an axonal, sensorimotor neuropathy caused by an immunomodulatory agent (e.g., thalidomide) or spindle poisons (e.g., vinca alkaloids or taxanes) (Chamberlain, 2010).

5.3   CHEMOTHERAPEUTIC DRUGS: CLASSES AND AGENTS

5.3.1   PLATINUM-BASED CHEMOTHERAPEUTIC AGENTS

The three most common platinum-based compounds used in chemotherapy in the United States are cisplatin, carboplatin, and oxaliplatin. They share structural similarities (Figure 5.3) but have certain pharmacokinetic and adverse event profile distinctions (Cavaletti and Marmiroli, 2004).

Platinum-based chemotherapeutic drugs cross the blood-brain barrier only poorly, but they gain access to dorsal root ganglia (DRG) through a more permeable barrier (Malik and Stillman, 2008). All of the platinum-based drugs are all known to affect DRG neurons. They cross-link and damage DNA; if sufficient damage occurs, apoptosis pathways are activated (Gill and Windebank, 1998a; Huang et al., 1995; Krarup-Hansen et al., 2007). Although apoptosis affects the entire sensory neuron, symptoms occur in the fields of distal axonal branches. Platinum-based compounds are unique among the chemotherapeutic agents discussed in this chapter, in that they cause sensory ganglionopathy (Windebank and Grisold, 2008). They are also associated with a phenomenon called coasting, in which neuronal damage continues after the drug is discontinued (Balmaceda and Korkin, 2003; Plotkin and Wen, 2003; van den Bent, 2005; Verstappen et al., 2005). It has been postulated that the mechanism of this delayed neuronal toxicity is platinum's avid binding to mitochondrial DNA (Podratz et al., 2007).

Thus the vulnerability of neurons to the destructive effects of platinum-based compounds depends, in part, on the blood supply to the particular neurons (Screnci et al., 2000) and the avid binding of these drugs to neuronal DNA (McDonald et al., 2005; Ta et al., 2006).

The chronic sensory neurotoxicity associated with platinum-based compounds is both cumulative and dose dependent (Lehky et al., 2004). However, the precise mechanisms are unclear (Cavaletti et al., 2001; Holmes et al., 1998; McKeage et al., 2001; Screnci et al., 2000).

5.3.1.1   Cisplatin

Cisplatin is the most highly protein bound of the platinum-based chemotherapeutic agents (Go and Adjei, 1999), and it is the most neurotoxic. Cisplatin is also known to

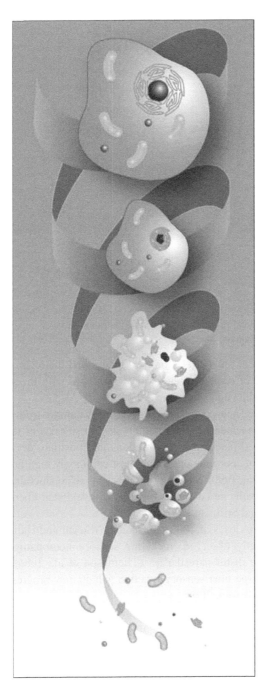

FIGURE 5.2   Apoptosis or programmed cell death is initiated by biochemical changes that alter cell morphology. These changes may include blebbing, loss of cell membrane asymmetry and attachment, cell shrinkage, nuclear fragmentation, chromatin condensation, and chromosomal DNA fragmentation.

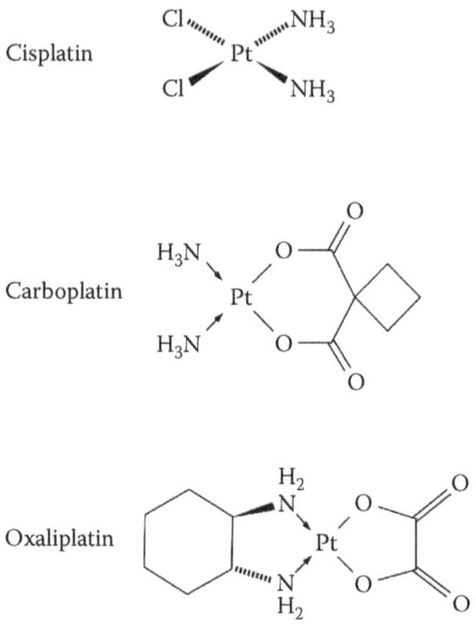

FIGURE 5.3 Chemical structure of three main platinum-based chemotherapeutic compounds currently used in the United States.

have dose-dependent toxic effects on the kidneys and the organ of Cori (Cvitkovic, 1998). The extent of cisplatin cytotoxicity correlates with the amount of its DNA cross-linkings (Oshita and Eastman, 1993).

Cisplatin-induced neuropathy is characterized by damage to large myelinated nerve fibers. Symptoms include tingling, numbness, paresthesias of the upper and lower extremities, reduced perception of vibrations and position, decreased deep-tendon reflexes, and lack of coordination, which most commonly manifests itself as gait disturbances (Mollman, 1990). Slowing of sensory nerve conduction velocity may occur along with axonopathy and damage to the large myelinated fibers and cell bodies of the DRG (Malik and Stillman, 2008).

With cumulative doses of 400 to 500 mg/m² (Siegal and Haim, 1990) symptoms are more commonly observed, including sensory neuropathy with initial complaints of extreme distal paresthesias (Thompson et al., 1984). The predominant aspect is loss of large-fiber sensory function, which may progress to sensory ataxia (Windebank and Grisold, 2008).

The disproportionate accumulation of platinum in peripheral sensory tissue may be a crucial point in understanding cisplatin-induced peripheral neuropathy:

- DNA-platinum binding in cisplatin-treated rats is greater in the DRG than in most other tissues (McDonald et al., 2005).
- Cisplatin induces apoptosis in DRG neurons *in vitro* and *in vivo* (Fischer et al., 2001a; Gill and Windebank, 1998a).
- Apoptosis occurs when high-affinity adducts are formed between cisplatin and either genomic or mitochondrial DNA. A simultaneous translocation

of the Bax (Bcl2-associated X protein) to the mitochondrion accompanies this platinum binding, along with a release of cytochrome c into the cytosol. This sequence of events has been associated with the initiation of apoptotic cell death (McDonald et al., 2005).

- Concomitant treatment with nerve growth factor (NGF) prevents cisplatin-mediated neuronal apoptosis *in vitro*, but does not reduce adduct formation (McDonald et al., 2005), nor was NGF able to alter the platination of DNA (Gill and Windebank, 1998a). These findings suggest that NGF may be able to interrupt the cisplatin toxicity process, but that this process occurs *after* adduct formation. NGF can protect from Bax redistribution after cisplatin treatment (McDonald et al., 2005), so it appears that the NGF-mediated protection from Bax distribution is not adduct formation, per se.

Cisplatin-induced neuronal apoptosis differs from cancer cell apoptosis, in that cisplatin-induced apoptosis is independent of Fas-receptor/Fas-ligand binding (Fischer et al., 2001b; McDonald and Windebank, 2002). *In vitro*, cisplatin has been reported to reduce fast axonal transport (Russell et al., 1995).

The paradox of cisplatin cytotoxicity is that differentiated neurons appear to be susceptible to cisplatin, an agent designed to damage DNA. It is known that platinum adduct formation and platinum accumulation are greater in DRG neurons than in rapidly dividing PC12 cell lines (cells derived from a pheochromocytoma of the rat adrenal medulla, useful for studies of neuronal differentiation) (McDonald et al., 2005). Likewise, there is a greater amount of platinum-DNA binding in DRG neurons than in cancer cell lines, which may be related to an increased platinum uptake, decreased platinum efflux, reduced platinum detoxification, decreased DNA adduct repair, or some combination of these.

It also has been suggested that cisplatin acts as a calcium channel blocker in neurons, altering intracellular calcium homeostasis that can in turn lead to apoptosis (Hartmann and Lipp, 2003). It also causes morphological changes in neurons (Barajon et al., 1996). Ultrasound examination of the basal ganglia of cisplatin-treated rats found shrunken neuronal soma, nuclei, and nucleoli and alterations in the rough endoplasmic reticulum and Golgi apparatus, all of which may be evidence of disrupted protein synthesis (Cece et al., 1995). These changes further imply damage to fast axonal transport of organelles (Russell et al., 1995).

Sex differences in cisplatin-induced neuropathy have been demonstrated in preclinical studies where certain effects were more severe in males (weight loss, prolonged nociceptive response latency, and lower muscle fiber conduction velocity), whereas other effects were more severe in females (reductions in myelinated fiber diameters, myelin thickness, and myelinated fiber density) (Wongtawatchai et al., 2009). Both sexes evidenced similar decreased levels of NGF. In cisplatin-treated patients, worse neurological outcomes occur, and occur more frequently, in men than women (Argyriou et al., 2005). The exact mechanisms behind gender differences in cisplatin-induced neuropathy are not known, but sex differences in nerve regeneration have been reported in preclinical studies (Jones, 1993; Kovacic et al., 2004; Kujawa et al., 1991).

Symptoms of testicular cancer patients treated with cisplatin ($n = 16$) are consistent with loss of large myelinated fibers in that patients lose distal tendon and Hoffman reflexes (H-reflexes, a reflectory reaction of muscles after sensory fiber stimulation) at cumulative doses over 300 mg/m^2 but not at lower doses. At doses of 400 to 700 mg/m^2, sensory nerve action potential conduction velocities decreased by 10 to 15% (Krarup-Hansen et al., 2007). In a larger study of testicular cancer patients ($n = 1814$), those treated with cisplatin were significantly more likely to report Raynaud-like symptoms (cold hands, fingers, and toes, and pain on exposure to cold) and paresthesia in hands and feet than were similar patients not treated with chemotherapy (Brydoy et al., 2009).

Cisplatin can induce sensory neuronopathy (Peltier and Russell, 2006), which is associated with neuronal cell death and, as such, is not reversible. Neurotoxicity occurs in a relatively large proportion (up to 30%) of patients treated with cisplatin (Ta et al., 2006). About 20% of patients taking cisplatin cannot complete a full course of treatment because of sensory neuropathy (McDonald et al., 2005).

Coasting, or emergence of symptoms 2 to 4 months after discontinuing treatment, is common for cisplatin (Cavaletti and Marmiroli, 2004). Furthermore, the neurotoxic effects of cisplatin may persist for years after treatment (Strumberg et al., 2002).

5.3.1.2   Carboplatin

At chemotherapeutic doses, carboplatin is generally considered to be less neurotoxic than the other platinum compounds (McKeage, 1995), with the prevalence of carboplatin-induced neuropathy around 4 to 6% (Hartmann and Lipp, 2003). However, carboplatin can produce peripheral neuropathy similar to, albeit not as severe as, that associated with cisplatin (Cavaletti et al., 1998a, 1998b). In fact, at high doses, carboplatin can be as toxic as cisplatin (Malik and Stillman, 2008). In carboplatin-induced peripheral neuropathy, the first signs are typically slowing of sensory nerve conduction velocity with reduced amplitude and prolonged, or even absent, H-reflexes. Axonopathy and neuronopathic damage of large myelinated fibers occurs, and there can also be damage to the cell bodies of the DRG (Malik and Stillman, 2008).

5.3.1.3   Oxaliplatin

Oxaliplatin is a platinum-based alkylating agent that forms interstrand and intrastrand cross-linking with DNA (Rosson, 2006) and in that way blocks DNA synthesis (Wiseman et al., 1999). *In vitro* studies in which oxaliplatin elicited cellular hyperexcitability in a dose-dependent fashion (Adelsberger et al., 2000) suggest that oxaliplatin interferes with axonal ion conduction and alters neural excitability (Quasthoff and Hartung, 2002). Its cancer-killing mechanism of action is not fully understood, but it has been suggested that an oxalate metabolite chelates free calcium and, in that way, affects sodium channels (Cavaletti and Marmiroli, 2004; Rosson, 2006). Oxalate interference with potassium or sodium channels in myelinated axons is thought to be the cause of a unique symptom of oxaliplatin-induced neuropathy, namely, cold-induced dyesthesias (Boughattas et al., 1994; Grolleau et al., 2001), which typically are not permanent (Cersosimo, 2005; Gamelin et al., 2002).

The inhibition of voltage-gated sodium currents may explain acute sensory neuropathy, which can develop as quickly as 60 seconds of onset of a course of oxaliplatin (Wilson et al., 2002), and usually develops in less than an hour (Extra et al., 1998). Acute neurotoxicity, which occurs in 85% or more of patients treated with oxaliplatin (Grothey, 2003), may manifest as cold-induced paresthesias or dysesthesia, laryngospasm, and muscle contractions resembling neuromyotonia, all of which may be associated with voltage-gated channelopathies (Krishnan et al., 2005; Lehky et al., 2004). Intravenous infusions of 100 mg calcium gluconate and 1,000 mg magnesium sulfate have been shown in some cases to improve oxaliplatin-induced neuropathy (Gamelin et al., 2002, 2004). The sodium channel blocker carbamazepine has been tried in oxaliplatin-induced neuropathy, but with equivocal results (Eckel et al., 2002).

Axonal refractoriness is associated with the inactivation of voltage-gated nodal sodium channels (Burke et al., 2001; Krishnan et al., 2008). The refractoriness of motor axons depends on impulse transmission through the neuromuscular junction, but high-frequency impulse trains may cause such transmissions to fail (Krishnan et al., 2009). Acute oxaliplatin exposure is associated with motor nerve hyperexcitability (Lehky et al., 2004; Wilson et al., 2002), which could underlie increased refractoriness in motor axons.

Acute sodium channel dysfunction in both motor and sensory axons (Krishnan et al., 2005) and refractoriness (Burke et al., 2001; Krishnan et al., 2008; Park et al., 2009) have been observed after a single oxaliplatin infusion. While motor and sensory axons respond differently to acute oxaliplatin exposure, the extent of oxaliplatin-induced abnormality in motor axons is proportional to the degree of change in sensory axons (Lehky et al., 2004; Wilson et al., 2002). Oxaliplatin has further been shown to slow sodium channel inactivation kinetics (Adelsberger et al., 2000), shift voltage dependence of activation and inactivation (Benoit et al., 2006; Webster et al., 2005), and reduce the overall sodium current (Benoit et al., 2006; Grolleau et al., 2001). Alterations in sodium channel properties may predispose to ectopic activity, which could lead to symptoms of paresthesia (Webster et al., 2005).

Sensory axons exposed to oxaliplatin likewise exhibit changes in refractoriness and superexcitability (Park et al., 2009), which are considered hallmarks of axonal hyperpolarization (Kiernan et al., 2000). Experimental models of axonal degeneration showed similar abnormalities (Moldovan and Krarup, 2004; Moldovan et al., 2009), suggesting that these changes reflect axonal damage in sensory neurons.

It thus appears that acute oxaliplatin-induced neuropathy is attributable to modulation of axonal membrane sodium channels, whereas chronic oxaliplatin-induced neuropathy is attributable to sensory axonal excitability, which requires cumulative exposure (Park et al., 2009). Acute oxaliplatin-induced neuropathy is common, but is usually self-limited (Grothey, 2003). Cumulative sensory peripheral neuropathy, which can be dose limiting, develops gradually and in some cases may be irreversible (Cassidy and Misset, 2002). About 10 to 15% of oxaliplatin-treated patients develop a moderate neuropathy, typically after cumulative intravenous doses of 700 to 800 mg/m^2 (Hartmann and Lipp, 2003), but other studies suggest the proportion of patients who develop oxaliplatin-induced peripheral neuropathy is much higher (Krishnan et al., 2005). Unlike platinum-based compounds that exhibit coasting, both acute and chronic oxaliplatin-induced neuropathy typically remit upon drug discontinuation.

Oxaliplatin is a planar coordination compound similar in structure to cisplatin (Figure 5.3), but oxaliplatin contains a nonleaving carrier ligand, that is, a diamminocyclohexane (DACH) ligand and a hydrolysable oxalate ligand (Ta et al., 2006; Woynarowski et al., 1998). Both oxaliplatin and cisplatin cause apoptosis of DRG neurons *in vitro*, but oxaliplatin forms fewer Pt-DNA adducts and is less neurotoxic to DRG neurons while being as cytotoxic to cancer cells as cisplatin (Ta et al., 2006). Since oxaliplatin forms fewer total adducts than cisplatin (Arnould et al., 2003), it is possible that the bulkier DACH-platinum adducts formed by oxaliplatin have a more disruptive effect on DNA structure than cisplatin-formed adducts (Rixe et al., 1996; Schmidt and Chaney, 1993; Ta et al., 2006).

The broad-spectrum capase inhibitor (z-VAD-fmk) suppresses cell death for up to 72 hours in treatments of oxaliplatin (Ta et al., 2006) and cisplatin (Gill and Windebank, 1998a). The fact that cell numbers can be preserved by z-VAD-fmk argues that capase-mediated cell death is a major pathway induced by oxaliplatin. Cisplatin-induced apoptosis in DRG involves Bax-mediated cytochrome c release from mitochondria (Gill and Windebank, 1998a).

It has been suggested that a hydrophobic DACH moiety in oxaliplatin might interact with hydrophobic binding pockets in certain groups of cellular proteins and disrupt the cell's protein formation (Ta et al., 2006). If these proteins are different than those that react with cisplatin, it could explain the disproportionate rates of cancer cell apoptosis with oxaliplatin versus cisplatin (Raymond et al., 1998).

Oxaliplatin can exert a cytotoxic effect by directly inducing mitochondrial-mediated apoptosis in cells without nuclear DNA (Gourdier et al., 2004). When oxaliplatin is applied to DRG neurons, sodium current increases and a shift in voltage response toward more negative membrane potentials occurs (Adelsberger et al., 2000; Grolleau et al., 2001). Oxaliplatin does not appear to affect sodium currents of hippocampal neurons, suggesting that the agent is restricted to one or more channel subtypes (Pasetto et al., 2006).

In an assessment of 16 patients who completed a course of oxaliplatin therapy, half developed neuropathic symptoms. In nerve conduction studies in the 50% of patients with chronic neuropathic symptoms ($n = 8$), abnormal conduction in the form of low sensory potentials was found (Krishnan et al., 2005). Refractoriness was significantly greater in symptomatic than asymptomatic patients ($p < 0.05$). At 12 months posttreatment, nerve conduction study abnormalities persisted, although some patients reported symptomatic improvement.

5.3.2 TAXANES

Taxane-induced peripheral neuropathy is dose related but rarely severe enough to be dose limiting (Postma et al., 1995). The antineoplastic action of taxane drugs relies on their ability to interfere with the mitotic spindle by increased aggregation of intracellular microtubules (Rowinsky and Donehower, 1996), which slows mitosis and results in disordered cell division and apoptosis of daughter cells (Windebank and Grisold, 2008). Receptors and mitochondria rely on microtubule-dependent axonal transport. Fast axonal transport, necessary for maintaining and replacing these components for proper nerve function, depends on the microtubule infrastructure, as does retrograde transport of trophic factors from the nerve terminal. Taxanes interfere with microtubule assembly, thereby disrupting axonal transport and, in that way, axonal functionality (Windebank and Grisold, 2008). Taxanes hyperstabilize microtubule subunit cross-linking, making their action distinct from the tubule interference of vinca compounds, which damage microtubules by destablizing them. By increasing microtubule stability, taxanes reduce the cell's ability to dynamically reorganize its cytoskeleton (Windebank and Grisold, 2008). Increased cross-linking by taxane compounds may produce crystalline arrays of microtubule subunits within the cell or axon, a process that also interferes with axonal transport (Apfel, 2000).

By promoting large, disordered arrays of microtubules in axons, Schwann cells, and DRG neurons, taxanes are associated with a predominantly sensory axonal neuropathy (Malik and Stillman, 2008). Taxanes are unable to cross the blood-brain barrier because of their relatively large molecular weight and because they are substrates of P-glycoprotein, which acts as a drug-efflux pump (Kemper et al., 2003).

In a preclinical study, taxanes caused significant dose-dependent reductions in nerve conduction velocity, but morphological measurements determined that the pathological changes induced by both paclitaxel and docetaxel were milder than anticipated in light of their concomitant neuropathy. It is thus speculated that taxane compounds may affect more than just the microtubular system (Persohn et al., 2005). However, it is unclear what these other targets or mechanisms might be.

Neurotoxicity from taxane compounds may occur with cumulative doses of 175 to 200 mg/m^2 (Malik and Stillman, 2008), which typically occurs in a dying-back pattern starting at distal nerve endings, followed by Schwann cells, with changes to neuronal body and axonal transport, and then disrupted cytoplasmatic flow (Argyriou et al., 2008). Taxanes affect all sensory neurons but preferentially thick myelinated nerve fibers associated with vibration sensation and proprioception (Montero et al., 2005). At doses over 200 mg/m^2, 16 out of 60 paclitaxel-treated patients developed a predominantly sensory neuropathy with electrophysiological data that suggested axonal degeneration and demyelination (Lipton et al., 1989).

The two main taxane chemotherapeutic compounds are paclitaxel (formerly called taxol) and docetaxel. The greater the duration of systemic exposure to paclitaxel, the greater its hematologic and neurologic toxicity (Mielke et al., 2005). Docetaxel has the same toxicity profile as paclitaxel, but spontaneous recovery is more common with docetaxel-induced peripheral neuropathy than with paclitaxel-induced peripheral neuropathy (New et al., 1996). When 100 mg/m^2 docetaxel was directly compared to 176 mg/m^2 paclitaxel over a 3-week course, the incidence of peripheral neuropathy was slightly higher with docetaxel than paclitaxel (7% versus 4%, respectively) but not statistically significant (Jones et al., 2005).

Although the clinical effectiveness of docetaxel and paclitaxel are comparable (Chon et al., 2009; Vahdat, 2008), patients in a weekly paclitaxel arm of a study developed grade 2, 3, or 4 peripheral neuropathy more frequently than similar patients on a 3-week schedule (27% versus 20%, respectively), but docetaxel-induced neuropathy occurred at a rate of 16% regardless of whether the administration was weekly or every 3 weeks (Vahdat, 2008). In a study of gastric cancer patients ($n = 66$), paclitaxel was associated with a higher rate of peripheral neuropathy (5%) than docelitaxel (2%) (Chon et al., 2009).

5.3.2.1 Paclitaxel

Paclitaxel binds to β-tubulin and stabilizes its polymerization, which disrupts the mitotic spindle and halts cell division (Schiff and Horwitz, 1981). Paclitaxel may increase or alter distribution of detyrosinated tubulin, which is considered a marker for stable microtubules (Laferriere et al., 1997). Paclitaxel is associated with dose-dependent, painful, sensory-predominant distal axonopathy (Peltier and Russell, 2006), but the mechanisms have not been determined.

At clinical doses, paclitaxel causes axonal degeneration, but not neuronal death (Melli et al., 2006). However, biopsies of human nerves following paclitaxel treatment showed that ganglionopathy, rather than axonopathy, was the most likely mechanism for paclitaxel-induced peripheral neuropathy (Sahenk et al., 1994). Preclinical studies suggest that paclitaxel-induced peripheral neuropathy is characterized by injury to the sensory neurons and their supporting cells, macrophage activation in the DRG, and combined peripheral nerve and microglial activation in the spinal cord (Jimenez-Andrade et al., 2006). Thus, paclitaxel may first interfere with axonal transport and, in that way, affect the function of the cells (Kimura, 2001), since survival and function of a peripheral neuron are closely dependent on axonal transport and signal transduction (Dustin, 1980).

Paclitaxel-induced toxicity may be multifaceted (Yang et al., 2009). Paclitaxel induces an increase in detyrosinated tubulin, resulting in a cold-stable microtubule assembly within the axons, which has been speculated to disrupt axonal transport in such a way that distal axons fail to receive vital nutrients (Melli et al., 2006; Shea, 1999). But in another study (Yang et al., 2009), investigators found blebs even on the most proximal segments of paclitaxel-treated axons. Axonal blebbing is often interpreted as a prelude to axonal degeneration (Johnson et al., 2004), and could be induced by local axonal activation of protein degradation pathways, e.g., involving capases or calpains.

Almost all microtubules in differentiated axons orient themselves such that their positive end faces toward the axonal tip. This polarity of orientation allows efficient organelle transport through the axon. Microtubules are not anchored in cell structures, and the mechanisms maintaining this polarity pattern have not been elucidated. Paclitaxel was found *in vitro* to lead to a massive destabilization of this polarization pattern, to the extent that axonal transport was interrupted (Shemesh and Spira, 2010). This disorganized polarity survived paclitaxel washout, and it is unclear if and how normal polarization patterns can be restored.

Paclitaxel acute pain syndrome has been described in the literature as aches and pains, often described as arthralgia and myalgia, that include pain in the large axial muscle and joints of the back, hips, shoulders, legs, and feet (Loprinzi et al., 2007; Onetto et al., 1993; Rowinsky et al., 1989; Wolf et al., 2008). Paclitaxel acute pain syndrome typically commences within 1 to 3 days of drug administration and resolves spontaneously within a week. About 58% of paclitaxel-treated patients develop this acute pain syndrome (Loprinzi et al., 2007). It has been theorized that paclitaxel acute pain syndrome might be distinct from paclitaxel-induced peripheral neuropathy because the former involves the sensitization of the nociceptors and their fibers (the spinothalamtic system) and is temporally limited (Loprinzi et al., 2007).

Cremophor EL, the vehicle compound for paclitaxel, has been reported to have neurotoxic properties (Gelderblom et al., 2001; Mielke et al., 2006). In fact, it has been speculated that paclitaxel-induced peripheral neuropathy might be due more to Cremophor EL than paclitaxel. In a study of advanced cancer patients ($n = 24$) randomized to receive a 12-week course of 1- or 3-hour infusions of 100 mg/m^2 paclitaxel, the majority of patients ($n = 14$) developed peripheral neuropathy (Mielke et al., 2005). Those patients who developed peripheral neuropathy were more likely to have more weeks of therapy ($p = 0.056$) and have significantly higher ($p < 0.05$) and greater overall systemic drug exposure, defined as weeks of therapy multiplied by the area under the curve (AUC) ($p < 0.05$), than those without peripheral neuropathy. Cremophor EL had no effect on neuropathy development, which is contrary to pre-clinical studies (Lesser et al., 1995; Windebank et al., 1994), but is consistent with the findings of two more recent human studies (Ibrahim et al., 2002; Kim et al., 2004).

5.3.2.2   Docetaxel

Docetaxel-induced peripheral neuropathy is dose dependent and characterized by sensory loss in the lower distal extremities and pain that can be severe enough to limit dosage (Roglio et al., 2009). In a preclinical study, docetaxel affected the gene expression in the spinal cord of calcitonin gene-related peptide (CGRP), such that a marked decrease in CGRP mRNA content in the lumbar spinal cord was determined (Roglio et al., 2009). Docetaxel in this study was also shown to affect the gene expression of myelin proteins (P0, PMP22, MAL, and 21.5 and 18.5 MBP isoforms) that occur in other forms of neuropathy, such as diabetic neuropathy (Leonelli et al., 2007; Roglio et al., 2008). There may be an association between these changes and dymyelination of Schwann cells (Quasthoff and Hartung, 2002; Windebank and Grisold, 2008). When docetaxel-induced peripheral neuropathy resolved following treatment, myelin protein mRNA levels were restored as well, except for MBP isoforms (Roglio et al., 2009).

In humans, docetaxel-induced neuropathic symptoms include paresthesia, weakness, itching or tingling, feelings of heaviness in the hands and feet, numbness, and loss of ankle and knee jerk, which can be manifested as loss of dexterity, gait unsteadiness, or clumsiness (Baker et al., 2009).

5.3.3   Vinca Alkaloids

The vinca alkaloid drugs (including vincristine, vinblastine, vindesine, and vinorelbine) inhibit the assembly of microtubules and promote their disassembly, thus disrupting axonal transport (Himes et al., 1976; Malik and Stillman, 2008). This interferes with mitotic spindle formation in cancer cells, slowing of mitosis, and disordering of cell division in such a way that daughter cells go into apoptosis (Windebank and Grisold, 2008). Vinca alkaloids do not readily cross the blood-brain barrier (Greig et al., 1990), but can access peripheral nerves where they act on the cell body (Pan et al., 2003). All of the vinca alkaloids are associated with dose-related sensorimotor neuropathy, which typically occurs within the first 3 months of treatment. Early symptoms frequently include pain in hands and feet (Windebank and Grisold, 2008).

Muscle weakness and cramping have also been reported, as has weakness in the wrist extensors and dorsiflexors (DeAngelis et al., 1991).

Vincristine may be the most neurotoxic of the vinca alkaloid agents (Malik and Stillman, 2008). It is believed to exhibit neurotoxic effects at cumulative doses above 4 mg/m². Vincristine is known to induce axonal neuropathy by disrupting the microtubular axonal transport system, evidenced by reduced compound muscle action potential and sensory nerve action potential amplitude (Malik and Stillman, 2008). Vincristine causes distal axonal degeneration, which may be reversible in mild cases (Peltier and Russell, 2006). Vincristine-induced peripheral neuropathy in preclinical studies has a prominent pain component (Tanner et al., 1998).

Vincristine binds with tubulin and blocks its polymerization into microtubules (Peltier and Russell, 2006). By binding intracellular tubulin and altering cellular microtubular structures, vincristine impedes both fast and slow axonal transport (Quasthoff and Hartung, 2002). Vincristine's disruption of axonal transport may cause distal axonopathy (Schaumberg et al., 2000). Ultrastructural changes in the cytoskeleton of large myelinated axons and the accumulation of neurofilaments in dorsal sensory ganglion neurons have been observed with vincristine (Topp et al., 2000).

5.3.4 SURAMIN

Suramin is a reverse transcriptase inhibitor with a long half-life (De Clercq, 1979). It is associated with demyelinating neuropathy and a dose-dependent axonal neuropathy (Malik and Stillman, 2008). Neurtoxic effects of suramin include dose-dependent axonal sensorimotor neuropathy and subacute demyelinating polyneuropathy similar to Gullain-Barré syndrome (Chaudhry et al., 1996), with elevated levels of cerebrospinal fluid protein (La Rocca et al., 1990). Signs of denervation rarely appear on the electromyogram, and nerve conduction velocity may or may not be blocked (Malik and Stillman, 2008).

Suramin-induced peripheral neuropathy has a few unique pathological features, including multilamellar inclusion bodies in neurons, axons, and Schwann cells (Windebank and Grisold, 2008). It has been proposed that these are associated with suramin's interference with intracellular lipid metabolism (Gill et al., 1995, 1996; Gill and Windebank, 1998b; Russell et al., 1994, 2001; Sun and Windebank, 1996).

5.3.5 THALIDOMIDE

Known for its antiangiogenic properties, thalidomide has also been associated with sensory and axonal neuropathy (Malik and Stillman, 2008). The rate of thalidomide-induced neuropathy may be as high at 20 to 50%, and its frequency has been associated with patient age, length of treatment, and possibly cumulative dose (Dimopoulos et al., 2004; Matthews and McCoy, 2003; Mazumder and Jagannath, 2006). Dose dependence in thalidomide-induced peripheral neuropathy is uncertain in that one study reported no correlation between thalidomide cumulative dose and peripheral neuropathy (Briani et al., 2004), whereas another found a dose-dependent relationship at higher doses (Cavaletti et al., 2004).

Thalidomide can cause both neuropathy and axonopathy (Chaudhry et al., 2002). Nerve conduction studies report that thalidomide is associated with reduced sensory nerve action potential and compound muscle action potential (Malik and Stillman, 2008). In one study of cancer patients treated with thalidomide ($n = 7$), 100% developed clinical and painful paresthesias or numbness (Chaudhry et al., 2002), but a clear relationship between dose, therapy duration, and neuropathy has not been established.

Thalidomide-induced neuropathy has been clinically described for decades (Fullerton and O'Sullivan, 1968), along with the fact that thalidomide-induced neuropathy is often irreversible (Gibbels et al., 1973). A recent study proposed that thalidomide-induced neuropathy is caused by length-dependent, primary sensory axonal neuropathy affecting the large and small nerve fibers (Chaudhry et al., 2002). This study found symptoms commenced in the lower limbs (distal sensory loss) and included the loss of ankle reflexes, suggesting a dying-back degeneration of sensory and motor nerves. Nevertheless, the exact mechanism behind thalidomide-induced neuropathy is not known.

5.4   SOME MAJOR UNANSWERED QUESTIONS

This chapter addresses the basic mechanisms recently thought to be involved in CIPN, but several important questions remain:

- Many cancers are treated with complex combinations of chemotherapeutic drugs. Such combination therapies are effective, but potentially could amplify the neurotoxicity of the drugs (Pignata et al., 2006), and it is not known if such neurotoxic effects would be additive or synergistic (Hilkens et al., 1997). Considerably more research should be done to better understand the potential neuropathic effects of combination chemotherapy.
- Very little conclusive information is available in the literature regarding the most advantageous routes of chemotherapy administration with respect to reducing the likelihood of CIPN, although there are suggestions that intrathecal administration and focal radiotherapy may increase neurotoxic effects (Windebank and Grisold, 2008). More research is needed to understand the best routes of administration to reduce the likelihood of developing CIPN.
- Treatments for CIPN are limited, yet it may be that neuroprotective agents can be identified to help reduce CIPN in chemotherapy patients.
- Since CIPN is associated with neuropathic pain in many chemotherapy patients, better pain management strategies should be identified. For example, there is a role for preemptive analgesia in patients undergoing chemotherapy.
- Emerging treatments for cancer pain and treatments for symptoms related to chemotherapy (Davis et al., 2007), such as neuropathic pain (Stillman and Cata, 2006), may be useful for CIPN patients or specific subsets of CIPN patients. However, more studies are required to determine if and to what extent these new agents may be appropriate.

5.5   CONCLUSION

Cancer chemotherapeutic drugs save lives. But no class of drugs is free of adverse effects. Since drugs used to treat cancer are by their very nature cytotoxic, it is not surprising that these drugs produce collateral damage to noncancerous cells. Although chemotherapeutic agents do not readily cross the blood-brain barrier, fenestrated capillaries near peripheral neurons permit exposure of these cells to chemotherapeutic drugs, with the result that some of the cytotoxicity of the chemotherapeutic agents inflicts damage, up to and including cell death, on bystander cells of the peripheral nervous system. The result is peripheral neuropathy, and neuropathic pain often ensues. If damage is mild, the CINP may be reversible (of variable duration). If the damage is more severe, the CINP may be long lasting or even permanent.

Although a great deal about CIPN is known, key pieces of information are lacking. In particular, the mechanisms are only partially understood. As a consequence, effective oncology might expose patients to the risk of neuropathic pain and potentially permanent neuropathy as part of successfully treating the cancer. Furthermore, in modern practice, chemotherapy drugs are often used in combination. The impact of this on CIPN is largely unknown.

Although CIPN is associated with neuropathic pain, there are few treatment strategies to help manage pain in CIPN patients. Cannabinoid neuromodulators are discussed in the literature as a treatment for chemotherapy-induced nausea and vomiting, but may have a role in pain management as well (Davis et al., 2007). However, current treatment options for the pain associated with CIPN are limited (Stillman and Cata, 2006). New agents (Rao et al., 2008) or established neuropathic treatments (Dray, 2008) may be useful, but remain to be evaluated for CIPN patients.

DECLARATIONS AND ACKNOWLEDGMENT

Dr. Raffa is a speaker, consultant, and basic science investigator for several pharmaceutical companies involved in analgesics research, but receives no royalty (cash or otherwise) from the sale of any product. Dr. Pergolizzi is a consultant for Grünenthal, Baxter, and Hospira. This article was prepared with editorial assistance from LeQ Medical, Angleton, Texas.

REFERENCES

Adelsberger H, Quasthoff S, Grosskreutz J, Lepier A, Eckel F, Lersch C. (2000). The chemotheapeutic oxaliplatin alters voltage-gated Na(+) channel kinetics on rat sensory neurons. *Eur J Pharmacol* 406(1):25–32.

Apfel S. (2000). Taxoids. In Schaumburg H, Spencer P (eds.), *Experimental and clinical neurotoxicology*, 1135–39. Oxford: Oxford University Press.

Argyriou AA, Koltzenburg M, Polychronopoulos P, Papapetropoulos S, Kalofonos HP. (2008). Peripheral nerve damage associated with administration of taxanes in patients with cancer. *Crit Rev Oncol Hematol* 66(3):218–28.

Argyriou AA, Polychronopoulos P, Koutras A, Iconomou G, Iconomou A, Kalofonos HP, et al. (2005). Peripheral neuropathy induced by administration of cisplatin- and paclitaxel-based chemotherapy. Could it be predicted? *Support Care Cancer* 13(8):647–51.

Arnould S, Hennebelle I, Canal P, Bugat R, Guichard S. (2003). Cellular determinants of oxaliplatin sensitivy in colon cancer cell lines. *Eur J Cancer* 39(1):112–19.

Authier N, Balayssac D, Marchand F, Ling B, Zangarelli A, Descoeur J, et al. (2009). Animal models of chemotherapy-evoked painful peripheral neuropathies. *Neurotherapeutics* 6(4):620–29.

Baker J, Ajani J, Scotte F, Winther D, Martin M, Aapro MS, et al. (2009). Docetaxel-related side effects and their management. *Eur J Oncol Nurs* 13(1):49–59.

Balmaceda C, Korkin E. (2003). Cancer and cancer treatment-related neuromuscular disease. In Schiff D, Wen P (eds.), *Cancer neurology in clinical practice*, 193–213. Totowa, NJ: Humana Press.

Barajon I, Bersani M, Quartu M, Fiacco MD, Cavaletti G, Holst J, et al. (1996). Neuropeptides and morphological changes in cisplatin-induced dorsal root ganglion neuronopathy. *J Exp Neurol* 138:93–104.

Benoit E, Brienza S, Dubois J. (2006). Oxaliplatin, an anticancer agent that affects both Na+ and K+ channels in frog peripheral myelinated axons. *Gen Physiol Biophys* 25:263–76.

Boughattas N, Hecquet B, Fournier C, Bruguerolle B, Trabelsi H, Bouzouita K, et al. (1994). Comparative pharmacokinetics of oxaliplatin (L-OHP) and carboplatin (CBDCA) in mice with reference to circadian dosing time. *Bipharm Drug Dispos* 15(9):761–63.

Briani C, Zara G, Rondinone R, Della Libera S, Ermani M, Ruggero S, et al. (2004). Thalidomide neurotoxicity: Prospective study in patients with lupus erythematosus. *Neurology* 62(12):2288–90.

Brydoy M, Oldenburg J, Klepp O, Bremnes RM, Wist EA, Wentzel-Larsen T, et al. (2009). Observational study of prevalence of long-term Raynaud-like phenomena and neurological side effects in testicular cancer survivors. *J Natl Cancer Inst* 101(24):1682–95.

Burke D, Kiernan M, Bostock H. (2001). Excitability of human axons. *Clin Neurophysiol* 112:1575–85.

Cassidy J, Misset JL. (2002). Oxaliplatin-related side effects: Characteristics and management. *Semin Oncol* 29(5 Suppl 15):11–20.

Cavaletti G, Bogliun G, Zincone A, Marzorati L, Melzi P, Frattola L, et al. (1998a). Neuro- and ototoxicity of high-dose carboplatin treatment in poor prognosis ovarian cancer patients. *Anti-Cancer Res* 18(5B):3797–802.

Cavaletti G, Broenio A, Reni L, Ghiglione E, Schenone A, Briani C, et al. (2004). Thalidomide sensory neurotoxicity: A clinical and neurophysilogic study. *Neurophysiology* 62(12):2291–93.

Cavaletti G, Fabbrica D, Minoia C, Frattola L, Tredici G. (1998b). Carboplatin toxic effects on the peripheral nervous system of the rat. *Ann Oncol* 9(4):443–47.

Cavaletti G, Frigeni B, Lanzani F, Mattavelli L, Susani E, Alberti P, et al. (2010). Chemotherapy-induced peripheral neurotoxicity assessment: A critical revision of the currently available tools. *Eur J Cancer* 46:479–94.

Cavaletti G, Marmiroli P. (2004). Chemotherapy-induced peripheral neurotoxicity. *Expert Opin Drug Saf* 3(6):535–46.

Cavaletti G, Marmiroli P. (2006). The role of growth factors in the prevention and treatment of chemotherapy-induced peripheral neurotoxicity. *Curr Drug Saf* 1(1):35–42.

Cavaletti G, Tredici G, Petruccioli MG, Donde E, Tredici P, Marmiroli P, et al. (2001). Effects of different schedules of oxaliplatin treatment on the peripheral nervous system of the rat. *Eur J Cancer* 37(18):2457–63.

Cece R, Petruccioli M, Cavaletti G, Barajon I, Tredici G. (1995). An ultrastructural study of neuronal changes in dorsal root ganglion (DRG) of rats after chronic cisplatin administrations. *Histol Histopathol* 10:837–45.

Cersosimo RJ. (2005). Oxaliplatin-associated neuropathy: A review. *Ann Pharmacother* 39(1):128–35.

Chamberlain M. (2010). Neurotoxicity of cancer treatment. *Curr Oncol Rep* 12:60–67.

Chaudhry V, Cornblath D, Corse A, Freimer M, Simmons-O'Brien E, Vogelsang G. (2002). Thalidomide-induced neuropathy. *Neurology* 59:1872–75.

Chaudhry V, Eisenberger MA, Sinibaldi VJ, Sheikh K, Griffin JW, Cornblath DR. (1996). A prospective study of suramin-induced peripheral neuropathy. *Brain* 119(Pt 6):2039–52.

Chon H, Rha S, Im C, Kim C, Hong M, Kim H, et al. (2009). Docetaxel versus paclitaxel combined with 5-FU and leucovorin in advanced gastric cancer: Combinated analysis of two phase II trials. *Cancer Res Treat* 41(4):196–204.

Cvitkovic E. (1998). Cumulative toxicities from cisplatin therapy and current cytoprotective measures. *Cancer Treat Rev* 24(4):265–81.

Davis M, Maida V, Daeninck P, Pergolizzi J. (2007). The emerging role of cannabinoid neuro-modulators in symptom management. *Support Care Cancer* 15:63–71.

DeAngelis LM, Gnecco C, Taylor L, Warrell RP Jr. (1991). Evolution of neuropathy and myopathy during intensive vincristine/corticosteroid chemotherapy for non-Hodgkin's lymphoma. *Cancer* 67(9):2241–46.

De Clercq E. (1979). Suramin: A potent inhibitor of the reverse transcriptase of RNA tumor viruses. *Cancer Lett* 8:9–22.

Dimopoulos MA, Eleutherakis-Papaiakovou V. (2004). Adverse effects of thalidomide admin-istration in patients with neoplastic diseases. *Am J Med* 117(7):508–15.

Dray A. (2008). Neuropathic pain: Emerging teatments. *Br J Anaesthesia* 101(1):48–58.

Dustin P. (1980). Microtubules. *Sci Am* 243:66–76.

Eckel F, Schmelz R, Adelsberger H, Erdmann J, Quasthoff S, Lersch C. (2002). Prevention of oxaliplatin-induced neuropathy by carbamazepine. A pilot study. *Dtsch Med Wochenschr* 127(3):78–82.

Extra J, Marty M, Brienza S, Misset J. (1998). Pharmacokinetics and safety profile of oxaliplatin. *Semin Oncol* 25:13–22.

Fischer S, McDonald E, Gross L, Windebank A. (2001a). Alterations in cell cycle regulation underlie cisplatin induced apoptosis of dorsal root ganglion neurons *in vivo*. *Neurobiol Dis* 8:1027–35.

Fischer S, Podratz J, Windebank A. (2001b). Nerve growth factor rescue of cisplatin neuro-toxicity is mediated through the high affinity receptor: Studies in PC12 cells and p75 null mouse dorsal root ganglia. *Neurosci Lett* 308:1–4.

Fullerton P, O'Sullivan D. (1968). Thalidomide neuropathy: A clinical electrophysiological and histological follow-up study. *J Neruol Neurosurg Psychiatry* 31:543–51.

Gamelin L, Boisdron-Celle M, Delva R, Guerin-Meyer V, Ifrah N, Morel A, et al. (2004). Prevention of oxaliplatin-related neurotoxicity by calcium and magnesium infusions: A retrospective study of 161 patients receiving oxaliplatin combined with 5-fluorouracil and leucovorin for advanced colorectal cancer. *Clin Cancer Res* 10(12 Pt 1):4055–61.

Gamelin E, Gamelin L, Bossi L, Quasthoff S. (2002). Clinical aspects and molecular basis of oxaliplatin neurotoxicity: Current management and development of preventive mea-sures. *Semin Oncol* 29:21–23.

Gelderblom H, Verweij J, Nooter K, Sparreboom A. (2001). Cremophor EL: The drawbacks and advantages of vehicle selection for drug formulation. *Eur J Cancer* 37(13):1590–98.

Gibbels E, Scheid W, Wieck HH, Kinzel W. (1973). Thalidomide neuropathy in the late stage. A clinical documentation. *Fortschr Neurol Psychiatr Grenzgeb* 41(7):378–417.

Gilbert M. (1998). The neurotoxicity of chemotherapy. *Neurologist* 4:43–53.

Gill J, Connolly D, McManus M, Maihle N, Windebank A. (1996). Suramin induces phos-phorylation of the high-affinity nerve growth factor receptor in PC12 cells and dorsal root ganglion neurons. *J Neurochem* 66:963–72.

Gill J, Hobday K, Windebank A. (1995). Mechanism of suramin toxicity in stable myelinating dorsal root ganglion cutlures. *Exp Neurol* 133:113–24.

Gill J, Windebank A. (1998a). Cisplatin-induced apoptosis in rat dorsal root ganglion neurons is associated with attempted entry into the cell cycle. *J Clin Invest* 101:2842–50.

Gill J, Windebank A. (1998b). Suramin induced ceramide accumulation leads to apoptotic cell death in dorsal root ganglion neurons. *Cell Death Diff* 5:876–83.

Go R, Adjei A. (1999). Review of the comparative pharmacology and clinical activity of cisplatin and carboplatin. *J Clin Oncol* 17(1):409–22.

Gourdier I, Crabbe L, Andreau K, Pau B, Kroemer G. (2004). Oxaliplatin-induced mitochonrdial apoptotic response of colon carcinoma cells does not require nuclear DNA. *Oncogene* 23(45):7449–57.

Greig N, Soncrant T, Shetty H, Momma S, Smith Q, Rapoport S. (1990). Brain uptake and anticancer activities of vincristine and vinblastine are restricted by their lower cerebrovascular permeability and binding to plasma constituents in rat. *Cancer Chemother Pharmacol* 26:263–68.

Grolleau F, Gamelin L, Boisdron-Celle M, Lapied B, Pelhate M, Gamelin E. (2001). A possible explanation for a neurotoxic effect of the anticancer agent oxaliplatin on neuronal voltage-gated sodium channels. *J Neurophysiol* 85(5):2293–97.

Grothey A. (2003). Oxaliplatin-safety profile: Neurotoxicity. *Semin Oncol* 30(4 Suppl 15):5–13.

Hartmann J, Lipp H. (2003). Toxicity of platinum compounds. *Expert Opin Pharmacother* 4(6):889–901.

Hilkens PH, Pronk LC, Verweij J, Vecht CJ, van Putten WL, van den Bent MJ. (1997). Peripheral neuropathy induced by combination chemotherapy of docetaxel and cisplatin. *Br J Cancer* 75(3):417–22.

Himes R, Kersey R, Heller-Bettinger I, Samson F. (1976). Action of the vinaca alkaloids vincristine, vinblastine, and desacetyl vinblastine amide on microtubules *in vitro*. *Cancer Res* 36:3798–802.

Holmes J, Stanko J, Varchenko M, Ding H, Madden V, Bagnell C, et al. (1998). Comparative neurotoxicity of oxaliplatin, cisplatin, and ormaplatin in a Wistar rat model. *Toxicol Sci* 46(2):342–51.

Huang H, Zhu L, Reid B, Drobny G, Hopkins P. (1995). Solution structure of a cisplatin-induced DNA interstrand cross-link. *Science* 270:1842–45.

Ibrahim NK, Desai N, Legha S, Soon-Shiong P, Theriault RL, Rivera E, et al. (2002). Phase I and pharmacokinetic study of ABI-007, a Cremophor-free, protein-stabilized, nanoparticle formulation of paclitaxel. *Clin Cancer Res* 8(5):1038–44.

Jimenez-Andrade JM, Peters CM, Mejia NA, Ghilardi JR, Kuskowski MA, Mantyh PW. (2006). Sensory neurons and their supporting cells located in the trigeminal, thoracic and lumbar ganglia differentially express markers of injury following intravenous administration of paclitaxel in the rat. *Neurosci Lett* 405(1–2):62–67.

Johnson M, Uhl C, Spittler K, Wang H, Gorres G. (2004). Mitochondrial injury and capase activation by the local anesthetic lidocaine. *Anesthesiology* 101:1184–94.

Jones K. (1993). Recovery from facial paralysis following crush injury of the facial nerve in hamsters: Differential effects of gender and androgen exposure. *Exp Neurol* 121:133–38.

Jones S, Erban J, Overmoyer B, Budd G, Hutchins L, Lower E, et al. (2005). Randomized phase III study of docetaxel compared with paclitaxel in metastatic breast cancer. *J Clin Oncol* 23:5542–51.

Kemper E, Zandbergen Av, Cleypool C, Mos H, Boogerd W, Beijnen J, et al. (2003). Increased penetration of paclitaxel into brain by inhibition of P-glycoprotein. *Clin Cancer Res* 9(7):2849–55.

Kiernan M, Burke D, Andersen K, Bostock H. (2000). Multiple measures of axonal excitability: A new approach in clinical testing. *Muscle Nerve* 23:399–409.

Kim T, Kim D, Chung J, Shin S, Kim S, Heo D, et al. (2004). Phase I and pharmacokinetic study of Genexol-PM, a cremophor-free, polymeric micelle-formulated paclitaxel, in patients with advanced malignancies. *Clin Cancer Res* 10:3708–16.

Kimura J. (2001). Electrodiagnosis in diseases of nerve and muscle, principles and practice. In *Polyneuropathies*, 669. 3rd ed. Oxford: Oxford University Press.

Kovacic U, Zele T, Osredkar J, Sketelj J, Bajrovic F. (2004). Sex-related differences in the regeneration of sensory axons and recovery of nociception after peripheral nerve crush in the rate. *Exp Neurol* 189:94–104.

Krarup-Hansen A, Helweg-Larsen S, Schmalbruch H, Rorth M, Krarup C. (2007). Neuronal involvement in cisplatin neuropathy: Prospective clinical and neurophysiological studies. *Brain* 130(Pt 4):1076–88.

Krishnan A, Lin C, Park S, Kiernan M. (2008). Assessment of nerve excitability in toxic and metabolic neuropathies. *J Peripher Nerv Syst* 13:7–26.

Krishnan A, Lin C, Reddel S, McGrath R, Kiernan M. (2009). Conduction block and impaired axonal function in tick paralysis. *Muscle Nerve* 40:358–62.

Krishnan AV, Goldstein D, Friedlander M, Kiernan MC. (2005). Oxaliplatin-induced neurotoxicity and the development of neuropathy. *Muscle Nerve* 32(1):51–60.

Kujawa K, Emeric E, Jones K. (1991). Testosterone differentially regulates the regenerative properties of injured hamster facial motoneurons. *J Neurosci* 11:3898–906.

Laferriere L, MacRae T, Brown D. (1997). Tubulin synthesis and assembly in differentiating neurons. *Biochem Cell Biol* 75:103–17.

La Rocca RV, Meer J, Gilliatt RW, Stein CA, Cassidy J, Myers CE, et al. (1990). Suramin-induced polyneuropathy. *Neurology* 40(6):954–60.

Lehky TJ, Leonard GD, Wilson RH, Grem JL, Floeter MK. (2004). Oxaliplatin-induced neurotoxicity: Acute hyperexcitability and chronic neuropathy. *Muscle Nerve* 29(3):387–92.

Leonelli E, Bianchi R, Cavaletti G, Caruso D, Crippa D, Garcia-Segura LM, et al. (2007). Progesterone and its derivatives are neuroprotective agents in experimental diabetic neuropathy: A multimodal analysis. *Neuroscience* 144(4):1293–304.

Lesser G, Grossman S, Eller S, Rowinsky E. (1995). The distribution of systemically administered [3H]-paclitaxel in rats: A quantitiative autoradiographic study. *Cancer Chemother Pharmacol* 37:173–78.

Lipton L, Apfel S, Dutcher J, Rosenberg R, Kaplan J, Berger A, et al. (1989). Taxol produces a predominantly sensory neuropathy. *Neurology* 39:368.

Loprinzi C, Maddocks-Christianson K, Wolf S, Rao R, Dyck P, Mantyh P, et al. (2007). The paclitaxel acute pain syndrome: Sensitization of nociceptors as the putative mechanism. *Cancer J* 13(6):399–403.

Malik B, Stillman M. (2008). Chemotherapy-induced peripheral neuropathy. *Curr Pain Headache Rep* 12(3):165–74.

Matthews S, McCoy C. (2003). Thalidomide: A review of approved and investigational uses. *Clin Ther* 25:342–95.

Mazumder A, Jagannath S. (2006). Thalidomide and lenalidomide in multiple myeloma. *Best Pract Res Clin Haematol* 19:769–80.

McDonald E, Randon K, Knight A, Windebank A. (2005). Cisplatin preferentially binds to DNA in dorsal root ganglion neurons *in vitro* and *in vivo*: A potential mechanism for neurotoxicity. *Neurobiol Dis* 18:305–13.

McDonald E, Windebank A. (2002). Cisplatin-induced apoptosis of DRG neurons involves Bax redistribution and cycochrome c release but not Fas receptor signaling. *Neurobiol Dis* 9:220–33.

McKeage M. (1995). Comparative adverse effect profiles of platinum drugs. *Drug Safety* 13:228–44.

McKeage M, Hsu T, Screnci D, Haddad G, Baguley B. (2001). Nucleolar damage correlates with neurotoxicity induced by different platinum drugs. *Br J Cancer* 85(8):1219–25.

Melli G, Jack C, Lambrinos G, Ringkamp M, Hoke A. (2006). Erythropoietin protects sensory axons against paclitaxel-induced distal degeneration. *Neurobiol Dis* 24:525–30.

Mielke S, Sparreboom A, Mross K. (2006). Peripheral neuropathy: A persisting challenge in paclitaxel-based regimes. *Eur J Cancer* 42(1):24–30.

Mielke S, Sparreboom A, Steinberg SM, Gelderblom H, Unger C, Behringer D, et al. (2005). Association of paclitaxel pharmacokinetics with the development of peripheral neuropathy in patients with advanced cancer. *Clin Cancer Res* 11(13):4843–50.

Moldovan M, Alvarez S, Krarup C. (2009). Motor axon excitability during Wallerian degeneration. *Brain* 132:511–23.

Moldovan M, Krarup C. (2004). Mechanisms of hyperpolarization in regenerated mature motor axons in cat. *J Physiol* 560:807–19.

Mollman J. (1990). Cisplatin neurotoxicity. *N Engl J Med* 322(2):126–27.

Montero A, Fossella F, Hortobagyi G, Valero V. (2005). Docetaxel for treatment of solid tumours: A systematic review of clinical data. *Lancet Oncol* 6(4):229–39.

New PZ, Jackson CE, Rinaldi D, Burris H, Barohn RJ. (1996). Peripheral neuropathy secondary to docetaxel (Taxotere). *Neurology* 46(1):108–11.

Onetto N, Canetta R, Winograd B, Catane R, Dougan M, Grechko J, et al. (1993). Overview of taxol safety. *J Natl Cancer Inst Monogr* 1993(15):131–39.

Oshita F, Eastman A. (1993). Gene-specific damage produced by cisplatin, ormaplatin and UV light in human cells are assayed by the polymerase chain reaction. *Oncol Res* 5:111–18.

Oztas E. (2003). Neuronal tacing. *Neuroanatomy* 2:2–5.

Pan Y, Misgeld T, Lichtman J, Sanes J. (2003). Effects of neurotoxic and neuroprotective agents on peripheral nerve regeneration assayed by time-lapse imaging *in vivo*. *J Neurosci* 23:11479–88.

Park SB, Lin CS, Krishnan AV, Goldstein D, Friedlander ML, Kiernan MC. (2009). Oxaliplatin-induced neurotoxicity: Changes in axonal excitability precede development of neuropathy. *Brain* 132(Pt 10):2712–23.

Pasetto LM, D'Andrea MR, Rossi E, Monfardini S. (2006). Oxaliplatin-related neurotoxicity: How and why? *Crit Rev Oncol Hematol* 59(2):159–68.

Peltier AC, Russell JW. (2006). Recent advances in understanding drug-induced neuropathies. *Drug Saf* 29(1):23–30.

Persohn E, Canta A, Schoepfer S, Traebert M, Mueller L, Gilardini A, et al. (2005). Morphological and morphometric analysis of paclitaxel and docetaxel-induced peripheral neuropathy in rats. *Eur J Cancer* 41:1460–66.

Pignata S, De Placido S, Biamonte R, Scambia G, Di Vagno G, Colucci G, et al. (2006). Residual neurotoxicity in ovarian cancer patients in clinical remission after first-line chemotherapy with carboplatin and paclitaxel: The Multicenter Italian Trial in Ovarian cancer (MITO-4) retrospective study. *BMC Cancer* 6:5.

Plotkin S, Wen P. (2003). Neurologic complications of cancer therapy. *Neurol Clin N Am* 21:279–318.

Podratz J, Schlattau A, Chen B, Knight A, Windebank A. (2007). Platinum adduct formation in mitochondrial DNA may underlie the phenomenon of coasting. *J Peripher Nerv Syst* 12:69.

Postma TJ, Vermorken JB, Liefting AJ, Pinedo HM, Heimans JJ. (1995). Paclitaxel-induced neuropathy. *Ann Oncol* 6(5):489–94.

Quasthoff S, Hartung HP. (2002). Chemotherapy-induced peripheral neuropathy. *J Neurol* 249(1):9–17.

Rao R, Flynn P, Sloan J, Wong G, Novotny P, Johnson D, et al. (2008). Efficacy of lamotrigine in the management of chemotherapy-induced peripheral neuropathy. *Cancer* 112:2802–8.

Raymond E, Chaney S, Taamma A, Cvitkovic E. (1998). Oxaliplatin: A review of preclinical and clinical studies. *Ann Oncol* 9:1053–71.

Reyes-Gibby CC, Morrow PK, Buzdar A, Shete S. (2009). Chemotherapy-induced peripheral neuropathy as a predictor of neuropathic pain in breast cancer patients previously treated with paclitaxel. *J Pain* 10(11):1146–50.

Rixe O, Ortuzar W, Alvarex M, Parker R, Reed E, Paull K, et al. (1996). Oxaliplatin, tetra-platin, cisplatin, and carboplatin: Spectrum of activity in drug-resistant cell lines in the cell lines of the National Cancer Institute's Anticancer Drug Screen panel. *Biochem Pharmacol* 52(12):1855–65.

Roglio I, Bianchi R, Camozzi F, Carozzi V, Cervellini I, Crippa D, et al. (2009). Docetaxel-induced peripheral neuropathy: Protective effects of dihydroprogesterone and progester-one in an experimental model. *J Peripher Nerv Syst* 14(1):36–44.

Roglio I, Bianchi R, Gotti S, Scurati S, Giatti S, Pesaresi M, et al. (2008). Neuroprotective effects of dihydroprogesterone and progesterone in an experimental model of nerve crush injury. *Neuroscience* 155(3):673–85.

Rosson GD. (2006). Chemotherapy-induced neuropathy. *Clin Podiatr Med* Surg 23(3):637–49.

Rowinsky E, Donehower R. (1996). Antimicrotubule agents. In Chabner B, Longo D (eds.), *Cancer chemotherapy and biptherapy*, 263–96. 2nd ed. Philadelphia: Lippincott-Raven Publishers.

Rowinsky EK, Burke PJ, Karp JE, Tucker RW, Ettinger DS, Donehower RC. (1989). Phase I and pharmacodynamic study of taxol in refractory acute leukemias. *Cancer Res* 49(16):4640–47.

Russell J, Windebank A, McNiven M, Brat D, Brimijoin W. (1995). Effect of cisplatin and ACTH4-9 on neural transport in cisplatin induced neurotoxicity. *Brain Res* 676(2):258–67.

Russell J, Windebank A, Podratz J. (1994). Role of nerve growth factor in suramin neuro-toxicity studied *in vitro. Ann Neurol* 197:71–80.

Russell JW, Gill JS, Sorenson EJ, Schultz DA, Windebank AJ. (2001). Suramin-induced neuropathy in an animal model. *J Neurol Sci* 192(1–2):71–80.

Sahenk Z, Barohn R, New P, Mendell J. (1994). Taxol neuropathy. Electrodiagnostic and sural nerve biopsy findings. *Arch Neurol* 51(7):726–29.

Schaumberg H, Ludolph A, Gold B. (2000). Tacrolimus. In Spencer P, Schaumberg H (eds.), *Experimental and clinical neurotoxicology*, 1131–33. New York: Oxford University Press.

Schiff P, Horwitz S. (1981). Taxol assembles tubulin in the absence of exogenous guanosine 5'-triphosphate or microtubule-associated proteins. *Biochemistry* 20:3247–52.

Schmidt W, Chaney S. (1993). Role of carrier ligand in platinum resistance of human carci-noma cell lines. *Cancer Res* 53(4):799–805.

Screnci D, McKeage M, Galettis P, Hambley T, Palmer B, Baguley B. (2000). Relationships between hedrophobicity, reactivity, accumulation, and peripheral nerve toxicity of a series of platinum drugs. *Br J Cancer* 82:966–72.

Shea T. (1999). Selective stabilization of microtubules within the proximal region of develop-ing axonal neurites. *Brain Res Bull* 48:255–61.

Shemesh O, Spira M. (2010). Paclitaxel induces axonal microtubules polar reconfiguration and impaired organelle transport: Implications for the pathogenesis of paclitaxel-induced polyneuropathy. *Acta Neuropathol* 119:235–48.

Siegal T, Haim N. (1990). Cisplatin-induced peripheral neuropathy. Frequent off-therapy dete-rioration, demyelinating syndromes, and muscle cramps. *Cancer* 66(6):1117–23.

Stillman M, Cata JP. (2006). Management of chemotherapy-induced peripheral neuropathy. *Curr Pain Headache Rep* 10(4):279–87.

Strumberg D, Brugge S, Korn MW, Koeppen S, Ranft J, Scheiber G, et al. (2002). Evaluation of long-term toxicity in patients after cisplatin-based chemotherapy for non-seminomatous testicular cancer. *Ann Oncol* 13(2):229–36.

Sun X, Windebank A. (1996). Calcium in suramin-induced rat sensory neuron toxicity *in vitro. Brain Res* 742:149–56.

Ta L, Espeset L, Podratz J, Windebank A. (2006). Neurotoxicity of oxaliplatin and cisplatin for dorsal root ganglion neurons correlates with platinum-DNA binding. *Neurotoxicology* 27:992–1002.

Tanner KD, Reichling DB, Levine JD. (1998). Nociceptor hyper-responsiveness during vincristine-induced painful peripheral neuropathy in the rat. *J Neurosci* 18(16):6480–91.

Thompson SW, Davis LE, Kornfeld M, Hilgers RD, Standefer JC. (1984). Cisplatin neuropathy. Clinical, electrophysiologic, morphologic, and toxicologic studies. *Cancer* 54(7):1269–75.

Topp KS, Tanner KD, Levine JD. (2000). Damage to the cytoskeleton of large diameter sensory neurons and myelinated axons in vincristine-induced painful peripheral neuropathy in the rat. *J Comp Neurol* 424(4):563–76.

Vahdat L. (2008). Choosing a taxane for adjuvant treatment of breast cancer: More than a flip of the coin? *Nat Clin Pract Oncol* 5(10):570–71.

van den Bent MJ (2005). Prevention of chemotherapy-induced neuropathy: Leukemia inhibitory factor. *Clin Cancer Res* 11(5):1691–93.

Verstappen CC, Koeppen S, Heimans JJ, Huijgens PC, Scheulen ME, Strumberg D, et al. (2005). Dose-related vincristine-induced peripheral neuropathy with unexpected off-therapy worsening. *Neurology* 64(6):1076–77.

Webster R, Brain K, Wilson R, Grem J, Vincenter A. (2005). Oxaliplatin induces hyperexcitabilty at motor and autonomic neuromuscular junctions through effects on voltage-gated sodium channels. *Br J Pharmacol* 146:1027–39.

Wilson RH, Lehky T, Thomas RR, Quinn MG, Floeter MK, Grem JL. (2002). Acute oxaliplatin-induced peripheral nerve hyperexcitability. *J Clin Oncol* 20(7):1767–74.

Windebank A, Blexrud M, Groen PD. (1994). Potential neurotoxicity of the solvent vehicle for cyclosporine. *J Pharmacol Exp Ther* 268:1051–56.

Windebank AJ, Grisold W. (2008). Chemotherapy-induced neuropathy. *J Peripher Nerv Syst* 13(1):27–46.

Wiseman L, Adkins J, Plosker G, Goa K. (1999). Oxaliplatin: A review of its use in the management of metastatic colorectal cancer. *Drugs Aging* 14:459–75.

Wolf S, Barton D, Kottschade L, Grothey A, Loprinzi C. (2008). Chemotherapy-induced peripheral neuropathy: Prevention and treatment strategies. *Eur J Cancer* 44(11):1507–15.

Wongtawatchai T, Agthong S, Kaewsema A, Chentanez V. (2009). Sex-related differences in cisplatin-induced neuropathy in rats. *J Med Assoc Thai* 92(11):1485–91.

Woynarowski J, Chapman W, Napier C, Herzig M, Juniewicz P. (1998). Sequence- and region-specificity of oxaliplatin adducts in naked and cellular DNA. *Mol Pharmacol* 54(5):770–77.

Yang IH, Siddique R, Hosmane S, Thakor N, Hoke A. (2009). Compartmentalized microfluidic culture platform to study mechanism of paclitaxel-induced axonal degeneration. *Exp Neurol* 218(1):124–28.

Zhou Y, Garcia MK, Chang DZ, Chiang J, Lu J, Yi Q, et al. (2009). Multiple myeloma, painful neuropathy, acupuncture? *Am J Clin Oncol* 32(3):319–25.

6 Bedside to Bench
Research on Chemotherapy-Induced Neuropathic Pain

Haijun Zhang, Juan P. Cata, and Patrick M. Dougherty

CONTENTS

6.1 Introduction 137
6.2 Chemotherapy-Induced Axon Injury 137
6.3 Sensitization of Primary Sensory Neurons in Dorsal Root Ganglia 139
6.4 Central Sensitization 140
6.5 Conclusion 142
References 142

6.1 INTRODUCTION

Chemotherapy-induced peripheral neuropathy (CIPN) is relatively common following the administration of chemotherapeutic drugs such as vinca alkaloids, taxanes, platinum-derived compounds, and thalidomide. It is also seen in patients receiving newer and more effective anticancer drugs, such as epothilones, bortezomib, and nano-albumin-bounded paclitaxel (Argyriou et al., 2007a, 2007b; Cata et al., 2007; Lee et al., 2006; Roy et al., 2009). Factors that could affect the incidence of CIPN include the type of drugs, dosages, duration of usage, and the pattern of administration (Augusto et al., 2008; Chaudhry et al., 2008; Nurgalieva et al., 2009; Richardson et al., 2006). Different animal models have been explored to mimic symptoms of CIPN in patients and provide a basis for investigation of the pathological processes of CIPN (Authier et al., 2009). This chapter will review progress in preclinical studies of the mechanisms underlying CIPN that may result in new therapeutic strategies for the treatment or prevention of CIPN.

6.2 CHEMOTHERAPY-INDUCED AXON INJURY

One of the common characteristics of CIPN is the stocking-and-glove distribution of sensory disturbances. This has led to the hypothesis that CIPN may result from the direct toxicity of chemotherapeutic drugs on axons of peripheral afferent fibers.

Antitubulins such as vincristine and paclitaxel are thought to disrupt axonal transport by interfering with neuronal microtubule functions (Hiser et al., 2008; Scuteri et al., 2006). Histological studies have found some structural abnormalities, such as defects at the microtubular level, axonal degeneration, demyelination of myelinated fibers, and morphological changes in Schwann cells from both animal and human biopsies (Cavaletti et al., 2007; Persohn et al., 2005; Topp et al., 2000). In agreement with these structural abnormalities, the impairment in conduction velocity of peripheral nerves also seems common in both animals and humans receiving these antitubulin drugs (Authier et al., 2000; Chaudhry et al., 1994; Rowinsky et al., 1993).

The studies mentioned above may be useful to examine the toxicity of antitubulins on nerve fibers, but one question remaining unclear is the neuropathic pain, one of the most disturbing symptoms of CIPN, since either no effect on pain perception or a decreased sensitivity to pain has been found in these studies (Polomano and Bennett, 2001). Recently, several studies have reported no apparent morphological changes in axons in rats that clearly show signs of neuropathic pain after a low-dose paclitaxel treatment (Flatters and Bennett 2006; Polomano et al., 2001). Direct exposure of dorsal root ganglia (DRG) neurons to paclitaxel *in vitro* at chemotherapeutic doses did not impair axonal transport (Horie et al., 1987). TZT-1027, a derivative of dolastatin that disrupts microtubule assembly, does not induce any morphological change in sensory nerves or hyperalgesia (Ogawa et al., 2001). Colchicine, which depolymerizes microtubules like vincristine (Archer et al., 1994; Dahlstrom, 1968), blocks neurogenic plasma extravasation following direct application to the sciatic nerve, yet does not induce neuropathic pain (Kingery et al., 1998; Younger et al., 1991). These data bring into question whether the effect of these drugs on microtubules in primary afferent fibers is the real cause of CIPN. Furthermore, chemotherapeutic drugs such as cisplatin, thalidomide, and bortezomib, which do not target microtubules, induce neuropathy with the same symptoms as antitubulins (Quasthoff and Hartung, 2002). All these studies have suggested mechanisms other than dysfunctions of microtubules in peripheral axons may account for the development of CIPN.

Mitochondrial dysfunction has been proposed as a possible cause of axonopathy induced by CIPN. Bortezomib and oxaliplatin cause mitochondrial injury through an increase in the production of reactive oxygen species and greater inner mitochondrial membrane potential (Joseph and Levine, 2009; Ling et al., 2003). The administration of bortezomib and paclitaxel causes significant increases in the prevalence of atypical (swelling and vacuolated) mitochondria in both myelinated and unmyelinated axons (Flatters and Bennett, 2004, 2006; Flatters et al., 2006; Jin et al., 2008). The application of drugs such as acetyl-L-carnitine and olesoxime, which are known to have mitochondrial protective effects, has proven effective in the treatment of vincristine- and paclitaxel-induced painful neuropathy in animals (Flatters et al., 2006). But in contrast to these studies, the application of inhibitors of the mitochondrial electron transport chain and antioxidants did not eliminate cisplatin-induced painful neuropathy (Flatters and Bennett, 2006; Joseph and Levine, 2009), indicating that dysfunction of mitochondria may be involved in some but not all CIPN.

Intraepidermal nerve fibers (IENFs) represent the free endings of Aδ- and C-fibers (Kalman and Levine, 2005). These IENFs can be immunohistochemically labeled with anti-PGP9.5 antibody recognizing a housekeeping enzyme, ubiquitin

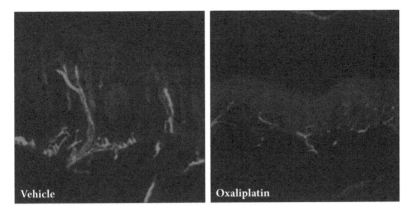

FIGURE 6.1 Loss of intraepidermal nerve endings (IENFs) of glabrous skin is induced by oxaliplatin. Skin tissues are taken from rats 15 days after they are treated with vehicle or oxaliplatin. IENFs are labeled by PGP9.5.

C-terminal hydrolase (Wilkinson et al., 1989), which is expressed at very similar levels by all afferent cell bodies in the DRG (Calzada et al., 1994). Recent studies have reported that degeneration of IENFs has been observed in glabrous skins of animals receiving chronic treatment of paclitaxel, vincristine, and oxaliplatin (Figure 6.1) (Boyette-Davis et al., 2011a; Boyette-Davis and Dougherty, 2011; Jin et al., 2008; Siau et al., 2006). Similar changes of IENF density have been found in patients receiving chronic chemotherapeutic treatment (Boyette-Davis et al., 2011b). Although studies have shown that early treatment with minocycline prevented the development of mechanical hypersensitivity and degeneration of IENFs in both paclitaxel- and oxaliplatin-treated rats (Boyette-Davis et al., 2011a; Boyette-Davis and Dougherty, 2011), it is still not clear whether the degeneration of IENFs is the cause or consequence of CIPN. The degeneration of IENFs seems more related to the status of chronic chemotherapeutic treatment since it is usually prominent around 2 to 3 weeks following chemotherapeutic treatment and persists for several weeks (Boyette-Davis et al., 2011a; Boyette-Davis and Dougherty, 2011; Jin et al., 2008; Siau et al., 2006), while chemotherapy-induced mechanical hypersensitivity (e.g., paclitaxel) in rats occurs as early as several hours (Dina et al., 2001) or 3 to 7 days (Cata et al., 2006a, 2008a; Polomano et al., 2001) after treatment and can last several weeks (Cata et al., 2008a; Dina et al., 2001; Polomano et al., 2001) to several months (Ledeboer et al., 2007). Furthermore, the degeneration of IENFs, which are mostly composed of Aδ- and C-fibers, cannot explain the prominent Aβ neuropathy induced by paclitaxel, though counts for myelinated fibers in dermal papillae also show depletion consistent with this latter sign (Dougherty et al., 2004).

6.3 SENSITIZATION OF PRIMARY SENSORY NEURONS IN DORSAL ROOT GANGLIA

A high incidence of abnormal spontaneous discharges in both myelinated and unmyelinated sensory neurons has been observed in animals treated with both paclitaxel and vincristine (Xiao and Bennett, 2008). A subset of spontaneously firing C-nociceptors shows increased responses to both mechanical and heat stimulation (Tanner et al., 1998). Although the origins (peripheral fiber terminals versus neuronal somata) of spontaneous discharges in primary afferents need to be elucidated, these data have clearly shown the sensitization of primary sensory neurons induced by chemotherapeutic drugs.

The activation of both primary sensory neurons and their supporting cells in DRG has been reported after paclitaxel treatment (Peters et al., 2007). Enhanced expression of voltage-dependent calcium channel $\alpha2\delta1$ subunit in DRG has been found after paclitaxel and oxaliplatin treatment (Gauchan et al., 2009). Targeting calcium channel $\alpha2\delta1$ subunit with gabapentin significantly reduced paclitaxel- and vincristine-induced mechanical allodynia (Matsumoto et al., 2006; Xiao et al., 2007). The administration of oxaliplatin has been shown to modulate the expression of sodium, potassium, and hyperpolarization-activated cyclic nucleotide-gated (HCN) channels in DRG neurons and, targeting HCN channels prevented oxaliplatin-induced hyperalgesia (Descoeur et al., 2011). The transient receptor potential vanilloid (TRPV) channels play important roles in sensing thermal, mechanical, and osmotic stimuli applied to nociceptors. It has been found that TPRV4, which is located in peripheral sensory neurons as a transducer of osmotic and mechanical stimuli, is involved in paclitaxel- and vincristine-induced hyperalgesia (Alessandri-Haber et al., 2008). Oxaliplatin-induced cold allodynia may involve TRPV1, TRPA1, and TRPM8 channels (Anand et al., 2010; Nassini et al., 2011; Ta et al., 2010).

Inflammation and proinflammatory cytokines may also contribute to the sensitization of DRG neurons. Infiltration of macrophages into DRG has been observed in animals receiving vincristine or paclitaxel treatment (Peters et al., 2007). Animals treated with cisplatin showed increased expression of matrix metallopeptidase-9 (MMP9), which is known to be involved in inflammation in DRG (Alaedini et al., 2008). Increased expression of proinflammatory cytokines such as tumor necrosis factor-α (TNFα), interleukin-1β (IL-1β), and interleukin-6 (IL-6) has been found in DRG after chemotherapy (Ledeboer et al., 2007; Ogura et al., 2000). Application of anti-inflammatory cytokine interleukin-10 (IL-10) or minocycline, an antimicrobial agent with anti-inflammatory effects, prevented paclitaxel- or oxaliplatin-induced CIPN (Boyette-Davis et al., 2011a; Boyette-Davis and Dougherty, 2011; Ledeboer et al., 2007).

6.4   CENTRAL SENSITIZATION

Compared to studies regarding the peripheral mechanisms of CIPN (Balayssac et al., 2011), the central mechanisms of CIPN have been less well studied. Previous studies have shown that wide-dynamic-range neurons in spinal dorsal horn display increased incidence of spontaneous activities, enhanced evoked responses to acute natural stimuli, and increased after discharges and windup in animals after treatment of various therapeutic drugs, including paclitaxel, vincristine, cisplatin, and thalidomide (Cata et al., 2004, 2006a, 2006b, 2008b). These data clearly indicate central sensitization can be induced by chemotherapeutic drugs. Several factors may

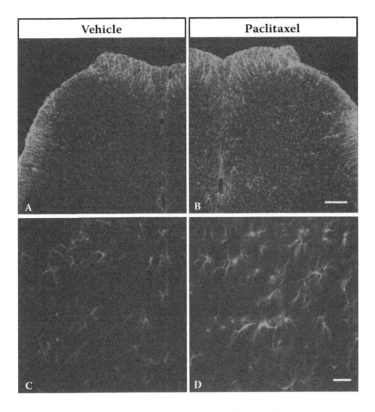

FIGURE 6.2 Paclitaxel induces more expression of glial fibrillary acidic protein (GFAP) (a marker for astrocytes) in the spinal cord indicating the activation of spinal astrocytes. Animals are treated with either paclitaxel (2 mg/kg, once every other day for 4 injections, i.p.) (B and D) or vehicle (A and C). Spinal cord tissues are collected 14 days after the treatment. Scale bar: 200 μm in A and B; 20 μm in C and D.

be involved in the development of central sensitization following chemotherapeutic treatment. It has been found that paclitaxel treatment induces the activation of spinal astrocytes (Figure 6.2) and downregulation of glial glutamate transporters GLAST and GLT-1 (Cata et al., 2006a; Weng et al., 2005). Glutamate is a major excitatory neurotransmitter released from primary afferent terminals and critical for spinal excitatory synaptic transmission. GLAST and GLT-1 are two types of glial glutamate transporters predominantly expressed on spinal astrocytes to uptake glutamate (Liaw et al., 2005; Yaster et al., 2011; Zhang et al., 2009). Blockade of GLAST and GLT-1 induces spontaneous nociceptive behaviors and hypersensitivity to both peripheral thermal and mechanical stimuli in rats (Liaw et al., 2005). Enhanced activities of neurons and excessive activation of postsynaptic AMPA and NMDA receptors in spinal dorsal horn can be induced by blocking GLAST and GLT-1 (Nie and Weng, 2009, 2010; Weng et al., 2007). Downregulation of GLAST and GLT-1 in spinal dorsal horn induced by peripheral nerve injury facilitates the development of neuropathic pain, which is reversed by restoring activity of glial glutamate transporters (Sung et al., 2003; Xin et al., 2009). Besides the impaired uptake of glutamate, increased expression of the voltage-dependent calcium channel $\alpha 2\delta 1$ subunit in spinal dorsal horn was found after treatment with several anticancer drugs (Xiao et al., 2007). The increase of 5-HT_{2A} receptor was also found throughout the dorsal horn after vincristine treatment (Thibault et al., 2008). There is an altered modulation of cannabinoid receptors by vincristine (Rahn et al., 2007). A dysfunction of the nitrous oxide-cyclic guanosine monophosphate (NO/cGMP) pathway could contribute to neuronal hyperexcitability in dorsal horn after chemotherapy (Bujalska and Gumulka, 2008). It is likely that different factors may contribute to the development of central sensitization simultaneously or at different stages during the development of CIPN.

6.5 CONCLUSION

The mechanism of chemotherapy-induced neuropathic pain remains unknown though significant progress has been made by preclinical studies in recent years. Although symptoms of CIPN induced by different types of chemotherapeutic drugs vary, suggesting different mechanisms, a certain identity in the clinical picture of CIPN among divergent chemotherapy drugs also suggests the possibility of some shared mechanisms. Further studies using proper animal models are needed to understand the complete picture of CIPN.

REFERENCES

Alaedini A, Xiang Z, Kim H, Sung YJ, Latov N. 2008. Up-regulation of apoptosis and regeneration genes in the dorsal root ganglia during cisplatin treatment. *Exp Neurol* 210(2):368–74.

Alessandri-Haber N, Dina OA, Joseph EK, Reichling DB, Levine JD. 2008. Interaction of transient receptor potential vanilloid 4, integrin, and SRC tyrosine kinase in mechanical hyperalgesia. *J Neurosci* 28(5):1046–57.

Anand U, Otto WR, Anand P. 2010. Sensitization of capsaicin and icilin responses in oxaliplatin treated adult rat DRG neurons. *Mol Pain* 6:82.

Archer DR, Dahlin LB, McLean WG. 1994. Changes in slow axonal transport of tubulin induced by local application of colchicine to rabbit vagus nerve. *Acta Physiol Scand* 150:57–65.

Argyriou AA, Polychronopoulos P, Iconomou G, Koutras A, Makatsoris T, Gerolymos MK, Gourzis P, Assimakopoulos K, Kalofonos HP, Chroni E. 2007a. Incidence and characteristics of peripheral neuropathy during oxaliplatin-based chemotherapy for metastatic colon cancer. *Acta Oncol* 46(8):1131–37.

Argyriou AA, Polychronopoulos P, Koutras A, Xiros N, Petsas T, Argyriou K, Kalofonos HP, Chroni E. 2007b. Clinical and electrophysiological features of peripheral neuropathy induced by administration of cisplatin plus paclitaxel-based chemotherapy. *Eur J Cancer Care (Engl)* 16(3):231–37.

Augusto C, Pietro M, Cinzia M, Sergio C, Sara C, Luca G, Scaioli V. 2008. Peripheral neuropathy due to paclitaxel: Study of the temporal relationships between the therapeutic schedule and the clinical quantitative score (QST) and comparison with neurophysiological findings. *J Neurooncol* 86(1):89–99.

Authier N, Balayssac D, Marchand F, Ling B, Zangarelli A, Descoeur J, Coudore F, Bourinet E, Eschalier A. 2009. Animal models of chemotherapy-evoked painful peripheral neuropathies. *Neurotherapeutics* 6(4):620–29.

Authier N, Gillet J-P, Fialip J, Eschalier A, Coudore F. 2000. Description of a short-term taxol-induced nociceptive neuropathy in rats. *Brain Res* 887(2):239–49.

Balayssac D, Ferrier J, Descoeur J, Ling B, Pezet D, Eschalier A, Authier N. 2011. Chemotherapy-induced peripheral neuropathies: From clinical relevance to preclinical evidence. *Expert Opin Drug Saf* 10(3):407–17.

Boyette-Davis J, Dougherty PM. 2011. Protection against oxaliplatin-induced mechanical hyperalgesia and intraepidermal nerve fiber loss by minocycline. *Exp Neurol* 229(2):353–57.

Boyette-Davis J, Xin W, Zhang H, Dougherty PM. 2011a. Intraepidermal nerve fiber loss corresponds to the development of taxol-induced hyperalgesia and can be prevented by treatment with minocycline. *Pain* 152(2):308–13.

Boyette-Davis JA, Cata JP, Zhang H, Driver LC, Wendelschafer-Crabb G, Kennedy WR, Dougherty PM. 2011b. Follow-up psychophysical studies in bortezomib-related chemoneuropathy patients. *J Pain* 12:1017–24.

Bujalska M, Gumulka SW. 2008. Effect of cyclooxygenase and nitric oxide synthase inhibitors on vincristine induced hyperalgesia in rats. *Pharmacol Rep* 60(5):735–41.

Calzada B, Naves FJ, Del Valle ME, Vega JA. 1994. Distribution of protein gene product 9.5 (PGP 9.5) immunoreactivity in the dorsal root ganglia of adult rat. *Ann Anat* 176(5):437–41.

Cata JP, Weng HR, Chen JH, Dougherty PM. 2006a. Altered discharges of spinal wide dynamic range neurons and down-regulation of glutamate transporter expression in rats with paclitaxel-induced hyperalgesia. *Neuroscience* 138(1):329–38.

Cata JP, Weng HR, Dougherty PM. 2004. Increased excitability of WDR neurons accompanies paclitaxel-induced hyperalgesia in rats. In *2004 abstract viewer/itinerary planner.* Program 982.4. Washington, DC: Society for Neuroscience.

Cata JP, Weng HR, Dougherty PM. 2008a. The effects of thalidomide and minocycline on taxol-induced hyperalgesia in rats. *Brain Res* 1229:100–10.

Cata JP, Weng H-R, Burton AW, Villareal H, Giralt S, Dougherty PM. 2007. Quantitative sensory findings in patients with bortezomib-induced pain. *J Pain* 8(4):296–306.

Cata JP, Weng H-R, Dougherty PM. 2006b. Clinical and experimental findings in humans and animals with chemotherapy-induced peripheral neuropathy. *Minerva Anes* 72:151–69.

Cata JP, Weng H-R, Dougherty PM. 2008b. Behavioral and electrophysiological studies in rats with cisplatin-induced chemoneuropathy. *Brain Res* 1230:91–98.

Cavaletti G, Gilardini A, Canta A, Rigamonti L, Rodriguez-Menendez V, Ceresa C, Marmiroli P, Bossi M, Oggioni N, D'Incalci M, De Coster R. 2007. Bortezomib-induced peripheral neurotoxicity: A neurophysiological and pathological study in the rat. *Exp Neurol* 204(1):317–25.

Chaudhry V, Cornblath DR, Polydefkis M, Ferguson A, Borrello I. 2008. Characteristics of bortezomib- and thalidomide-induced peripheral neuropathy. *J Peripher Nerv Syst* 13(4):275–82.

Chaudhry V, Rowinsky EK, Sartorius SE, Donehower RC, Cornblath DR. 1994. Peripheral neuropathy from taxol and cisplatin combination chemotherapy: Clinical and electrophysiological studies. *Ann Neurol* 35:304–11.

Dahlstrom A. 1968. Effect of colchicine on transport of amine storage granules in sympathetic nerve of rat. *Eur J Pharmacol* 5:111–13.

Descoeur J, Pereira V, Pizzoccaro A, Francois A, Ling B, Maffre V, Couette B, Busserolles J, Courteix C, Noel J, Lazdunski M, Eschalier A, Authier N, Bourinet E. 2011. Oxaliplatin-induced cold hypersensitivity is due to remodelling of ion channel expression in nociceptors. *EMBO Mol Med* 3(5):266–78.

Dina OA, Chen X, Reichling D, Levine JD. 2001. Role of protein kinase C[epsi] and protein kinase A in a model of paclitaxel-induced painful peripheral neuropathy in the rat. *Neuroscience* 108(3):507–15.

Dougherty PM, Cata JP, Cordella JV, Burton A, Weng H-R. 2004. Taxol-induced sensory disturbance is characterized by preferential impairment of myelinated fiber function in cancer patients. *Pain* 109:132–42.

Flatters SJ, Bennett GJ. 2006. Studies of peripheral sensory nerves in paclitaxel-induced painful peripheral neuropathy: Evidence for mitochondrial dysfunction. *Pain* 122(3):245–57.

Flatters SJ, Xiao WH, Bennett GJ. 2006. Acetyl-L-carnitine prevents and reduces paclitaxel-induced painful peripheral neuropathy. *Neurosci Lett* 397(3):219–23.

Flatters SJL, Bennett GJ. 2004. Ethosuximide reverses paclitaxel- and vincristine-induced painful peripheral neuropathy. *Pain* 109(1–2):150–61.

Gauchan P, Andoh T, Ikeda K, Fujita M, Sasaki A, Kato A, Kuraishi Y. 2009. Mechanical allodynia induced by paclitaxel, oxaliplatin and vincristine: Different effectiveness of gabapentin and different expression of voltage-dependent calcium channel alpha(2) delta-1 subunit. *Biol Pharm Bull* 32(4):732–34.

Hiser L, Herrington B, Lobert S. 2008. Effect of noscapine and vincristine combination on demyelination and cell proliferation *in vitro*. *Leuk Lymphoma* 49(8):1603–9.

Horie H, Takenaka T, Ito S, Kim SU. 1987. Taxol counteracts colchicine blockade of axonal transport in neurites of cultured dorsal root ganglion cells. *Brain Res* 420:144–46.

Jin HW, Flatters SJ, Xiao WH, Mulhern HL, Bennett GJ. 2008. Prevention of paclitaxel-evoked painful peripheral neuropathy by acetyl-L-carnitine: Effects on axonal mitochondria, sensory nerve fiber terminal arbors, and cutaneous Langerhans cells. *Exp Neurol* 210(1):229–37.

Joseph EK, Levine JD. 2009. Comparison of oxaliplatin- and cisplatin-induced painful peripheral neuropathy in the rat. *J Pain* 10(5):534–41.

Kalman M, Levine A. 2005. The skin and other diffuse sensory system. In *Atlas of the sensory organs, functional and clinical anatomy*, ed. Csillag A. Totowa: Humana Press.

Kingery WS, Guo T-Z, Poree LR, Maze M. 1998. Colchicine treatment of the sciatic nerve reduces neurogenic extravasation, but does not affect nociceptive thresholds or collateral sprouting in neuropathic rats. *Pain* 74(1):11–20.

Ledeboer A, Jekich BM, Sloane EM, Mahoney JH, Langer SJ, Milligan ED, Martin D, Maier SF, Johnson KW, Leinwand LA, Chavez RA, Watkins LR. 2007. Intrathecal interleukin-10 gene therapy attenuates paclitaxel-induced mechanical allodynia and proinflammatory cytokine expression in dorsal root ganglia in rats. *Brain Behav Immun* 21:686–98.

Lee JJ, Low JA, Croarkin E, Parks R, Berman AW, Mannan N, Steinberg SM, Swain SM. 2006. Changes in neurologic function tests may predict neurotoxicity caused by ixabepilone. *J Clin Oncol* 24(13):2084–91.

Liaw WJ, Stephens RL Jr., Binns BC, Chu Y, Sepkuty JP, Johns RA, Rothstein JD, Tao YX. 2005. Spinal glutamate uptake is critical for maintaining normal sensory transmission in rat spinal cord. *Pain* 115(1–2):60–70.

Ling YH, Liebes L, Zou Y, Perez-Soler R. 2003. Reactive oxygen species generation and mitochondrial dysfunction in the apoptotic response to bortezomib, a novel proteasome inhibitor, in human H460 non-small cell lung cancer cells. *J Biol Chem* 278(36):33714–23.

Matsumoto M, Inoue M, Hald A, Xie W, Ueda H. 2006. Inhibition of paclitaxel-induced A-fiber hypersensitization by gabapentin. *J Pharmacol Exp Ther* 318(2):735–40.

Nassini R, Gees M, Harrison S, De Siena G, Materazzi S, Moretto N, Failli P, Preti D, Marchetti N, Cavazzini A, Mancini F, Pedretti P, Nilius B, Patacchini R, Geppetti P. 2011. Oxaliplatin elicits mechanical and cold allodynia in rodents via TRPA1 receptor stimulation. *Pain* 152(7):1621–31.

Nie H, Weng HR. 2009. Glutamate transporters prevent excessive activation of NMDA receptors and extrasynaptic glutamate spillover in the spinal dorsal horn. *J Neurophysiol* 101(4):2041–51.

Nie H, Weng HR. 2010. Impaired glial glutamate uptake induces extrasynaptic glutamate spillover in the spinal sensory synapses of neuropathic rats. *J Neurophysiol* 103:2570–80.

Nurgalieva Z, Xia R, Liu CC, Burau K, Hardy D, Du XL. 2009. Risk of chemotherapy-induced peripheral neuropathy in large population-based cohorts of elderly patients with breast, ovarian, and lung cancer. *Am J Ther* 17:148–58.

Ogawa T, Mimura Y, Isowa K, Kato H, Mitsuishi M, Toyoshi T, Kuwayama N, Morimoto H, Murakoshi T, Nakayama T. 2001. An antimicrotubule agent, TZT-1027, does not induce neuropathologic alterations, which are detected after administration of vincristine or paclitaxel in animal models. *Toxicol Lett* 121:97–106.

Ogura K, Ohta S, Ohmori T, Takeuchi H, Hirose T, Horichi N, Okuda K, Ike M, Ozawa T, Siba K, Kasahara K, Sasaki Y, Nakajima H, Adachi M. 2000. Vinca alkaloids induce granulocyte-macrophage colony stimulating factor in human peripheral blood mononuclear cells. *Anticancer Res* 20(4):2383–88.

Persohn E, Canta A, Schoepfer S, Traebert M, Mueller L, Gilardini A, Galbiati S, Nicolini G, Scuteri A, Lanzani F, Giussani G, Cavaletti G. 2005. Morphological and morphometric analysis of paclitaxel and docetaxel-induced peripheral neuropathy in rats. *Eur J Cancer* 41(10):1460–66.

Peters CM, Jimenez-Andrade JM, Jonas BM, Sevcik MA, Koewler NJ, Ghilardi JR, Wong GY, Mantyh PW. 2007. Intravenous paclitaxel administration in the rat induces a peripheral sensory neuropathy characterized by macrophage infiltration and injury to sensory neurons and their supporting cells. *Exp Neurol* 203(1):42–54.

Polomano RC, Bennett GJ. 2001. Chemotherapy-evoked painful peripheral neuropathy. *Pain Med* 2(1):8–14.

Polomano RC, Mannes AJ, Clark US, Bennett GJ. 2001. A painful peripheral neuropathy in the rat produced by the chemotherapeutic drug, paclitaxel. *Pain* 94(3):293–304.

Quasthoff S, Hartung H-P. 2002. Chemotherapy-induced peripheral neuropathy. *J Neurol* 249:9–17.

Rahn EJ, Makriyannis A, Hohmann AG. 2007. Activation of cannabinoid CB1 and CB2 receptors suppresses neuropathic nociception evoked by the chemotherapeutic agent vincristine in rats. *Br J Pharmacol* 152(5):765–77.

Richardson PG, Briemberg H, Jagannath S, Wen PY, Barlogie B, Berenson J, Singhal S, Siegel DS, Irwin D, Schuster M, Srkalovic G, Alexanian R, Rajkumar SV, Limentani S, Alsina M, Orlowski RZ, Najarian K, Esseltine D, Anderson KC, Amatruda T. 2006. Frequency, characteristics, and reversibility of peripheral neuropathy during treatment of advanced multiple myeloma with bortezomib. *J Clin Oncol* 24:3113–20.

Rowinsky EK, Chaudry V, Cornblath DR, Donehower RC. 1993. Neurotoxicity of taxol. *J Natl Cancer Inst Monogr* 15:107–15.

Roy V, LaPlant BR, Gross GG, Bane CL, Palmieri FM. 2009. Phase II trial of weekly nab (nanoparticle albumin-bound)-paclitaxel (nab-paclitaxel) (Abraxane) in combination with gemcitabine in patients with metastatic breast cancer (N0531). *Ann Oncol* 20(3):449–53.

Scuteri A, Nicolini G, Miloso M, Bossi M, Cavaletti G, Windebank AJ, Tredici G. 2006. Paclitaxel toxicity in post-mitotic dorsal root ganglion (DRG) cells. *Anticancer Res* 26(2A):1065–70.

Siau C, Xiao W, Bennett GJ. 2006. Paclitaxel- and vincristine-evoked painful peripheral neuropathies: Loss of epidermal innervation and activation of Langerhans cells. *Exp Neurol* 201:507–14.

Sung B, Lim G, Mao J. 2003. Altered expression and uptake activity of spinal glutamate transporters after nerve injury contribute to the pathogenesis of neuropathic pain in rats. *J Neurosci* 23(7):2899–910.

Ta LE, Bieber AJ, Carlton SM, Loprinzi CL, Low PA, Windebank AJ. 2010. Transient receptor potential vanilloid 1 is essential for cisplatin-induced heat hyperalgesia in mice. *Mol Pain* 6:15.

Tanner KD, Reichling DB, Levine JD. 1998. Nociceptor hyper-responsiveness during vincristine-induced painful peripheral neuropathy in the rat. *J Neurosci* 18(16):6480–91.

Thibault K, Van Steenwinckel J, Brisorgueil MJ, Fischer J, Hamon M, Calvino B, Conrath M. 2008. Serotonin 5-HT2A receptor involvement and Fos expression at the spinal level in vincristine-induced neuropathy in the rat. *Pain* 140(2):305–22.

Topp KS, Tanner KD, Levine JD. 2000. Damage to the cytoskeleton of large diameter sensory neurons and myelinated axons in vincristine-induced painful peripheral neuropathy in the rat. *J Comp Neurol* 424:563–76.

Weng HR, Aravindan N, Cata JP, Chen JH, Shaw AD, Dougherty PM. 2005. Spinal glial glutamate transporters downregulate in rats with taxol-induced hyperalgesia. *Neurosci Lett* 386:18–22.

Weng HR, Chen JH, Pan ZZ, Nie H. 2007. Glial glutamate transporter 1 regulates the spatial and temporal coding of glutamatergic synaptic transmission in spinal lamina II neurons. *Neuroscience* 149(4):898–907.

Wilkinson KD, Lee KM, Deshpande S, Duerksen-Hughes P, Boss JM, Pohl J. 1989. The neuron-specific protein PGP 9.5 is a ubiquitin carboxyl-terminal hydrolase. *Science* 246(4930):670–73.

Xiao WH, Bennett GJ. 2008. Chemotherapy-evoked neuropathic pain: Abnormal spontaneous discharge in A-fiber and C-fiber primary afferent neurons and its suppression by acetyl-L-carnitine. *Pain* 135(3):262–70.

Xiao W, Boroujerdi A, Bennett GJ, Luo ZD. 2007. Chemotherapy-evoked painful peripheral neuropathy: Analgesic effects of gabapentin and effects on expression of the alpha-2-delta type-1 calcium channel subunit. *Neuroscience* 144(2):714–20.

Xin WJ, Weng HR, Dougherty PM. 2009. Plasticity in expression of the glutamate transporters GLT-1 and GLAST in spinal dorsal horn glial cells following partial sciatic nerve ligation. *Mol Pain* 5(1):15.

Yaster M, Guan X, Petralia RS, Rothstein JD, Lu W, Tao YX. 2011. Effect of inhibition of spinal cord glutamate transporters on inflammatory pain induced by formalin and complete Freund's adjuvant. *Anesthesiology* 114(2):412–23.

Younger DS, Mayer SA, Weimer LH, Alderson LM, Seplowitz AH, Lovelace RE. 1991. Colchicine-induced myopathy and neuropathy. *Neurology* 41:943–44.

Zhang HJ, Xin WJ, Dougherty PM. 2009. Synaptically evoked glutamate transporter currents in spinal dorsal horn astrocytes. *Mol Pain* 5:36.

7 *In Vivo* Models and Assessment of Pharmacotherapeutics for Chemotherapy-Induced Neuropathic Pain

Sara Jane Ward

CONTENTS

7.1 Introduction 147
7.2 Models 148
7.3 Pharmacotherapeutics: Preclinical Assessment 150
    7.3.1 Ca^{2+} and Na^+ Channel Blockers 151
    7.3.2 Cytokines and Glial Modulators 152
    7.3.3 Acetyl L-Carnitine 153
    7.3.4 Cannabinoids 153
7.4 Conclusion 157
References 158

7.1 INTRODUCTION

Many chemotherapeutic agents produce significant neuropathies that can lead to cessation of treatment, even in the absence of alternate therapy. Symptoms are typically peripheral and sensory, consisting of mechanical, heat, and cold sensitivities with ongoing burning pain, tingling, and numbness in a glove and stocking distribution. In the worst cases damage can be permanent. There are no Food and Drug Administration (FDA)-approved drugs for the treatment of such neuropathies (chemotherapy-induced peripheral neuropathies [CIPNs]), and mechanisms by which chemotherapeutics induce CIPN remain under investigation. For example, they can affect cellular microtubules and alter axonal transport, disrupt mitochondrial function, or impair DNA synthesis, all of which lead to damage to peripheral nerves. This distal peripheral nerve injury leads to sensitization and spontaneous activity of these fibers. Such nerve injury also leads to hyperexcitability in the dorsal column of the spinal cord and induces infiltration of activated microglia and proinflammatory cytokines, leading to ascending pain pathway sensitization and related changes in substance P and glutamate release. There are also functional changes to the descending inhibitory pain pathway, such as a loss of GABA-releasing neurons and alterations in serotonin and norepinephine signaling, further amplifying the effects of central sensitization. On the basis of these mechanisms, potential therapeutic targets for treatment of CIPN include sodium and calcium channels, GABA receptors, serotonin and norepinephine receptors, N-methyl-aspartic acid (NMDA) receptors, cannabinoid receptors, and agents that suppress cytokine release and activation of microglia, among others. *In vivo* models of chemotherapy-induced neuropathy are currently being used to continue the study into the mechanisms of neurotoxicity and to evaluate the efficacy of putative pharmacotherapies to reverse or prevent CIPN.

7.2   MODELS

In vivo models of CIPN involve the induction of neuropathy in laboratory animals, primarily rats but also mice, by administration of a chemotherapeutic agent. These models are used successfully to study clinically relevant features of neuropathy over a relatively long time course in order to investigate basic mechanisms underlying neuropathy and to test the efficacy of putative therapeutic agents.

The majority of rodent models of CIPN employ repeated systemic injection of the taxane chemotherapeutic agent paclitaxel to induce changes in mechanical or thermal pain threshold. Relatively low doses can be used that do not result in systemic toxicity or motor impairment. In a common dosing regimen in rats, paclitaxel is administered at a dose of 0.5 to 2.0 mg/kg every other day for a total of four doses, producing a neuropathy characterized by heat hyperalgesia, mechanical allodynia and hyperalgesia, and cold allodynia (Polomano et al., 2001; Flatters and Bennett, 2004). On average, changes in sensory sensitivity are detectable by day 5 and can persist for several weeks after the last dose of paclitaxel. Rat models employing higher cumulative doses of paclitaxel have also been used, with the most striking difference being the presence of thermal hypoalgesia which results from a loss of thermal sensation from higher paclitaxel doses (Authier et al., 2000a). Anatomical and functional peripheral nerve fiber abnormalities are also reported at these higher dosing regimens, including sciatic nerve edema (Cavaletti et al., 1995), alterations in myelination (Kilpatrick et al., 2001), and decreases in sensory nerve conduction velocity (Bárdos et al., 2003). Therefore it is important to note that behavioral changes in sensitivity to mechanical and thermal stimuli manifest at lower doses than are required to produce significant anatomical and electrophysiological deficits in these models.

Neuropathies in rodents have also been characterized following systemic administration of platinum agents (e.g., cisplatin, oxaliplatin) and intravenous administration of the vinca alkaloids (e.g., vincristine). For example, rat models of cisplatin-induced neuropathy use a range of low cumulative doses (7.5 to 20 mg/kg) to produce changes in electrophysiological and anatomical properties of sensory nerves and increased sensory sensitivity (Authier et al., 2000b, 2003). Changes in sensory threshold are reported to include mechanical hyperalgesia and allodynia, cold hyperalgesia and allodynia, and thermal hypoalgesia. Higher cumulative doses of cisplatin can also produce alterations in proprioceptive function (Chattopadhyay et al., 2004). In contrast to paclitaxel- and cisplatin-induced neuropathies, a single intravenous dose of vincristine (50 to 200 µg/kg) causes a rapid onset, long-lasting painful peripheral neuropathy in rats characterized by mechanical hyperalgesia and allodynia (Joseph and Levine, 2003). Repeated administration leads to increased sensory sensitivity with additional electrophysiological and anatomical alterations.

These rodent models of CIPN have made a positive impact on both our understanding of the etiology underlying CIPN induced by several chemotherapeutic agents and the directions we have taken clinically for its treatment. However, aspects of the most commonly applied versions of these animal models could be improved along several dimensions. For example, male rats are used almost exclusively in these models (e.g., Pascual et al., 2005; Costa et al., 2007; Comelli et al., 2008; Rahn et al., 2008; Tatsushima et al., 2011; but see Joseph and Levine, 2003), while CIPN is often a particular treatment risk for women, as agents such as paclitaxel are so often the first-line treatment for late-stage gynecological cancers. It is therefore vital to model this neuropathy in female rodents, given the significant sex difference regarding increased rates of neuropathic pain in women versus men, coupled with our current understanding of the presence of sex differences in pharmacological effects of other drugs. Furthermore, while rats are the dominant species used to model CIPN (but see Smith et al., 2004), mice represent the primary species used in genetic animal models for biomedical research, including those of key interest to the present topic. A wider characterization of CIPN behaviors across mouse strains will strengthen efforts to determine key mechanisms underlying successful preclinical treatment outcomes. Last, we are unaware of any publications describing the sensory, anatomical, or functional effects of chemotherapy administration or reversal effects of potential pharmacotherapies using *in vivo* mouse cancer models. Given the global impact that cancer has on multiple organ systems, including the immune and nervous systems, the most accurate modeling of CIPN for further understanding its causes and treatment should incorporate cancer presence.

Behavioral measurements to characterize sensory neuropathy in rodent models of CIPN have relied predominantly on traditional allodynia and algesia measurements, such as sensitivity to mechanical stimulation with von Frey filaments or to thermal stimuli such as a hot plate or application of acetone (cold). These measurements fall into the category of pain-stimulated behaviors (Negus et al., 2010), and while they can be very valuable, their exclusive use has many recognized shortcomings, including poor correlation with verbal reports of pain in sufferers of chronic or neuropathic pain (Skljarevski and Ramadan, 2002). Our laboratory has also begun to characterize the effects of paclitaxel on pain-depressed behavior, defined as "any behavior that decreases in rate, frequency, duration or intensity in response to a noxious stimulus" (Negus et al., 2010, 79–80). We have established a *CIPN-induced decrease in food motivation* procedure, wherein mice trained to respond for a sweet food (vanilla Ensure) under a progressive ratio (PR) schedule of reinforcement are treated with saline or an 8.0 mg/kg × 4 injections paclitaxel regimen. We have observed in this model that paclitaxel significantly suppressed PR responding for Ensure, indicative of a decreased motivation for reward in the paclitaxel-treated mice (Figure 7.1). The paclitaxel-induced decrease in food responding is likely not due to anorexic effects,

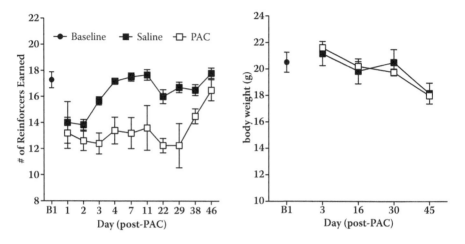

FIGURE 7.1 Effects of paclitaxel on food motivation and body weight in female C57Bl/6 mice. Female mice ($N = 8$/group) were trained to respond for liquid Ensure under a progressive ratio schedule of reinforcement as described in Ward and Dykstra (2005). Following stable PR responding, mice were treated i.p. with saline or 8.0 mg/kg paclitaxel on days 1, 3, 5, and 7, while daily performance on PR responding continued to be assessed. Two-way analysis of variance (ANOVA) revealed a significant effect of treatment and time, and no significant interaction. Bonferroni posttest revealed a significant effect of treatment on days 3 to 29.

in that these mice maintain normal body weight and home cage food consumption throughout the course of treatment. In addition, Porreca and colleagues have also adapted a place conditioning procedure to measure spontaneous pain and negative affect components of neuropathic pain (King et al., 2009; Qu et al., 2011). Therefore we have also established a *CIPN-induced place conditioning* procedure to assess whether paclitaxel treatment induces an aversive state that can be reversed by pain relief, and results of these studies will be discussed in Section 7.3.4.

7.3 PHARMACOTHERAPEUTICS: PRECLINICAL ASSESSMENT

Peripheral neuropathies induced by chemotherapeutic agents are often resistant to standard analgesics. To date, no one drug or drug class is considered to be both a safe and effective analgesic in the treatment of CIPN. The following drugs are used clinically for the treatment of CIPN, although overall results are equivocal for each drug, pain relief, when observed, is generally modest, and side effects can be significant: tricyclic antidepressants (Wolfe et al., 2002), opioids (Levy, 1996), and gabapentin (Bosnjak et al., 2002; Rao et al., 2007). In light of the present lack of a clearly identified safe and effective pharmacotherapy for the treatment or prevention of CIPN, it is obvious that continued efforts to identify such compounds using *in vivo* models of CIPN are critical. It is also important to note, however, that while these *in vivo* models fit the criteria for both face and possibly construct validity, predictive validity of the above-mentioned models remains undetermined. Last, it is also necessary to assess in parallel the potential impact that a putative pharmacotherapy may have on the antitumor efficacy of the chemotherapy itself. The following is an overview of the most promising potential pharmacotherapies currently being investigated in pre-clinical models of CIPN, with most attention paid to cannabinoid-based treatments. Other chapters in this book are dedicated to discussions of pharmacotherapies that have been more thoroughly characterized in human chemotherapy patients.

7.3.1 Ca²⁺ and Na⁺ Channel Blockers

Flatters and Bennett (2004) reported on the first study examining the effect of systemic analgesics on established chemotherapy-induced mechanical sensitivity in rats. In this study, the T-type calcium channel antagonist and antiepileptic drug ethosuximide reversed paclitaxel-induced mechanical allodynia and hyperalgesia and cold allodynia, and vincristine-induced mechanical allodynia and hyperalgesia. The calcium channel antagonist nimodipine also showed neuroprotective effects in a rat CIPN model. More recently, a highly selective Ca(v)3.2 T-type calcium channel antagonist, NNC 55-0396, was reported to reverse paclitaxel-induced mechanical hypersensitivity (Okubo et al., 2011). The neurosteroid and progesterone metabolite allopregnanolone also interact with calcium channels and various other targets, including $GABA_A$ receptors. Allopregnanolone has been shown to exert neuroprotective and analgesic effects, and so it has also been investigated as a potential CIPN treatment. In rats treated with vincristine, alloregnanolone attenuated alterations in nerve conduction velocity while having no impact on antitumor effects of vincristine (Meyer et al., 2010). Importantly, however, the safety of using neurosteroids in patients with hormone-sensitive cancers has been questioned. The antiepileptic drug gabapentin, which blocks the α2-δ ligand of the calcium channel and putatively decreases the firing of sensitized nociceptive neurons, is effective in treating many forms of neuropathy. In rats, repeated administration of gabapentin significantly reduced paclitaxel- and vincristine-induced mechanical sensitivity (Xiao et al., 2007). Xiao et al. (2007) also reported that paclitaxel-induced neuropathy was associated with increased expression of the α2-δ1 subunit that was normalized by repeated gabapentin injections. However, despite the fact that gabapentin is widely used in clinical practice for treatment of CIPN, there is no convincing clinical study evidence to show that it is effective. Pregabalin, also an antiepileptic with a mechanism similar to that of gabapentin, significantly decreased vincristine-induced mechanical allodynia in rats (Nozaki-Taguchi et al., 2001). Pregabalin is a more potent binder to the presynaptic calcium channel and also is effective at treating a wide range of peripheral neuropathies in humans. To date, one small human trial revealed an improvement in oxaliplatin-induced sensory neuropathy in almost 50% of patients that received pregabalin (Saif et al., 2010).

Preclinical studies have also been carried out to investigate the efficacy of systemic administration of sodium channel blockers. Carbamazepine is an antiepileptic drug that blocks voltage-gated sodium channels, and administration in rats has been shown to decrease vincristine-induced mechanical allodynia (Lynch et al., 2004) and paclitaxel-induced thermal and mechanical hyperalgesia (Chogtu et al., 2011). Also, mice treated with the sodium channel blocker mexiletine showed less vincristine-induced thermal hyperalgesia (Kamei et al., 2006). Another study reported that both mexiletine and lidocaine attenuated mechanical allodynia and cold hyperalgesia in oxaliplatin-treated rats (Egashira et al., 2010). The tocainide analog NeP1 was recently identified as a potent blocker of hNav1.4 and hNav1.7 sodium channels that also significantly reduced hyperalgesia in oxaliplatin-treated rats (Ghelardini et al., 2010). Last, the anticonvulsant valproate, which has been demonstrated to be effective in treating diabetic neuropathy in humans, also improved sensory nerve conduction and DRG neuronal survival while also attenuating sensory sensitivity in rats treated with cisplatin (Rodriguez-Menendez et al., 2008). Valproate enhances neurotransmission of GABA by inhibiting GABA transaminase, but it also blocks the voltage-gated sodium channels and T-type calcium channels.

7.3.2 CYTOKINES AND GLIAL MODULATORS

Erythropoietin (EPO) is a cytokine involved in erythropoiesis with clinical utility in the treatment of certain types of anemia. Because other research has also suggested that EPO has neuroprotective and neurotropic effects, the effect of EPO on prevention or treatment of CIPN in animal models has been characterized in several studies. EPO treatment was reported to prevent cisplatin-induced neuropathy in rats by several mechanisms, including prevention of nerve fiber damage, as well as promoting myelination (Orhan et al., 2004). In another study, EPO treatment attenuated cisplatin-induced reduction in sensory nerve conduction velocity and nerve fiber density (Bianchi et al., 2006). Unfortunately, significant concerns regarding the safety of EPO treatment in cancer patients exist and decrease the therapeutic potential of this treatment in humans. As mentioned above, one mechanism by which chemotherapeutic agents likely induced peripheral neuropathy is through activation of microglia and release of several proinflammatory cytokines. Therefore, the ability of the anti-inflammatory cytokine interleukin-10 (IL-10) to reduce CIPN in rats has also been investigated. Ledeboer et al. (2007) reported that paclitaxel treatment induced mRNA expression of the proinflammatory cytokines IL-1 and tumor necrosis factor (TNF), and microglia markers in the dorsal root ganglia (DRG). Intrathecal IL-10 gene therapy prevented paclitaxel-induced mechanical allodynia and increased levels of IL-10 while decreasing levels of IL-1 and TNF in the DRG. They also reported that intrathecal administration of an IL-1 antagonist was able to attenuate paclitaxel-induced mechanical allodynia. Interleukin-6 (IL-6) expression has been associated with repair of damaged nerve fibers and the promotion of axonal growth. It has also been shown that IL-6 administration protected against the development of diabetic neuropathy in streptozotoxin rats (Andriambeloson et al., 2006). Therefore, the potential neuroprotective effect of IL-6 on CIPN has also been investigated in rats (cisplatin and vincristine) and mice (paclitaxel) (Callizot et al., 2008). IL-6 treatment prevented CIPN-induced allodynia produced by all three agents as well as pathological changes in peripheral nerves. Importantly, they also demonstrated that IL-6 did not inhibit the antitumor efficacy of chemotherapy treatment or stimulate tumor growth on its own. Last, the effect of glial cell modulation on CIPN in animals has also been investigated. For example, daily i.p. administration of the glial modulating agent propentofylline attenuated mechanical allodynia induced by vincristine administration. In addition, propentofylline was found to decrease spinal microglial and astrocytic activation also associated with vincristine treatment (Sweitzer et al., 2006). The effect of the glial cell suppressor AV411 (ibudilast) on paclitaxel-induced mechanical allodynia (and other models of neuropathic pain) was also tested in rats (Ledeboer et al., 2007). Repeated administration of AV411 was able to both reverse and prevent paclitaxel-induced allodynia.

7.3.3 Acetyl L-Carnitine

Acetyl L-carnitine (ALC) is synthesized in the mitochondria and has been shown to increase nerve conduction velocity and promote nerve regeneration (Chiechio et al., 2007). It has also shown some efficacy for treatment of diabetic neuropathy and HIV-associated neuropathy in humans, and has been investigated in preclinical studies of CIPN. In an initial report, ALC significantly reduced both cisplatin and paclitaxel neurotoxicity in rats, and this effect was correlated with a modulation of the plasma levels of nerve growth factor (NGF) in the cisplatin-treated animals (Pisano et al., 2003). They also demonstrated that across tumor models ALC did not interfere with the antitumor effects of cisplatin and paclitaxel. ALC was able to positively modulate NGFI-A expression, a gene relevant in the rescue from tissue-specific toxicity. Finally, the transcriptionally ALC-mediated effects were correlated to an increase in histone acetylation. Ghirardi et al. (2005) went on to extend these findings and reported that ALC treatment prevented the onset of mechanical allodynia when coadministered with cisplatin, paclitaxel, or vincristine in rats. They also demonstrated that ALC did not interfere with the antitumor effects of vincristine. Several additional studies have followed to further characterize the mechanisms underlying ALC protection from CIPN in rodents, including its effects on spontaneous discharge in A- and C-fibers of rats treated with chemotherapeutics (Xiao and Bennett, 2008) and neuroprotective effects on axonal mitochondria (Jin et al., 2008). ALC for the treatment of CIPN is also under investigation in clinical trials, and so far results have been encouraging (Bianchi et al., 2005; Maestri et al., 2005).

7.3.4 Cannabinoids

Both licit and illicit cannabinoid-based therapies play a well-established role as adjuncts to cancer chemotherapy treatment, mainly as agents to enhance appetite and reverse chemotherapy-induced nausea and vomiting. In addition, the cannabinoid system is one of several endogenous systems involved in pain modulation, with both natural and synthetic cannabinoids being able to reduce nociceptive behavior in acute pain models and allodynia and hyperalgesia in inflammatory and neuropathic pain models. For example, the nonselective CB1/CB2 agonist delta-9-tetrahydrocannabinol (THC), the main psychoactive ingredient of *Cannabis sativa*, produces robust, long-lasting analgesia, as measured by latency to flick a tail from a noxious stimulus in rats (Lichtman and Martin, 1991), while also significantly reducing mechanical allodynia and thermal hyperalgesia in the rat chronic constriction injury model of neuropathic pain (De Vry et al., 2004). The effects of activation of CB1 and CB2 receptors by synthetic cannabinoid agonists on rodent models of

CIPN have also recently been investigated. In an initial study, Pascual et al. (2005) reported that the nonselective CB agonist WIN 55,212-2 reduced thermal hyperalgesia and mechanical allodynia induced by paclitaxel administration in rats, and that this effect was at least in part CB1 receptor mediated, as the CB1-selective antagonist SR141716 blocked the efficacy of WIN 55,212-2. Subsequently, WIN 55,212-2 was also demonstrated to attenuate vincristine-induced mechanical allodynia in rats (Rahn et al., 2007). This study also investigated the role of CB1 and CB2 receptors in this effect, and found that both CB1- and CB2-selective antagonism alone could partially reverse WIN-induced antiallodynia, and that combined CB1/CB2 antagonism fully blocked the efficacy of WIN-55,212-2 to attenuate mechanical allodynia in vincristine-treated rats. However, it has also been demonstrated that selective activation of CB2 receptors with either AM1241 or AM1714 is sufficient to attenuate paclitaxel-induced mechanical allodynia, an effect blocked by CB2-selective but not CB1-selective antagonism (Rahn et al., 2008). Therefore, activation of either CB1 or CB2 receptors may successfully treat or prevent CIPN. The current understanding of the localization of CB1 versus CB2 receptors is that CB1 receptors are primarily localized to the CNS, while CB2 receptors are most often associated with immune cells, but growing evidence suggests meaningful exceptions to both generalizations. Therefore more work is necessary to identify site(s) and mechanism(s) of action for CB1 or CB2 agonists in ameliorating CIPN. In any case, the potential for successful development of CB receptor agonists is hampered by their association with *Cannabis* and potential unwanted psychoactive effects.

The phytocannabinoid-based pharmacotherapy Sativex, a buccal spray formulation of a 1:1 combination of THC and the nonpsychoactive cannabinoid cannabidiol (CBD), is approved in the EU and Canada for the treatment of multiple sclerosis spasticity with a license in Canada for neuropathic pain as well. In a recent United Kingdom multicenter, double-blind, randomized, placebo-controlled, parallel-group study of Sativex in patients with intractable cancer-related pain, THC:CBD significantly reduced pain scores and was well tolerated (Johnson et al., 2010). Sativex has recently received the attention of the USFDA, who has fast-tracked it directly into several late-stage trials because of its promising efficacy and safety profiles. The addition of CBD in Sativex was primarily intended to attenuate the psychoactive effects of THC and increase patient compliance, but a substantial amount of preclinical evidence now demonstrates that CBD possesses potent antinociceptive, anti-inflammatory, and neuroprotective effects of its own (e.g., Klein, 2005; Jan et al., 2007). For example, daily oral treatment with cannabidiol reduced mechanical and thermal hyperalgesia in rat models of neuropathic (sciatic nerve chronic constriction) and inflammatory (complete Freund's adjuvant intraplantar injection) pain in rats (Costa et al., 2007). In addition to attenuating neuropathic pain states, CBD also inhibits microglial proliferation and proinflammatory cytokine production, including TNF-α and interferon-gamma (IFN-γ), in several *in vivo* mouse models (Carrier et al., 2006; Toth et al., 2010). Furthermore, CBD treatment increased levels of the anti-inflammatory cytokine IL-10 in a murine model of autoimmune diabetes (Weiss et al., 2008) and in response to delayed-type hypersensitivity reactions (Liu et al., 2010). We recently reported that coadministration of CBD prevents the onset of paclitaxel-induced mechanical and cold allodynia in female C57Bl/6 mice (Ward et al., 2011), and we are currently investigating pharmacological and immunomodulatory mechanisms underlying this effect. As mentioned above, CBD is a potent inhibitor of proinflammatory cytokine release and also increases IL-10 in rodent neuropathic pain models. Initial experiments from our laboratory also demonstrate that CBD increases IL-10 levels in paclitaxel-treated mice. CBD exerts many pharmacological actions, but surprisingly, receptor mechanisms underlying its anti-inflammatory, antiallodynic, and neuroprotective effects are largely unconfirmed. For example, CBD exhibits moderate to high affinity for several receptors involved in analgesic actions along the descending pain pathway. While a cannabinoid by name, CBD has no appreciable affinity for CB1 or CB2 receptors. In a recent study in anesthetized rats, however, CBD-induced descending pathway activation and tail flick analgesia were blocked by coadministration of the CB1 antagonist SR141716. CBD binds with μM affinity to the TRPV1 receptor (Bisogno et al., 2001), a mediator of noxious heat and inflammation primarily localized to sensory neurons (Levine and Alessandri-Haber, 2007) that is also an important modulator of descending pain inhibition. Recent studies have identified a role for TRPV1 receptors in CIPN. For example, paclitaxel-induced sensory hypersensitivity was associated with sensitization of the TRPV1 receptor in rats (Chen et al., 2011). Some of CBD's pain-related effects are reversed by the TRPV1 antagonist capsazepine (Costa et al., 2007; Comelli et al., 2008), while others are not (for example, Bitencourt et al., 2008; Maione et al., 2011). CBD has also been well characterized as a direct agonist at serotonin 5-HT$_{1A}$ receptors (Russo et al., 2005; Alves et al., 2010; Gomes et al., 2012; Soares et al., 2010). CBD modulates activity of neurons in the rostroventromedial medulla (RVM) of the descending pain pathway, and this effect was blocked by the 5-HT$_{1A}$ antagonist WAY 100635 (Maione et al., 2011). Adenosine A1 receptors, with established involvement in neuropathic pain by Eisenach and colleagues (Gomes et al., 1999; Zhang et al., 2005), have recently been linked to CBD's pharmacological effects, including descending pain modulation (Maione et al., 2011). CBD indirectly increases adenosine signaling by decreasing adenosine uptake, a potential mechanism by which the adenosine system plays a role in CBD anti-inflammation (Carrier et al., 2006). To date, we have determined that the preventive effects of CBD in our mouse model of paclitaxel-induced neuropathic pain can be blocked by antagonism of 5-HT1A receptors, while CB1 receptor activation is not involved. It remains to be determined whether TRPV1 or A2A receptor activation also plays a role in CBD's positive effects in a CIPN animal model (Figure 7.2) (Ward et al., in preparation).

As mentioned toward the beginning of this chapter, we believe it is also important to consider alternate animal models of CIPN that do not rely on responses to applied mechanical or thermal stimuli. In the CIPN-induced decrease in food motivation model described above (Figure 7.1), administering CBD following the observed decrease in motivation significantly reverses the paclitaxel-induced reduction in responding. Also mentioned above, we have established a CIPN-induced place conditioning procedure to assess whether paclitaxel treatment induces an aversive state that can be reversed by pain relief. In the CIPN-induced place conditioning procedure, mice are treated with either vehicle or the four-injection paclitaxel regimen. Following the onset of mechanical allodynia in the paclitaxel-treated group, mice are conditioned in standard mouse conditioning chambers with alternating injections

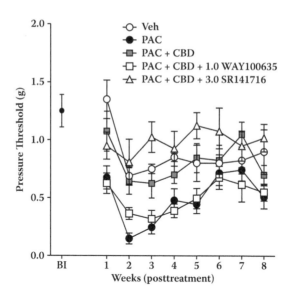

FIGURE 7.2 5-HT$_{1A}$-selective antagonism, and not CB1 antagonism, blocks CBD prevention of paclitaxel-induced mechanical allodynia in female C57Bl/6 mice. Female mice (N = 8/group) were treated with cremophor vehicle, 8.0 mg/kg PAC, 8.0 mg/kg PAC + 5.0 CBD, 8.0 mg/kg PAC + 5.0 CBD + 1.0 mg/kg WAY 100635, or 8.0 mg/kg PAC + 5.0 CBD + 3.0 mg/kg SR141716 on days 1, 3, 5, and 7. All treatment groups received three i.p. injections. Mechanical allodynia was measured prior to treatment and weekly after initiation of treatment. PAC-treated mice demonstrated a robust mechanical allodynia that was prevented by coadministration of CBD. Additional administration of WAY 100635 blocked this prevention, while SR141716 was without effect. Two-way ANOVA revealed significant effects of treatment and time and no interaction. Bonferroni posttests revealed a significant decrease in PAC versus Veh, a significant increase in CBD versus PAC, and a significant decrease in WAY versus Veh and WAY versus CBD on mechanical sensitivity.

of vehicle or 5.0 mg/kg CBD. We observed that on test day, paclitaxel-treated mice spent significantly more time in the CBD-paired compartment than vehicle-treated controls, demonstrating that CBD is not rewarding in saline-treated mice but is rewarding to mice experiencing CIPN. Taken together, both models represent novel ways to characterize CIPN and measure the efficacy of novel pharmacotherapies such as CBD.

Perhaps the most unique and exciting aspect of cannabinoid-based adjuncts to cancer chemotherapy treatment as antineuropathic agents is the parallel attention natural and synthetic cannabinoids have long received as antineoplastic agents in their own right (see Oesch and Gertsch, 2009, for review). Administration of cannabinoid agonists, including THC to rats or mice, has been shown, for example, to induce the regression of lung adenocarcinomas (Munson et al., 1975), gliomas (Galve-Roperh et al., 2000), thyroid epitheliomas (Bifulco et al., 2001), lymphomas (McKallip et al., 2002), skin carcinomas (Casanova et al., 2003), and breast carcinomas (Caffarel et al., 2006). Moreover, the CB agonist anandamide synergistically enhances paclitaxel-induced apoptosis on a gastric cancer cell line (Miyato et al., 2009), while the CB agonist HU 210, in combination with the antimetabolite chemotherapeutic agent 5-flourouracil (5-FU), produces synergistic cytotoxic effects in colorectal carcinoma cells (Gustafsson et al., 2009). Taken together, these data all point to the prospect of a combined chemotherapeutic regimen including a CB receptor-targeted treatment that possesses the added benefit of counteracting potential neurotoxic effects of another chemotherapeutic, such as paclitaxel.

The nonpsychoactive phytocannabinoid CBD has also been demonstrated to produce antitumor activity (Ligresti et al., 2006; McAllister et al., 2007, 2011). For example, CBD can reduce glioma cell viability *in vitro* (Jacobsson et al., 2000) and *in vivo* (Massi et al., 2004). CBD also reduces the growth of aggressive human breast cancer cells and breast cancer cell invasiveness *in vitro* and attenuates primary tumor growth as well as metastasis into the lung in an *in vivo* mouse model of breast cancer (McAllister et al., 2007, 2011). There are several other examples of CBD's antiproliferative and antimetastasis effects on other cancer types in the literature as well. Interestingly, CBD and THC were also found to act synergistically to inhibit cell proliferation in two glioblastoma cell lines, and each agent alone was shown to work through a distinct mechanism, suggesting again that CBD is not working through CB receptors (Marcu et al., 2010). Last, we have also now observed that CBD and paclitaxel can work synergistically to inhibit the viability of 4T1 breast cancer cells *in vitro* (Ward et al., in preparation). Again these data strongly suggest that a CBD component to a combination chemotherapy regimen can augment antineoplastic efficacy while preventing CIPN induced by many commonly used chemotherapeutics.

7.4 CONCLUSION

Over the last decade, *in vivo* rodent models of CIPN have been established for the most common neurotoxic chemotherapeutic agents, including paclitaxel, cisplatin, oxaliplatin, and vincristine. These animal models seem to accurately mimic the sensory abnormalities associated with CIPN induced by select agents and have shed light on underlying alterations in structure and function of the nervous system. Furthermore, several drugs that interact with specific channels, receptors, or immune system actions have shown positive results in these models by reversing or preventing sensory, physiological, or immune abnormalities. To date, the most effective preclinical interventions include calcium and sodium channel blockers, glial- or cytokine-directed therapies, acetyl L-carnitine, and cannabinoids. Some of these therapies are associated with concerns over potential negative interactions with cancer activity (allopregnanolone, EPO), while other compounds have been tested preclinically and show no negative impact on tumor activity (ALC, IL-6), and still other agents have demonstrated potent antineoplastive properties in their own right (cannabinoids). However, preclinical assessments using these models also seem to lead to some false positives, suggesting that improvements along many dimensions can be made. For example, more CIPN modeling should incorporate female rodent models, given the increased sensitivity of females to neuropathic pain states and the known differential effects some pharmacotherapies can have in males versus females. CIPN effects in mouse models should also be more extensively characterized, which will increase our ability to determine mechanisms of action using mutant mouse models and to assess putative CIPN treatments in mouse cancer models. Last, measurements of CIPN should extend from stimulus-evoked withdrawal reflexes to include assessment of chemotherapy-induced pain-depressed behaviors and changes in affect, and the reestablishment of healthy behaviors by successful treatments.

REFERENCES

Alves FH, Crestani CC, Gomes FV, Guimarães FS, Correa FM, Resstel LB. (2010). Cannabidiol injected into the bed nucleus of the stria terminalis modulates baroreflex activity through 5-HT1A receptors. *Pharmacol Res* 62(3):228–36.

Andriambeloson E, Baillet C, Vitte PA, Garotta G, Dreano M, Callizot N. (2006). Interleukin-6 attenuates the development of experimental diabetes-related neuropathy. *Neuropathology* 26(1):32–42.

Authier N, Gillet JP, Fialip J, Eschalier A, Coudore F. (2000a). Description of a short-term taxol-induced nociceptive neuropathy in rats. *Brain Res* 887:239–49.

Authier N, Fialip J, Eschalier A, Coudore F. (2000b). Assessment of allodynia and hyperalgesia after cisplatin administration to rats. *Neurosci Lett* 291:73–76.

Authier N, Gillet JP, Fialip J, Eschalier A, Coudore F. (2003). An animal model of nociceptive peripheral neuropathy following repeated cisplatin injections. *Exp Neurol* 182:12–20.

Bárdos G, Móricz K, Jaszlits L, Rabioczky G, Tory K, Racz I, Berman S, Sumegi B, Farkas B, Literáti-Nagi B, Literáti-Nagi P. (2003). BGP-15, a hydroximic acid derivative, protects against cisplatin- or taxol-induced peripheral neuropathy in rats. *Toxicol Appl Pharmacol* 190:9–16.

Bianchi et al. (2005). Symptomatic and neurophysiological responses of paclitaxel- or cisplatin-induced neuropathy to oral acetyl-L-carnitine. *Eur J Cancer* 41:1746–50.

Bianchi R, Brines M, Lauria G, Savino C, Gilardini A, Nicolini G, Rodriguez-Menendez V, Oggioni N, Canta A, Penza P, Lombardi R, Minoia C, Ronchi A, Cerami A, Ghezzi P, Cavaletti G. (2006). Protective effect of erythropoietin and its carbamylated derivative in experimental cisplatin peripheral neurotoxicity. *Clin Cancer Res* 12(8):2607–12.

Bifulco M, Laezza C, Portella G, Vitale M, Orlando P, De Petrocellis L, Di Marzo V. (2001). Control by the endogenous cannabinoid system of ras oncogene-dependent tumor growth. *FASEB J* 15(14):2745–47.

Bisogno T, Hanus L, De Petrocellis L, Tchilibon S, Ponde DE, Brandi I, Moriello AS, Davis JB, Mechoulam R, Di Marzo V. (2001). Molecular targets for cannabidiol and its synthetic analogues: Effect on vanilloid VR1 receptors and on the cellular uptake and enzymatic hydrolysis of anandamide. *Br J Pharmacol* 134(4):845–52.

Bitencourt RM, Pamplona FA, Takahashi RN. (2008). Facilitation of contextual fear memory extinction and anti-anxiogenic effects of AM404 and cannabidiol in conditioned rats. *Eur Neuropsychopharmacol* 18(12):849–59.

Bosnjak S, Jelik S, Susnjar S, Lukic V. (2002). Gabapentin for relief of neuropathic pain related to anticancer treatment: A preliminary study. *J Chemother* 14:214–19.

Caffarel MM, Sarrió D, Palacios J, Guzmán M, Sánchez C. (2006). Delta9-tetrahydrocannabinol inhibits cell cycle progression in human breast cancer cells through Cdc2 regulation. *Cancer Res* 66(13):6615–21.

Callizot N, Andriambeloson E, Glass J, Revel M, Ferro P, Cirillo R, Vitte PA, Dreano M. (2008). Interleukin-6 protects against paclitaxel, cisplatin and vincristine-induced neuropathies without impairing chemotherapeutic activity. *Cancer Chemother Pharmacol* 62(6):995–1007.

Carrier EJ, Auchampach JA, Hillard CJ. (2006). Inhibition of an equilibrative nucleoside transporter by cannabidiol: A mechanism of cannabinoid immunosuppression. *Proc Natl Acad Sci USA* 103(20):7895–900.

Casanova ML, Blázquez C, Martínez-Palacio J, Villanueva C, Fernández-Aceñero MJ, Huffman JW, Jorcano JL, Guzmán M. (2003). Inhibition of skin tumor growth and angiogenesis *in vivo* by activation of cannabinoid receptors. *J Clin Invest* 111(1):43–50.

Cavaletti G, et al. (1995). Experimental peripheral neuropathy induced in adult rats by repeated administration of taxol. *Exp Neurol* 133:64–72.

Chattopadhyay M, Goss J, Wolfe D, Goins WC, Huang S, Glorioso JC, Mata M, Fink DJ. (2004). Protective effect of herpes simplex virus-mediated neurotrophin gene transfer in cisplatin neuropathy. *Brain* 127:929–39.

Chen Y, Yang C, Wang ZJ. (2011). Proteinase-activated receptor 2 sensitizes transient receptor potential vanilloid 1, transient receptor potential vanilloid 4, and transient receptor potential ankyrin 1 in paclitaxel-induced neuropathic pain. *Neuroscience* 13(193):440–51.

Chiechio S, Copani A, Gereau RW 4th, Nicoltti F. (2007). Acetyl-L-carnitine in neuropathic pain: Experimental data. *CNS Drugs* 21(Suppl 1):31–38.

Chogtu B, Bairy KL, Smitha D, Dhar S, Himabindu P. (2011). Comparison of the efficacy of carbamazepine, gabapentin and lamotrigine for neuropathic pain in rats. *Indian J Pharmacol* 43(5):596–98.

Comelli F, Giagnoni G, Bettoni I, Colleoni M, Costa B. (2008). Antihyperalgesic effect of a *Cannabis sativa* extract in a rat model of neuropathic pain: Mechanisms involved. *Phytother Res.* 22(8):1017–24.

Costa B, Trovato AE, Comelli F, Giagnoni G, Colleoni M. (2007). The non-psychoactive *Cannabis* constituent cannabidiol is an orally effective therapeutic agent in rat chronic inflammatory and neuropathic pain. *Eur J Pharmacol* 556(1–3):75–83.

De Vry J, Denzer D, Reissmueller E, Eijckenboom M, Heil M, Meier H, Mauler F. (2004). 3-[2-Cyano-3-(trifluoromethyl)phenoxy]phenyl-4,4,4-trifluoro-1-butanesulfonate (BAY 59–3074): A novel cannabinoid Cb1/Cb2 receptor partial agonist with antihyperalgesic and antiallodynic effects. *J Pharmacol Exp Ther* 310(2):620–32.

Egashira N, Hirakawa S, Kawashiri T, Yano T, Ikesue H, Oishi R. (2010). Mexiletine reverses oxaliplatin-induced neuropathic pain in rats. *J Pharmacol Sci* 112:473–76.

Flatters SJ, Bennett GJ. (2004). Ethosuxamide reverses paclitaxel- and vincristine-induced painful peripheral neuropathy. *Pain* 109:150–61.

Galve-Roperh I, Sánchez C, Cortés ML, Gómez del Pulgar T, Izquierdo M, Guzmán M. (2000). Anti-tumoral action of cannabinoids: Involvement of sustained ceramide accumulation and extracellular signal-regulated kinase activation. *Nat Med* 6(3):313–19.

Ghelardini C, Desaphy JF, Muraglia M, Corbo F, Matucci R, Dipalma A, Bertucci C, Pistolozzi M, Nesi M, Norcini M, Franchini C, Camerino DC. (2010). Effects of a new potent analog of tocainide on hNav1.7 sodium channels and *in vivo* neuropathic pain models. *Neuroscience* 169(2):863–73.

Ghirardi O, Vertechy M, Vesci L, Canta A, Nicolini G, Galbiati S, Ciogli C, Quattrini G, Pisano C, Cundari S, Rigamonti LM. (2005). Chemotherapy-induced allodinia: Neuroprotective effect of acetyl-L-carnitine. *In Vivo* 19(3):631–37.

Gomes FV, Reis DG, Alves FH, Corrêa FM, Guimares FS, Resstel LB. (2012). Cannabidiol injected into the bed nucleus of the stria terminalis reduces the expression of contextual fear conditioning via 5-HT1A receptors. *J Psychopharmacol* 26(1):104–13.

Gomes JA, Li X, Pan HL, Eisenach JC. (1999). Intrathecal adenosine interacts with a spinal noradrenergic system to produce antinociception in nerve-injured rats. *Anesthesiology* 91(4):1072–79.

Gustafsson SB, Lindgren T, Jonsson M, Jacobsson SO. (2009). Cannabinoid receptor-independent cytotoxic effects of cannabinoids in human colorectal carcinoma cells: Synergism with 5-fluorouracil. *Cancer Chemother Pharmacol* 63(4):691–701.

Jacobsson SO, Rongård E, Stridh M, Tiger G, Fowler CJ. (2000). Serum-dependent effects of tamoxifen and cannabinoids upon C6 glioma cell viability. *Biochem Pharmacol* 60(12):1807–13.

Jan TR, Su ST, Wu HY, Liao MH. (2007). Suppressive effects of cannabidiol on antigen-specific antibody production and functional activity of splenocytes in ovalbumin-sensitized BALB/c mice. *Int Immunopharmacol* 7(6):773–80.

Jin HW, Flatters SJ, Xiao WH, Mulhern HL, Bennett GJ. (2008). Prevention of paclitaxel-evoked painful peripheral neuropathy by acetyl-L-carnitine: Effects on axonal mitochondria, sensory nerve fiber terminal arbors, and cutaneous Langerhans cells. *Exp Neurol* 210:229–37.

Johnson JR, Burnell-Nugent M, Lossignol D, Ganae-Motan ED, Potts R, Fallon MT. (2010). Multicenter, double-blind, randomized, placebo-controlled, parallel-group study of the efficacy, safety, and tolerability of THC:CBD extract and THC extract in patients with intractable cancer-related pain. *J Pain Symptom Manage* 39(2):167–79.

Joseph EK, Levine JD. (2003). Sexual dimorphism for protein kinase c epsilon signaling in a rat model of vincristine-induced painful peripheral neuropathy. *Neuroscience* 119(3):831–38.

Kamei J, Nozaki C, Saitoh A. (2006). Effect of mexilietine on vincristine-induced painful neuropathy in mice. *Eur J Pharmacol* 536:123–27.

King T, Vera-Portocarrero L, Gutierrez T, Vanderah TW, Dussor G, Lai J, Fields HL, Porreca F. (2009). Unmasking the tonic-aversive state in neuropathic pain. *Nat Neurosci* 12(11):1364–66.

Kilpatrick TJ, Phan S, Reardon K, Lopes EC, Cheema SS. (2001). Leukemia inhibitory factor abrogates paclitaxel-induced axonal atrophy in the Wistar rat. *Brain Res* 911:163–67.

Klein TW. (2005). Cannabinoid-based drugs as anti-inflammatory therapeutics. *Nat Rev Immunol* 5(5):400–11.

Ledeboer A, Jekich BM, Sloane EM, Mahoney JH, Langer SJ, Milligan ED, Martin D, Maier SF, Johnson KW, Leinwand LA, Chavez RA, Watkins LR. (2007). Intrathecal interleukin-10 gene therapy attenuates paclitaxel-induced mechanical allodynia and proinflammatory cytokine expression in dorsal root ganglia in rats. *Brain Behav Immun* 21(5):686–98.

Levine JD, Alessandri-Haber N. (2007). TRP channels: Targets for the relief of pain. *Biochim Biophys Acta* 1772(8):989–1003.

Levy MH. (1996). Drug therapy: Pharmacological treatment of cancer pain. *New Engl J Med* 335:1124–32.

Lichtman AH, Martin BR. (1991). Spinal and supraspinal components of cannabinoid-induced antinociception. *J Pharmacol Exp Ther* 258(2):517–23.

Ligresti A, Moriello AS, Starowicz K, Matias I, Pisanti S, De Petrocellis L, Laezza C, Portella G, Bifulco M, Di Marzo V. (2006). Antitumor activity of plant cannabinoids with emphasis on the effect of cannabidiol on human breast carcinoma. *J Pharmacol Exp Ther* 318:1375–87.

Liu DZ, Hu CM, Huang CH, Wey SP, Jan TR. (2010). Cannabidiol attenuates delayed-type hypersensitivity reactions via suppressing T-cell and macrophage reactivity. *Acta Pharmacol Sin* 31(12):1611–17.

Lynch JJ 3rd, Wade CL, Zhong CM, Mikusa JP, Honore P. (2004). Attenuation of mechanical allodynia by clinically utilized drugs in a rat chemotherapy-induced neuropathic pain model. *Pain* 110(1–2):56–63.

Maestri A, De Pasquale Ceratti A, Cundari S, Zanna C, Cortesi E, Crino L. (2005). A pilot study on the effect of acetyl-L-carnitine in paclitaxel- and cisplatin- induced peripheral neuropathy. *Tumori* 91:135–38.

Maione S, Piscitelli F, Gatta L, Vita D, De Petrocellis L, Palazzo E, de Novellis V, Di Marzo V. (2011). Non-psychoactive cannabinoids modulate the descending pathway of antinociception in anaesthetized rats through several mechanisms of action. *Br J Pharmacol* 162(3):584–96.

Marcu JP, Christian RT, Lau D, Zielinski AJ, Horowitz MP, Lee J, Pakdel A, Allison J, Limbad C, Moore DH, Yount, GL, Desprez PY, McAllister SD. (2010). Cannabidiol enhances the inhibitory effects of Delta9-tetrahydrocannabinol on human glioblastoma cell proliferation and survival. *Mol Cancer Ther* 9(1):180–89.

Massi P, Vaccani A, Ceruti S, Colombo A, Abbracchio MP, Parolaro D. (2004). Antitumor effects of cannabidiol, a nonpsychoactive cannabinoid, on human glioma cell lines. *J Pharmacol Exp Ther* 308(3):838–45.

McAllister SD, Christian RT, Horowitz MP, Garcia A, Desprez PY. (2007). Cannabidiol as a novel inhibitor of Id-1 gene expression in aggressive breast cancer cells. *Mol Cancer Ther* 6:2921–27.

McAllister SD, Murase R, Christian RT, Lau D, Zielinski AJ, Allison J, Almanza C, Pakdel A, Lee J, Limbad C, Liu Y, Debs RJ, Moore DH, Desprez PY. (2011). Pathways mediating the effects of cannabidiol on the reduction of breast cancer cell proliferation, invasion, and metastasis. *Breast Cancer Res Treat* 129(1):37–47.

McKallip RJ, Lombard C, Fisher M, Martin BR, Ryu S, Grant S, Nagarkatti PS, Nagarkatti M. (2002). Targeting CB2 cannabinoid receptors as a novel therapy to treat malignant lymphoblastic disease. *Blood* 100(2):627–34.

Meyer L, Patte-Mesah C, Taleb O, Mensah-Nyagan AG. (2010). Cellular and functional evidence for a protective action of neurosteroids against vincristine chemotherapy-induced painful neuropathy. *Cell Mol Life Sci* 67:3017–34.

Miyato H, Kitayama J, Yamashita H, Souma D, Asakage M, Yamada J, Nagawa H. (2009). Pharmacological synergism between cannabinoids and paclitaxel in gastric cancer cell lines. *J Surg Res* 155(1):40–7.

Munson AE, Harris LS, Friedman MA, Dewey WL, Carchman RA. (1975). Antineoplastic activity of cannabinoids. *J Natl Cancer Inst* 55(3):597–602.

Negus SS, Bilsky EJ, Do Carmo GP, Stevenson GW. (2010). Rationale and methods for assessment of pain-depressed behavior in preclinical assays of pain and analgesia. *Methods Mol Biol* 617:79–91.

Nozaki-Taguchi N, Chaplan SR, Higuera ES, Ajakwe RC, Yaksh TL. (2001). Vincristine-induced allodynia in the rat. *Pain* 93:69–76.

Oesch S, Gertsch J. (2009). Cannabinoid receptor ligands as potential anticancer agents—High hopes for new therapies? *J Pharm Pharmacol* 61(7):839–53.

Okubo K, Takahashi T, Sekiguchi F, Kanaoka D, Matsunami M, Ohkubo T, Yamazaki J, Fukushima N, Yoshida S, Kawabata A. (2011). Inhibition of T-type calcium channels and hydrogen sulfide-forming enzyme reverses paclitaxel-evoked neuropathic hyperalgesia in rats. *Neuroscience* 188:148–56.

Orhan B, Yalcin S, Nurlu G, Zeybek D, Muftuoglu S. (2004). Erythropoietin against cisplatin-induced peripheral neurotoxicity in rats. *Med Oncol* 21(2):197–203.

Pascual D, Goicoechea C, Suardíaz M, Martín MI. (2005). A cannabinoid agonist, WIN 55,212-2, reduces neuropathic nociception induced by paclitaxel in rats. *Pain* 118(1–2):23–34.

Pisano C, Pratesi G, Laccabue D, Zunino F, Lo Giudice P, Bellucci A, Pacifici L, Camerini B, Vesci L, Castorina M, Cicuzza S, Tredici G, Marmiroli P, Nicolini G, Galbiati S, Calvani M, Carminati P, Cavaletti G. (2003). Paclitaxel and cisplatin-induced neurotoxicity: A protective role of acetyl-L-carnitine. *Clin Cancer Res* 9(15):5756–67.

Polomano RC, Mannes AL, Clark US, Bennett GJ. (2001). A painful peripheral neuropathy in the rat produced by the chemotherapeutic drug paclitaxel. *Pain* 94:293–304.

Qu C, King T, Okun A, Lai J, Fields HL, Porreca F. (2011). Lesion of the rostral anterior cingulate cortex eliminates the aversiveness of spontaneous neuropathic pain following partial or complete axotomy. *Pain* 152(7):1641–48.

Rahn EJ, Makriyannis A, Hohmann AG. (2007). Activation of cannabinoid CB1 and CB2 receptors suppresses neuropathic nociception evoked by the chemotherapeutic agent vincristine in rats. *Br J Pharmacol* 152(5):765–77.

Rahn EJ, Zvonok AM, Thakur GA, Khanolkar AD, Makriyannis A, Hohmann AG. (2008). Selective activation of cannabinoid CB2 receptors suppresses neuropathic nociception induced by treatment with the chemotherapeutic agent paclitaxel in rats. *J Pharmacol Exp Ther* 327(2):584–91.

Rao RD, Michalak JC, Sloan JA, Loprinzi CL, Soori GS, Mikcevich DA, Warner DO, Novotny P, Kutteh LA, Wong GY; North Central Cancer Treatment Group. (2007). North Central Cancer Treatment Group. Efficacy of gabapentic in the management of chemotherapy-induced neuropathic peripheral neuropathy: A phase 3 randomized, double-blind, placebo controlled crossover trial (N00C3). *Cancer* 110:2110–18.

Rodriguez-Menendez V, Gilardini A, Bossi M, Canta A, Oggioni N, Carozzi V, Tremolizzo L, Cavaletti G. (2008). Valproate protective effects on cisplatin-induced peripheral neuropathy: An *in vitro* and *in vivo* study. *Anticancer Res* 28(1A):335–42.

Russo EB, Burnett A, Hall B, Parker KK. (2005). Agonistic properties of cannabidiol at 5-HT1a receptors. *Neurochem Res* 30(8):1037–43.

Saif MW, Syrigos K, Kaley K, Isufi I. (2010). Role of pregabalin in treatment of oxaliplatin-induced sensory neuropathy. *Anticancer Res* 30:2927–33.

Skljarevski V, Ramadan NM. (2002). The nociceptive flexion reflex in humans—Review article. *Pain* 96(1–2):3–8.

Smith SB, Crager SE, Mogil JS. (2004). Paclitaxel-induced neuropathic hypersensitivity in mice: Responses in 10 inbred mouse strains. *Life Sci* 74(21):2593–604.

Soares Vde P, Campos AC, Bortoli VC, Zangrossi H Jr, Guimarães FS, Zuardi AW. (2010). Intra-dorsal periaqueductal gray administration of cannabidiol blocks panic-like response by activating 5-HT1A receptors. *Behav Brain Res* 213(2):225–29.

Sweitzer SM, Pahl JL, DeLeo JA. (2006). Propentofylline attenuates vincristine-induced peripheral neuropathy in the rat. *Neurosci Lett* 400(3):258–61.

Tatsushima Y, Egashira N, Kawashiri T, Mihara Y, Yano T, Mishima K, Oishi R. (2011). Involvement of substance P in the peripheral neuropathy induced by paclitaxel but not by oxaliplatin. *J Pharmacol Exp Ther* 337(1):226–35.

Toth CC, Jedrzejewski NM, Ellis CL, Frey WH 2nd. (2010). Cannabinoid-mediated modulation of neuropathic pain and microglial accumulation in a model of murine type I diabetic peripheral neuropathic pain. *Mol Pain* 6:16.

Ward SJ, Dykstra LA. (2005). The role of CB1 receptors in sweet versus fat reinforcement: Effect of CB1 receptor deletion, CB1 receptor antagonism (SR141716A) and CB1 receptor agonism (CP-55940). *Behav Pharmacol* 16(5–6):381–88.

Ward SJ, Ramirez MD, Neelakantan H, Walker EA. (2011). Cannabidiol prevents the development of cold and mechanical allodynia in paclitaxel-treated female C57Bl6 mice. *Anesth Analg* 113(4):947–50.

Ward SJ, Walker EA, Neelakantan H, McAllister SD. Cannabidiol (CBD) for prevention of paclitaxel-induced neuropathic pain: Efficacy, mechanisms and safety in mice. *J Pharmacol Exp Ther*, in preparation.

Weiss L, Zeira M, Reich S, Slavin S, Raz I, Mechoulam R, Gallily R. (2008). Cannabidiol arrests onset of autoimmune diabetes in NOD mice. *Neuropharmacology* 54(1):244–49.

Wolfe GI, Hotz SE, Barohn RJ. (2002). Treatment of painful peripheral neuropathy. *J Clin Neuromuscul Dis* 4(2):50–59.

Xiao W, Boroujerdi A, Bennett GJ, Luo ZD. (2007). Chemotherapy-evoked painful peripheral neuropathy: Analgesic effects of gabapentin and effects on expression of the alpha-2-delta type-1 calcium channel subunit. *Neuroscience* 144(2):714–20.

Xiao WH, Bennett GJ. (2008). Chemotherapy-evoked neuropathic pain: Abnormal spontaneous discharge in A-fiber and C-fiber primary afferent neurons and its suppression by acetyl-L-carnitine. *Pain* 135(3):262–70.

Zhang Y, Conklin DR, Li X, Eisenach JC. (2005). Intrathecal morphine reduces allodynia after peripheral nerve injury in rats via activation of a spinal A1 adenosine receptor. *Anesthesiology* 102(2):416–20.

8 Drug Treatment for Chemotherapy-Induced Neuropathic Pain
Amitriptyline as an Example

Eija Kalso

CONTENTS

8.1 Introduction 163
8.2 Pharmacology of Tricyclic Antidepressants 164
    8.2.1 Mechanisms of Action of Tricyclic Antidepressants in the Management of Neuropathic Pain 164
    8.2.2 Clinical Pharmacology of Tricyclic Antidepressants 165
8.3 Efficacy of Tricyclic Antidepressants in the Management of Neuropathic Pain 165
8.4 Amitriptyline in the Management and Prevention of CIPN 165
    8.4.1 Amitriptyline and Nortriptyline in the Management of CIPN 165
    8.4.2 Amitriptyline in the Prevention of CIPN 166
8.5 A Look to the Future 167
References 168

8.1 INTRODUCTION

Several pharmacological alternatives are currently available for the management of chronic neuropathic pain. The two major classes of drugs that have been studied in randomized and controlled trials (RCTs) are antidepressants and anticonvulsants. Systematic reviews and meta-analyses indicate that tricyclic antidepressants are the most effective class of drugs studied in neuropathic pain (Finnerup et al., 2010). Most of the studies on tricyclic antidepressants are relatively old, and the total number of patients studied is small. Tricyclic antidepressants have several pharmacological actions that may explain their efficacy. However, some of the adverse effects of this class of drugs make them problematic to use, particularly in the elderly.

Tricyclic antidepressants, like other drugs used in the management of neuropathic pain, have been mainly studied in chronic diabetic polyneuropathy and postherpetic neuralgia. Very few studies have addressed the possibility to prevent the development of chronic neuropathic pain (Bowsher, 1997). Studies could be conducted in the prevention of postherpetic neuralgia, postsurgery neuropathic pain, and neuropathic pain due to neurotoxic agents.

Another important question is whether efficacy data from one condition (e.g., diabetic polyneuropathy) can be applied to other conditions (e.g., posttraumatic neuropathic pain or chemotherapy-induced pain). Regardless of the cause of neuropathy (infection, trauma, toxic agents), neuropathic pain has several different components that can make drug responses unpredictable even within the same disease entity (e.g., diabetic polyneuropathy).

The two interesting questions regarding the role of tricyclic antidepressants in the management of chemotherapy-induced neuropathic pain (CIPN) are whether tricyclics are as efficacious in CIPN as in other conditions where they have been studied and whether they can be used to prevent CIPN.

8.2 PHARMACOLOGY OF TRICYCLIC ANTIDEPRESSANTS

8.2.1 MECHANISMS OF ACTION OF TRICYCLIC ANTIDEPRESSANTS IN THE MANAGEMENT OF NEUROPATHIC PAIN

Tricyclic antidepressants (TCAs) were among the first drugs to be tried and studied in the alleviation of neuropathic pain. The early studies showed that the efficacy of TCAs was not dependent on their antidepressant effect, as they worked also in nondepressed patients (Max et al., 1987), and the analgesic effects started early (within a week) and at low doses that are not adequate in the management of depression (McQuay et al., 1992, 1993). In fact, TCAs are the only group of antidepressants and antiepiletics that provides analgesia at doses that are lower than those needed to relieve depression or anxiety.

Amitriptyline inhibits the uptake of 5-HT (serotonin) and norepinephrine equally well (Baldessarini, 1984). This has been considered to be the main mechanism of action of the dual-action antidepressants in the relief of neuropathic pain. However, several other mechanisms have been suggested to explain the superior efficacy of amitriptyline, including effects on 5-HT3-receptors, α_1- and α_2- adrenergic receptors, and adenosine availability (Micó et al., 2006).

Sodium channels have a central role in nerve function, and sodium channel blockers such as intravenous lidocaine have been shown to be effective in neuropathic pain (Kalso et al., 1998). The current evidence suggests that amitriptyline is a potent sodium channel blocker. It has been shown to cause nerve block (Gerner et al., 2001) and inhibit voltage-gated sodium channels at concentrations that are effective for treating neuropathic pain. Amitriptyline also shows a higher affinity for inactivated sodium channels and use-dependent binding of sodium channels (Dick et al., 2007). Other TCAs studied show similar but lesser effects on the sodium channels (Dick et al., 2007).

Other effects of amitriptyline that may play a role in analgesia include blocking of NMDA receptor-mediated synaptic responses (Watanabe et al., 1993) and inhibition of glia (Obuchowicz et al., 2006). Amitriptyline has also been reported to induce synthesis of glial cell line-derived neuropatrophic factor (GDNF) (Hisaoka et al., 2001).

Amitriptyline has significant anticholinergic effects and it blocks H_1-receptors. Anticholinergic adverse effects (e.g., dry mouth, constipation, cognitive impairment) are the main reason for discontinuation or contraindication of therapy. The anti-histaminergic effect causes sedation, which can be a benefit if it improves sleep. Some patients can gain weight due to the anti-H_1-effect.

8.2.2 Clinical Pharmacology of Tricyclic Antidepressants

Amitriptyline is metabolized to nortriptyline via CYP2D6-catalized metabolism. Nortriptyline is also active as an antidepressant and analgesic. It is a stronger norepi-nephrine reuptake inhibitor than amitriptyline. As CYP2D6 is polymorphic and also inhibited by many drugs, the plasma concentrations of amitriptyline and notriptyline can vary 30-fold, even though the dose is the same.

8.3 EFFICACY OF TRICYCLIC ANTIDEPRESSANTS IN THE MANAGEMENT OF NEUROPATHIC PAIN

According to a recent review (Finnerup et al., 2010) about 11 positive RCTs have been published on amitriptyline in painful polyneuropathy and 4 in postherpetic neuralgia. The number needed to treat (NNT) for 50% pain relief was about 2. One of the two studies in peripheral nerve injury was positive, whereas the other one was negative. The positive study indicated significant dose-dependent analgesia with 25–100 mg amitripty-line compared with placebo in a crossover study on postmastectomy pain (Kalso et al., 1995). Interestingly, both studies on amitriptyline in HIV neuropathy were negative. The combined number needed to harm (NNH), indicating how many patients had to withdraw from the study due to adverse effects, was 16 (11–26) (Finnerup et al., 2010).

8.4 AMITRIPTYLINE IN THE MANAGEMENT AND PREVENTION OF CIPN

Amitriptyline and its metabolite nortriptyline have been studied in three RCTS: one trial evaluated the efficacy of nortriptyline in the alleviation of symptoms of cis-platinum-induced peripheral neuropathy (Hammack et al., 2002), another studied amitriptyline in the management of neuropathic symptoms after different chemotherapeutic agents, and the third evaluated the possibility to prevent chemo-therapy-induced neuropathic symptoms with amitriptyline. All studies turned out to be negative regarding the first outcome variable. However, it is important to consider why these studies failed. Were the trials negative because of methodological prob-lems or is amitriptyline not effective in chemotherapy-induced neuropathic pain?

8.4.1 Amitriptyline and Nortriptyline in the Management of CIPN

Forty-four patients with chemotherapy-induced neuropathy with a severity of at least ≥3/10 participated in an 8-week, double-blind, randomized, placebo-controlled parallel group study. The treatment was started with 10 mg/day and the dose was increased by 10 mg per week up to the target maximum dose of 50 mg/day if tolerated (Kautio et al., 2008). The same physician saw the patients at the beginning of the study and at 8 weeks. The patients kept a diary and they were also contacted by phone. The various assessments included a neurological examination and assessment of sleep, physical activity, and neuropathic symptoms using the National Cancer Institute Common Toxicity Criteria (NCI-CTC) (Postma and Heimans, 2000). Quality of life was assessed with the European Organization for Research and Treatment of Cancer Quality of Life Questionnaire (EORTC-C30 questionnaire) (Ford et al., 2001). On the final visit, the patients assessed the global improvement of neuropathic symptoms by the study drug using a 5-point verbal rating scale. The primary endpoint was relief of neuropathic symptoms with amitriptyline compared with placebo.

Amitriptyline (50 mg/day) was well tolerated, but the study found no statistically significant differences in the severity of the neuropathic symptoms between the amitriptyline and placebo groups. However, amitriptyline significantly improved the quality of life of the patients compared with placebo.

The main reason for this study failing is likely the small number of patients, as the target of 120 included patients was not achieved. Also, the study lacked in sensitivity, as the most common neuropathic symptoms were paresthesia and mild tingling, whereas pain played a minor role. In addition, the symptoms were relatively mild. The patients received different types of chemotherapeutic drugs (vinca alkaloids, platinum derivatives, taxanes) or their combinations. It also seems that the dose of amitriptyline was too low, at least in some of the patients, as the total combined plasma concentration of amitriptyline and nortriptyline varied from below 100 to 845 nmol/L (median, 151 nmol/L).

The efficacy of nortriptyline in relieving neuropathic symptoms due to cis-platin was studied in a randomized, double-blind, placebo-controlled, crossover trial in 51 patients. The study consisted of two 4-week phases separated by a 1-week wash-out period. The dose of nortriptyline was increased from 25 to 100 mg/day if tolerated. Patients filled in weekly questionnaires assessing the severity of paresthesiae, hours of sleep, quality of life, and adverse effects.

Most patients were able to tolerate nortriptyline $\geq$ 75 mg/day. However, nortriptyline caused only a very moderate relief of cis-platin-induced paresthesiae. The average reduction of paresthesiae by nortriptyline was only 5% more than with placebo. Hours of sleep increased significantly ($p = 0.02$) due to nortriptyline compared with placebo.

Also, this study suffered from low power and sensitivity, as symptoms were mild. Paresthesiae and other neuropathic symptoms may be more difficult to treat with amitriptyline, or any other antidepressant used in neuropathic pain, than pain itself. The study also suffered from the crossover design because of the carryover effect. There were significant interindividual differences in the responses to both nortriptyline and placebo. Plasma concentrations of nortriptyline were not measured.

8.4.2 AMITRIPTYLINE IN THE PREVENTION OF CIPN

This study was placebo-controlled RCT where the dose of amitriptyline was gradually increased from 25 mg/day to 100 mg/day at a week's interval. Amitriptyline or placebo was started with the chemotherapy and continued during the whole chemo-therapy period, after which the patients were followed for a median of 20 weeks. Only patients who had no previous neuropathy were included. Chemotherapy-induced neu-ropathic symptoms were evaluated by neurological examination, with a patient diary, and the symptoms were scored according to the NCI-CTC (Postma and Heimans, 2000). Quality of life (QoL) was assessed with the EORTC-C30 questionnaire (Ford et al., 2001). During the visits the patients assessed the sensory and motor symptoms on a 4-point verbal scale. The primary endpoint was the appearance or progression of neuropathic symptoms based on the diary data. There were no significant differ-ences between the amitriptyline and the placebo groups regarding the amount and severity of neuropathic symptoms.

Why did this study fail? The most important reason is likely to be low sensitivity. Sensory neuropathy was seen in 61% of the patients after three cycles and 76% after nine cycles. However, patients in both study groups reported very low neuropathy scores, and the most prominent symptoms of chemotherapy-induced neuropathy were paresthesia, dysesthesia, and numbness, not pain. The study was terminated when 120 patients had been recruited. The planned study size had been 250. The patients had several different types of cancer and consequently received different chemotherapeutic agents (i.e., vinca alkaloids, platinum derivatives, taxanes) and their combinations. The mechanisms of neuropathy vary depending on the drug.

The study provides some useful data, though. The majority of patients (40 out of 54) were able to take the target dose of 100 mg of amitriptyline. However, the plasma concentrations varied significantly. The total combined concentration of amitripty-line and nortriptyline ranged from below 100 to 1,068 nmol/L (median, 317 nmol/L), indicating the great interindividual variation in the pharmacokinetics of amitriptyline due to CYP2D6 polymorphism. Interestingly, the severities of most adverse effects were very similar with both placebo and the high dose of amitriptyline. Only dry mouth and tremor were rated as significantly more severe with amitriptyline.

8.5 A LOOK TO THE FUTURE

The three small RCTs that have been conducted with amitriptyline/nortriptyline in the treatment or prevention of chemotherapy-induced neuropathic pain have failed due to methodological issues. However, the pharmacological profile of amitripty-line still remains interesting regarding both prevention and treatment of chemo-therapy-induced neuropathic pain. Amitriptyline is a well-known and cheap drug and it has been well tolerated. Much larger studies with higher sensitivity (patients having more severe pain) are needed. Patients at high risk (e.g., those who have risk factors for the development of neuropathic pain) should be included. Subgroup analyses for different chemotherapeutic agents should be performed. The dosing of amitriptyline should be based on monitoring the plasma concentrations of ami-triptyline and nortriptyline.

Amitriptyline is of particular interest in the neuroprotection during chemother-apy, as it may also have a supportive role in cancer treatment (Kulaksiz-Erkmen et al., 2011).

REFERENCES

Baldessarini RJ. Treatment of depression by altering monoamine metabolism: Precursors and metabolic inhibitors. *Psychopharmacol Bull* 1984;20:224–39.

Bowsher D. The effects of pre-emptive treatment of postherpetic neuralgia with amitriptyline: A randomized, double-blind, placebo-controlled trial. *J Pain Symptom Manage* 1997;13:327–31.

Dick IE, Brochu RM, Purohit Y, Kaczorowski GJ, Martin WJ, Priest BT. Sodium channel blockade may contribute to the analgesic efficacy of antidepressants. *J Pain* 2007;8:315–24.

Finnerup NB, Sindrup SH, Jensen TS. The evidence for pharmacological treatment of neuropathic pain. *Pain* 2010;150:573–81.

Ford ME, Havstad SL, Kart CS. Assessing the reliability of the EORTC QLQ-C30 in a sample of older African-American and Caucasian adults. *Qual Life Res* 2001;10:533–41.

Gerner P, Mujtaba M, Sinnott CJ, Wang GK. Amitriptyline versus bupivacaine in rat sciatic nerve blockade. *Anesthesiology* 2001;94:661–67.

Hammack J, Michalak JC, Loprinzi CL, Sloan JA, Novotny PJ, Soori GS, Tirona MR, Rowland KM, Stella PJ, Johnson JA. Phase III evaluation of nortriptyline for alleviation of symptoms of cis-platinum-induced peripheral neuropathy. *Pain* 2002;98:195–203.

Hisaoka K, Nishida A, Koda T, Miyata M, Zensho H, Morinobu S, Ohta M, Yamawaki S. Antidepressant drug treatment induce glial cell-line derived neuropatrophic factor (GDNF) synthesis and release in rat C6 glioblastoma cells. *J Neurochem* 2001;79:25–34.

Kalso E, Tasmuth T, Neuvonen PJ. Amitriptyline effectively relieves neuropathic pain following treatment of breast cancer. *Pain* 1995;64:293–302.

Kalso E, Tramèr MR, McQuay HJ, Moore RA. Systemic local-anaesthetic-type drugs in chronic pain: A systematic review. *Eur J Pain* 1998;2:3–14.

Kautio A-L, Haanpää M, Saarto T, Kalso E. Amitriptyline in the treatment of chemotherapy-induced neuropathic symptoms. *J Pain Symptom Manage* 2008;35:31–39.

Kulaksiz-Erkmen G, Dalmizrak O, Dincsoy-Tuna G, Dogan A, Ogus H, Ozer N. Amitriptyline may have a supportive role in cancer treatment by inhibiting glutathione S-transferase pi (GST-π) and a (GST-α). *J Enzyme Inhib Med Chem* 2011 (Epub ahead of print).

Max MB, Culnane M, Schafer SC, Gracely RH, Walther DJ, Smoller B, Dubner R. Amitriptyline relieves diabetic neuropathy pain in patients with normal or depressed mood. *Neurology* 1987;37:589–96.

McQuay HJ, Carroll D, Glynn CJ. Low dose amitriptyline in the treatment of chronic pain. *Anaesthesia* 1992;47:646–52.

McQuay HJ, Carroll D, Glynn CJ. Dose-response for analgesic effect of amitriptyline in chronic pain. *Anaesthesia* 1993;48:281–85.

Micó JA, Ardid D, Berrocoso E, Eschalier A. Antidepressants and pain. *Trends in Pharmacological Sciences* 2006 (July);27(7):348–54.

Obuchowicz E, Kowalski J, Labuzek K, Krysiak R, Pendzich J, Herman ZS. Amitriptyline and nortriptyline inhibit interleukin-1 release by rat mixed glial and microglial cell cultures. *Int J Psychopharmacol* 2006;9:27–35.

Postma TJ, Heimans JJ. Grading chemotherapy-induced peripheral neuropathy. *Ann Oncol* 2000;11:509–13.

Watanabe Y, Saito H, Abe K. Tricyclic antidepressants block NMDA receptor-mediated synaptic responses and induction of long-term potentiation in rat hippocampal slices. *Neuropharmacology* 1993;32:479–86.

9 Experimental Design and Analysis of Drug Combinations Applicable to Chemotherapy-Induced Neuropathic Pain

Ronald J. Tallarida

CONTENTS

9.1   Introduction 169
9.2   Dose-Effect Analysis.. 170
9.3   Isoboles 172
9.4   Application: Testing Drugs for Neuropathic Pain 174
9.5   Curved Isoboles 176
9.6   Analysis on the Effect Scale 178
9.7   Conclusion 179
References... 180

9.1   INTRODUCTION

Neuropathic pain may occur from numerous situations such as accidental nerve trauma, cancer chemotherapy, diabetes, and so on. These conditions involve varying anatomic sites and therefore require various treatment approaches. In this section we discuss the testing of agonist drug combinations and the analysis of data from these tests that may provide effective treatments. Our interest is in agonist drugs that are overtly similar in that they produce the same effect. In most cases these are agents that work through different mechanisms. It is well known that the treatment of neuropathic pain is difficult and the proper drug combination for any patient is often determined empirically (Fields et al., 1999). The main focus in this chapter is the experimental design and associated data analysis to assess whether certain drug combinations produce effects that differ from the expected effects, that is, is there synergism? Our main application, which follows from the theory, is drawn from a preclinical pain model in rodents. The drugs we discuss here to illustrate the methodology and analysis include tramadol, a *mu* opioid with concomitant action of blocking serotonin and norepinephrine (Codd et al., 1995), and one or more anticonvulsant agents since these agents have been shown to have efficacy in relieving neuropathic pain (Blackburn-Munro and Erichsen, 2005). However, the methodology presented here is broadly applicable. Our aim is a demonstration of the mathematical theory that underlies this approach and its use in guiding combination drug testing.

This methodology requires complete dose-effect data for each of the constituents used individually. The effect is always some measurable change in the subject receiving a dose of the drug. In rodent models these are often metrics that represent the tolerated time on a heated surface or the paw withdrawal threshold due to pressure at a paw that was previously damaged, for example, by ligation of lumbar spinal nerve, as described by Kim and Chung (1992). The dose of drug is therefore associated with such metrics and the resulting dose-effect data are determined and modeled as described below.

9.2 DOSE-EFFECT ANALYSIS

Analysis of dose-effect data is a key aspect of the analysis of drug combination data, and thus we begin our discussion with this topic. The most common model for describing dose-effect relations is the hyperbolic model given by $E = E_{max}D/(D + C)$, where D is the dose, E is the effect, and E_{max} is the maximum effect produced by the drug. The constant C is seen to be numerically equal to the dose that yields an effect = $\frac{1}{2} E_{max}$ for the drug, and thus it is a measure of the drug's potency. E_{max} indicates the efficacy. When discussing two different agonist drugs (say, drugs A and B) we use subscripts in the equations that denote each: $E = E_A\, a/(a + C_A)$, for drug A with dose a, maximum effect E_A, and potency C_A. The corresponding values for drug B are b, E_B, and C_B. The shape of a representative dose-effect curve that fits this model is illustrated in Figure 9.1, which is a graph of the mean effect at each dose and its standard error (not real data).

The smooth curve shown in Figure 9.1 is obtained by nonlinear regression, a standard mathematical procedure that minimizes the squared value of the vertical deviations. Parameters of the smoothed curve are assumed to be reliable indicators of the mean effect at each dose. Thus, the value of the ordinate (effect) at each dose is taken to be the value from the curve, rather than the value of the effect point that is plotted since each of those plotted effect points has an error shown by the vertical bars. The theoretical maximum effect for the data plotted here is 51.5 ± 1.5, and the potency index (C) is 11.5 ± 1.2. This potency value is often referred to as the D_{50} or ED_{50}. Dose-effect data are also sometimes plotted as effect against log(dose), a procedure that produces a sigmoid shape that is approximately linear in the mid-range and gives $\log(ED_{50})$ from which an estimate of the ED_{50} is obtained as the antilog. Because of the limited mid-range data used, the ED_{50} from the log dose plot may not be identical to that obtained from nonlinear regression of the complete dose-effect data set, but in most cases these values are acceptably close. (For the data illustrated in Figures 9.1 and 9.2, the nonlinear fit gives $ED_{50} = 11.5 ± 1.2$, whereas the log dose linear plot leads to $ED_{50} = 11.5 ± 0.24$.) In earlier times the linear log plot was a computational convenience. But today there are numerous statistical computer packages available that make it now feasible to use nonlinear regression in describing dose-effect data. The mathematical aspects of regression methods are well known

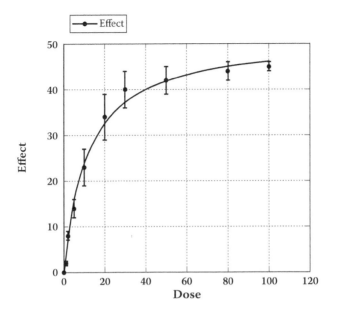

FIGURE 9.1 Dose-effect curve fitted to $E = E_{max}D/(D + C)$, where $E_{max} = 51.5 \pm 1.5$, and $C = ED_{50} = 11.5 \pm 1.2$.

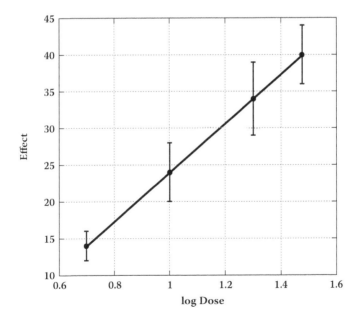

FIGURE 9.2 Linear regression for data in the mid-range of that in Figure 9.1, based on E versus log dose (x), and given by $E = 25.75 + m\ (x - C)$, where $m = 33.7 \pm 1.04$ and $C = \log (ED_{50}) = 1.06 \pm 0.0093$, from which $ED_{50} = 11.5 \pm 0.24$.

and computer programs are plentiful for performing this calculation. Further details of the theory and computation are contained in Tallarida (2000).

9.3   ISOBOLES

The common method for determining whether a drug combination is superadditive (synergistic), subadditive, or simply additive is the method of isoboles introduced by Loewe (1927, 1928, 1953). An isobole is a curve in rectangular coordinates whose points indicate dose pairs (a of drug A and b of drug B) that are expected to give a specified effect level (usually 50% of the maximum effect) when there is no inter-action between the two drugs. In other words this is a situation in which the actions are independent and thus the combination effects follow from each drug's potency.

The illustration in Figure 9.3 shows graphically how the isobole is determined, that is, how to get the dose pairs (a,b) that comprise its points. To illustrate we have constructed the dose-effect curves for drugs A and B. We show graphically how these curves lead to an isobole. Toward that end we have chosen the 50% effect level (with E_{max} based on the higher efficacy drug). In the dosage range shown, drug A has not yet achieved that effect level, but it may do so at higher doses indicated by the broken extension of the curve. Drug B may also increase further as shown by its broken line. Our concern is with the 50% level of effect, and thus in this illustration we are interested only in the pieces of the curves below this level. The graph illustrates how dose a of drug A leads to dose b of drug B, thereby providing a point on the 50% isobole. The aim of the combination analysis is to convert dose a into its equivalent of drug B so that the sum of dose b and that equivalent equals the ED_{50} of drug B. Because this procedure adds b_{eq} and the needed b we call the isobole additive. In the graph it is seen that the required b is the distance between b_{eq} and the ED_{50} of drug B. As a increases b_{eq} also increases, and thus the needed b (arrow length) becomes less. It follows therefore that the isobole is generally a

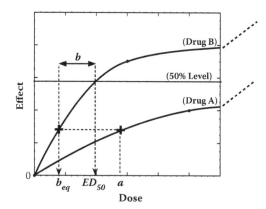

FIGURE 9.3   Illustration showing how points (a,b) of an isobole are determined from the individual dose-effect curves. Dose a of drug A is equally effective with a quantity of drug B denoted by b_{eq}, and therefore this equivalent must be added to dose b of drug B to reach the ED_{50} and thereby attain the 50% effect level.

monotone decreasing curve, that is, as a increases, b decreases (and vice versa). An exception is that situation in which drug A lacks efficacy, which means $b_{eq} = 0$, so that b for any a is a constant equal to its ED_{50}, which results in a horizontal line isobole. In the more usual case the isobole is a decreasing curve that may be linear or nonlinear.

A *linear* isobole results only if the individual dose-effect curves attain the same maximum and also have a constant potency ratio. That situation applies if each curve is expressed as $E = E_{max} D/(D + C_A)$ for drug A and $E = E_{max} D/(D + C_B)$ for drug B, for in this case the potency ratio is C_A/C_B. (In the log dose plot this means that the regression lines are parallel.) The isobole in this case is linear, as we show in a derivation given in the next section, and this is shown as an illustration in Figure 9.4. An *isobologram* is a graph consisting of the additive isobole and the experimentally determined dose combination that gives the specified effect. That experimental point is almost always determined by testing with a fixed ratio combination of the two drugs and obtaining the dose combination that gives the effect level. On the isobologram the fixed ratio dose combination is indicated by the broken radial lines of Figure 9.4, which show that the observed dose combination, which is somewhere on the radial line, may be on or off the isobole for the dose ratio tested. If that point is significantly below the isobole, then the interaction is synergistic. This means that the effects are enhanced and thus lower doses in the combination reach the effect

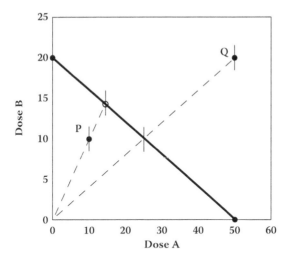

FIGURE 9.4   Illustration (not real data) of a linear isobole for effect = 50% of the maximum that is derived from drugs having a constant potency ratio with $C_A = 50$, the ED_{50} of drug A, and $C_B = 20$, the ED_{50} of drug B. A fixed dose ratio combination (1:1) is found to attain this effect with quantities (10,10) shown as point P, which is below the isobole, a finding that indicates synergism. Also shown is the result of another fixed dose ratio combination (5:2) in which the specified effect was achieved with dose combination (50,20) shown as point Q above the isobole, thereby indicating subadditivity. The terms *below* and *above* require appropriate statistical testing, for example, to distinguish between the value observed (e.g., point P) and the value on the isobole (open circle) for the fixed drug ratio used.

level. In contrast, the observed point (dose combination) may be located above the isobole, a situation that denotes subadditivity. An observed point on the isobole indicates simple additivity, that is, a situation where there is no interaction and the drugs, in combination, act in accord with their individual potencies. Figure 9.4 shows the isobole as the downward sloping line given by

$$\frac{a}{A} + \frac{b}{B} = 1 \tag{9.1}$$

where $A = ED_{50}$ of drug A and $B = ED_{50}$ of drug B. This equation follows from the fact that $b + b_{eq} = B$, where b_{eq} for dose $a = \dfrac{a}{A/B}$; thus $b + \dfrac{a}{A/B} = B$, which simplifies to Equation 9.1.

The expected dose combination is the intersection of the additive isobole and the radial line that defines the dose combination ratio that is used in testing. At this intersection the coordinates add to a total for the combination that we denoted by Z_{add}. This intersection point on the isobole has coordinates whose sum, Z_{add}, may be expressed in terms of the fractions, f of A and $(1 - f)$ of B,

$$Z_{add} = fA + (1 - f)B \tag{9.2}$$

One needs to have the standard error of Z_{add}, and this can be approximated by

$$[SE(Z_{add})]^2 = [f^2 V(A) + (1 - f)^2 V(B)] \tag{9.3}$$

where $V(A)$ and $V(B)$ are the variances of A (= ED_{50} of drug A) and B (= ED_{50} of drug B), respectively, that were previously determined from the individual dose-effect data (see Section 9.2). This standard error is needed in a statistical test to distinguish between Z_{add} and the observed total dose that arises from the experiment, a statistical topic that is described in Tallarida (2000, pp. 60–64). The expression given by Equation 9.3 is usually an acceptable approximation, although a more precise estimate of the standard error is obtained from the use of proportions p_1 of drug A and p_2 of drug B that are used in the combination. That calculation is made from Equation 9.4:

$$[SE(Z_{add})]^2 = \frac{p_1^2}{A^4}(Z_{add})^4 V(A) + \frac{p_2^2}{B^4}(Z_{add})^4 V(B) \tag{9.4}$$

9.4   APPLICATION: TESTING DRUGS FOR NEUROPATHIC PAIN

Tramadol is a weak *mu* opioid agonist that blocks the reuptake of norepinephrine and serotonin and also stimulates the release of serotonin (Raffa et al., 1992; Driessen and Reimann, 1992). Certain anticonvulsants that are sodium channel blockers have been used to treat neuropathic pain (Blackburn-Munro and Erichsen, 2005). These agents are believed to stabilize membranes and attenuate the firing of pain signals. These facts suggested that a combination of tramadol and certain anticonvulsants might be useful in treating neuropathic pain. In this regard we tested certain combinations and present here, as an illustration of the methodology, the results of our preclinical tests of tramadol and the anticonvulsant topiramate. This information, taken from the study by Codd et al. (2008), provides a typical example of the use of isobolographic analysis.

In this study Sprague-Dawley rats, 200 g, were used and subjected to ligation of the dorsal root ganglion prior to entrance into the sciatic nerve, a procedure resulting in allodynia in the left hind paw. The metric was derived from the paw withdrawal threshold as determined with the use of von Frey filaments. From this measure the paw withdrawal threshold was expressed as a percent of the maximum possible effect, and from this the percent effect was measured as a function of graded doses of drug or drug combination. All measurements were made at the time of peak effect, and it was found that each drug alone was capable of producing 100% effects with comparable ED_{50} values. These were 94.5 ± 5.3 mg/kg for tramadol and 98.0 ± 6.7 mg/kg for topiramate based on oral dosing.

These ED_{50} values are shown as the axial intercepts of the isobologram of Figure 9.5. Several fixed dose ratios of these drugs were used to assess combination effects, and we include in this illustration the results from dose ratios 3:1 and 1:1 (tramadol:topiramate). The first dose combination attained the selected effect (50% E_{max}) with the combination values 14.7 ± 4.2:4.9 ± 1.4, while the second yielded values 14.25 ± 0.92:14.25 ± 0.92, as shown on the isobologram. The corresponding additive values (on the line) are (71.5 ± 3.2:23.8 ± 1.1) for the first and (48.1 ± 2.1:48.1 ± 2.1) for the second. Each observed total is significantly less than the additive total, thereby indicating synergism for both combinations. A third

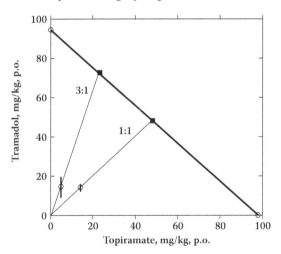

FIGURE 9.5 Isobologram for the combination of tramadol and topiramate in two different dose ratios (3:1 and 1:1, as shown by the radial lines) using an antiallodynic effect = 50% E_{max} in the rat paw. The additive isobole is the solid line with intercepts that denote the individual drugs' ED_{50} values. The open circles are the observed dose combinations that are seen to be below the isobole, thereby indicating synergism. (Data from Codd EE. et al., *Pain* 134:254–262, 2008.)

dose combination (1:3, tramadol:topiramate, data not shown) was also found to be synergistic, but the difference between the observed and additive totals was not as pronounced. These results demonstrate that synergism is not merely a property of the two drugs; it also depends on the dose ratio of the constituents. This same study (Codd et al., 2008) examined combinations of tramadol and lamotrigine and tramadol and gabapentin. Each of these combinations was found to be synergistic, but in contrast to the combination with topiramate, the synergism was seen only at certain dose ratios. In this same study we examined tramadol and gabapentin, and this test was rather interesting in that synergism was detected in a 9/1 ratio of the respective ED_{50} values (tramadol/gabapentin), but a pronounced subadditivity was found at 1/1 and 1/9 ratios. Because of the marked synergism that occurred with tramadol and topiramate in the spinal ligation model, we extended the testing by including a standard nociceptive pain model, the mouse 48°C hot-plate test. In this test topiramate had no significant antinociceptive effect. However, its presence along with tramadol resulted in a marked enhancement of tramadol's potency. Taken together these findings show that synergism is not only a property of the drugs and the dose ratio, but also depends on the test and the species that are used.

The finding of synergism and subadditivity described here is based on isobolographic analysis and the more fundamental concept of dose equivalence. The outcome of these tests (which are numerical) says nothing about the mechanism that underlies the finding. Nevertheless, the detection of synergism has often been shown to be the first step in exploring mechanism (Tallarida and Raffa, 2010). Results such as these, which are based on animal models, provide a guide for exploring mechanism, clinical testing, and ultimate drug development.

9.5　CURVED ISOBOLES

As we showed previously, the linear isobole is a consequence of a situation in which the two drugs have a constant potency ratio. Therefore, when their maximum effects differ the potency ratio is necessarily variable, and consequently the isobole is curvilinear (Grabovsky and Tallarida, 2004). In this case the dose-effect relations may be described by $E = E_B\, b/(b + C_B)$ and $E = E_A\, a/(a + C_A)$, with $E_B > E_A$, which means that drug B is the higher-efficacy drug. In this case the drug B equivalent of dose a is given by

$$b_{eq}(a) = \frac{C_B}{\left(\dfrac{E_B}{E_A}\right)\left(1 + \dfrac{C_A}{a}\right) - 1}$$

and therefore the expression $b + b_{eq}(a) = C_B$ leads to the isobole given by Equation 9.5:

$$b = C_B - \frac{C_B}{\left(\dfrac{E_B}{E_A}\right)\left(1 + \dfrac{C_A}{a}\right) - 1} \tag{9.5}$$

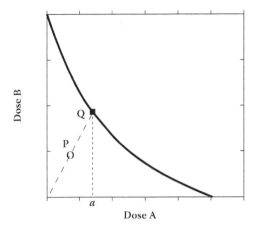

FIGURE 9.6   A curved isobole (for effect = 50% of E_{max}) is shown and represents the additive dose combinations for the case in which the individual drugs produce different maximum effects. These individual curves are given by $E = E_{max}b/(b + C_B)$ for drug B and $E = E_A \, a/(a + C_A)$ for drug A. The intercepts of the isobole denote the doses of each agent that individually give the specified effect, which is ½ E_{max}. The vertical intercept denotes the ED_{50} of drug B (higher efficacy drug), which equals C_B. The intercept on the horizontal is the dose of drug A that gives effect = ½ E_{max}, but in this case, it is not C_A because drug A does not reach E_{max} at any dose. The observed point (P) is to be compared with the corresponding additive point (Q), and that comparison requires the mean values of their heights (b values) and the variances of each b value. The variance for point P comes from the combination experiment, whereas the variance for the expected point (Q) is calculated from Equation 9.6 by use of the abscissa value a at point Q and the previously determined variances for C_A and C_B that arise from the dose-effect curves of drugs A and B.

Equation 9.5 produces a curved isobole of additivity. The fact that an isobole can be curved was recognized by Loewe (1953), but he did not provide a mathematical justification and used a complicated notation in his description. Most applications of isobolographic methods continued to use the linear form, which therefore make the tacit assumption of a constant potency ratio of the drugs. Yet it is clear that the concept of dose equivalence, which is also the basis of the isobole, leads to the nonlinear term for b_{eq} and the consequent nonlinear isobole of Equation 9.5 that is illustrated in Figure 9.6. It follows, therefore, that theoretical models of drug interactions that use the linear isobole (Equation 9.1) will not be generally applicable.

The curved isobole leads to a more complicated formula to estimate the variance (square of standard error) of a point on the line. To provide these we first write the isobole equation (9.5) in a simplified form:

$$b = C_B - \frac{C_B}{f(a)}$$

and from this we express the variance of b for a specified a as given by Equation 9.6:

$$V(b) = \left(1 - \frac{1}{f(a)}\right)^2 V(C_B) + \left(\frac{g}{a}\frac{C_B}{f(a)^2}\right)^2 V(C_A) \tag{9.6}$$

where $g = E_B/E_A$. With the calculation of variance from Equation 9.6 one may apply a statistical test to determine whether the b value from the isobole at a given a value differs from the observed b dose at that a value. Examples of curved isoboles are few because this theory and analysis are relatively recent (Grabovsky and Tallarida, 2004). A further discussion with details and an application is contained in Tallarida (2006, 2007).

9.6 ANALYSIS ON THE EFFECT SCALE

The method of isoboles is the common way to analyze and test drug combinations for synergism and antagonism. Yet a view from the effect scale may be more revealing than the isobole since an isobole is based on a single specified effect. Intuitively it seems reasonable to compare the individual effects and their sum with the effect of a combination that uses the same doses. But this is incorrect, as is easily demonstrated by a situation in which a dose a of drug A gives, say, 70% of E_{max}, and a dose b of drug B gives 60% of E_{max}. The simple addition of these percents is without meaning. Thus, we ask, how is the analysis performed? This is answered by employment of the concept of dose equivalence, the same concept that is the basis of isobolographic analysis. Toward that end let us suppose that the dose-effect curve of drug B is modeled in the common way: $E = E_{max}b/(b + C_B)$ for drug B and $E = E_{max}a/(a + C_A)$ for drug A. From these relations we wish to get the expected effect of the combination (a,b). For convenience in illustrating the approach we have used the same maximum for both drugs, and therefore any dose a has its drug B equivalent dose given by $b_{eq} = a\,C_B/C_A$. This equivalent of dose a adds to dose b so that the expected effect of the combination a,b is given by $E_{ab} = E_{max}(b + b_{eq})/(b + b_{eq} + C_B)$. This applies to every a,b combination and results in a complete combination dose-effect relation based on additivity. Because E_{ab} is a function of two variables, a and b, its graph is a surface whose height above the a,b coordinate plane indicates the effect magnitude. For this reason, this approach is termed a response surface method. Further details on this approach are contained in Tallarida et al. (1999).

The variance of E_{ab} is given by

$$V(E_{ab}) = (bE_{max})^2 \left(\frac{C_A^4}{T^4}\right) V(C_B) + (aE_{max})^2 \left(\frac{C_B^4}{T^4}\right) V(C_A) \tag{9.7}$$

where

$$T = bC_A + aC_B + C_A C_B$$

With E_{ab} and its variance calculated as described above we can statistically compare this expected effect with effects that are experimentally determined and thereby detect synergism from the effect values of any dose combination. This method, which is different from (but theoretically equivalent to) isobolar methods, was used in our study of dopamine release (the effect) due to combinations of cocaine and the cocaine analog, WIN 35,428 (Tanda et al., 2009). This alternate method, besides its intuitive appeal, may require fewer subjects for testing than the number needed in an isobolographic approach.

The expected effect of a combination dose is easily calculated as shown above. Clearly, a point on the isobole is a dose combination that must give the effect that characterizes that isobole. For example, if the effect is 50% of the maximum, then the dose pair (a,b) on the isobole must give 50%, and it does when computed as described above. This is easily seen as we now show for an example of drug A whose dose-effect equation is $E = 100\,a/(a + 100)$ and for drug B with equation $E = 100\,b/(b + 20)$. Clearly, the dose B–equivalent of any dose a is $1/5\,a$. Now take a point on the 50% isobole such as $(a = 50, b = 10)$. The drug B equivalent of $a = 50$ is 10. Therefore, dose B plus its equivalent is $10 + 10 = 20$. Insertion of that in drug B's dose-effect equation gives an effect of 50%. An alternate calculation known as "Bliss Independence" (Bliss, 1939) purports to get the combination expected effect from the following formula:

$$F_{ab} = F_a + F_b - (F_a \cdot F_b)$$

where F_a and F_b denote the fractions of the maximum effects, respectively, and F_{ab} is the fraction of the expected effect of the combination. This formula, presented in Bliss (1939) with no derivation and no extended explanation, is inconsistent with the isobole method as is easily illustrated for the dose combination (50,10) used above because it leads to $F_{ab} = 0.333 + 0.333 - (0.333)\,(0.333) = 0.555$. This is 55.5%, *not* 50%, and therefore, the Bliss formula is inconsistent with the isobole and the concept of dose equivalence that is the theoretical basis of the isobole.

9.7   CONCLUSION

The treatment of neuropathic pain with opioids and nonsteroidal anti-inflammatory drugs (NSAIDs) is generally limited. This condition seems to respond more favorably to anticonvulsants that block the brain's neurotransmitters. Thus, drug combinations such as those mentioned here hold promise for treating this condition. The development of effective drug combinations begins with preclinical testing of these combinations, and the quest is to find drug and dose combinations that are synergistic. Combination testing for synergism requires experimental designs and analysis that begin with a determination of the individual drugs' dose-effect relations. The most appropriate modeling, usually with the common hyperbolic dose-effect equation, then allows the test for synergy. Most often this test produces an isobole, a curve of dose pairs that are expected to give the desired effect. The plot of the observed dose combination and the isobole provide a view that determines whether interaction is superadditive, subadditive, or simply additive. An associated statistical test is needed to show whether the observed drug combination dose pair is off the isobole, and this is applicable to both the desired and undesired effects. Ideally the dose combination for the desired effect level (usually 50% E_{max}) should be below the isobole, and the dose combination for an adverse effect should be above the isobole. These determinations require statistical testing using the variance formulas given here. The linear isobole is a consequence of drug combinations that exhibit a constant potency ratio. Therefore, the linear form is not an appropriate starting part of any model that applies to drug interactions. Synergism and subadditivity can also be tested by an alternate method that examines the expected effect of a dose combination. This method, also based on dose equivalence, is an acceptable alternate way to detect departures from simple additivity. The applications mentioned here make clear that preclinical testing of combinations is useful as a guide to clinical testing and development, but the results of testing drug combinations in the laboratory also depend on the dose ratio and the animal model used.

REFERENCES

Blackburn-Munro G, Erichsen HK. (2005). Antiepileptics and the treatment of neuropathic pain: Evidence from animal models. *Curr Pharm Design* 11:2961–76.

Bliss CI. (1939). The toxicity of poisons applied jointly. *Annals of Appl Biol* 26:585–615.

Codd EE, Martinez RP, Molino L, Rogers KE, Stone DJ, Tallarida RJ. (2008). Tramadol and several anticonvulsants synergize in attenuating nerve injury-induced allodynia. *Pain* 134:254–62.

Codd EE, Shank RP, Schupsky JJ, Raffa RB. (1995). Serotonin and norepinephrine uptake inhibiting activity of centrally acting analgesics: Structural determinants and role in antinociception. *J Pharmacol Exp Ther* 274:1263–70.

Driessen B, Reimann W. (1992). Interaction of the central analgesic, tramadol, with the uptake and release of 5-hydroxytryptamine in the rat brain *in vitro*. *Brit J Pharmacol* 105:147–51.

Fields HL, Baron R, Rowbotham MC. (1999). Peripheral neuropathic pain: An approach to management. In Wall PD, Melzack R (eds.), *Text book of pain*, 1523–33. Churchill Livingstone, Philadelphia.

Grabovsky Y, Tallarida RJ. (2004). Isobolographic analysis for combinations of a full and partial agonist: Curved isoboles. *J Pharmacol Exp Ther* 310:981–86.

Kim SH, Chung JM. (1992). An experimental model for peripheral neuropathy produced by segmental spinal nerve ligation in the rat. *Pain* 50:355–63.

Loewe S. (1927). Die Mischiarnei. *Klin Wochenschr* 6:1077–85.

Loewe S. (1928). Die quantitativen Probleme der Pharmakologie. *Ergebn Physiol* 27:47–187.

Loewe S. (1953). The problem of synergism and antagonism of combined drugs. *Arzneimittel-forschung* 3:285–90.

Raffa RB, Friderichs E, Reimann W, Shank RP, Codd EE, Vaught JL. (1992). Opioid and nonopioid components independently contribute to the mechanism of action of tramadol, an 'atypical' opioid. *J Pharmacol Exp Ther* 260:275–85.

Tallarida RJ. (2000). *Drug synergism and dose-effect data analysis* (monograph). CRC/Chapman-Hall, Boca Raton, FL.

Tallarida RJ. (2006). An overview of drug combination analysis with isobolograms. Perspectives in pharmacology. *J Pharmacol Exp Ther* 319:1–7.

Tallarida RJ. (2007). Interactions between drugs and occupied receptors. *Pharmacol Ther* 113:197–209.

Tallarida RJ, Raffa RB. (2010). The application of drug dose equivalence in the quantitative analysis of receptor occupation and drug combinations. *Pharmacol Ther* 127:165–74.

Tallarida RJ, Stone DJ, McCary JD, Raffa RB. (1999). A response surface analysis of synergism between morphine and clonidine. *J Pharmacol Exp Ther* 289:8–13.

Tanda G, Hauck Newman A, Ebbs AL, Valeria Tronci V, Green J, Tallarida RJ, Katz JL. (2009). Combinations of cocaine with other dopamine uptake inhibitors: Assessment of additivity. *J Pharmacol Exp Ther* 330:802–9.

10 Central Neuromodulation for Chemotherapy-Induced Neuropathic Pain

Helena Knotkova, Dru J. Nichols,
and Ricardo A. Cruciani

CONTENTS

10.1 Introduction 181
10.2 Neuromodulatory Techniques.. 183
    10.2.1 Invasive Approach 183
        10.2.1.1 Deep Brain Stimulation (DBS) 183
        10.2.1.2 Motor Cortex Stimulation (MCS) 184
    10.2.2 Noninvasive Approach.. 186
        10.2.2.1 Transcranial Magnetic Stimulation (TMS)....................... 186
        10.2.2.2 Transcranial Direct Current Stimulation (tDCS).............. 187
10.3 Conclusion 189
References... 189

10.1 INTRODUCTION

Although significant progress has been made in pain management over the past decades, many patients with chronic pain do not respond to conventional treatment strategies, and do not experience adequate pain relief despite numerous courses of pharmacologic and nonpharmacologic treatment.

In recent years, advances in diagnostic methods, including neuroimaging, have yielded new findings regarding the mechanisms underlying the development and maintenance of chronic pain. Consequently, cutting-edge neuromodulatory techniques, such as transcranial magnetic stimulation (TMS), transcranial direct current stimulation (tDCS), deep brain stimulation (DBS), and epidural motor cortex stimulation (MCS), have been explored as novel treatment strategies for chronic pain. The foundations for the use of central neuromodulation (i.e., neuromodulation targeting brain structures) in the treatment of pain are based on the following:

1. Patients with chronic pain syndromes present with pathological changes of neural excitability and somatotopic organization in cortical and subcortical regions (such as the somatosensoric and motor cortices or thalamus), as well as other brain structures belonging to the pain processing network (the pain matrix) (Cohen et al., 1991; Elbert et al., 1994; Banati et al., 2002; Chen et al., 2002; Flor, 2003; Drewes et al., 2005; Eisenberg et al., 2005).
2. Research findings indicate that there is a functional link between the neuroplastic changes and pain (Flor et al., 1995, 1997; Tinazzi et al., 2000; Flor, 2000; Karl et al., 2001).
3. The neuroplastic changes in chronic pain can be modified/reverted (Garcia-Larrea et al., 1999; Bittar et al., 2005; Johnson et al., 2006).
4. There is a functional link between the reversal of the neuroplastic changes and pain relief (Birbaumer et al., 1997; Canavero et al., 2002; Flor, 2002; Maihöfner et al., 2004; Pleger et al., 2005).

Clinical observations and controlled trials indicate that neuromodulation has clinical potential in the treatment of neuropathic chronic pain, and both invasive and noninvasive neuromodulatory approaches have been explored in various settings, treatment protocols, and patient populations (Migita et al., 1995; Nguyen et al., 2000; Lefaucheur et al., 2001a, 2001b; Khedr et al., 2005; Fregni et al., 2006a, 2006b; Knotkova et al., 2010). Typically, neuropathic pain presents with some or all of the following abnormal sensory symptoms and signs:

- *Hyperalgesia*: An exaggerated pain response to mildly noxious (mechanical or thermal) stimuli applied to the symptomatic area.
- *Allodynia*: Pain elicited by nonnoxious stimuli. Allodynia may be static mechanical (induced by a light pressure) or dynamic mechanical (induced by moving a soft brush) or thermal (induced by a nonpainful cold or warm stimulus).
- *Paresthesia*: Spontaneous, intermittent, and painless abnormal sensation.
- *Dysesthesia*: Spontaneous or evoked unpleasant sensations, such as annoying sensations elicited by cold stimuli.
- *Hyperpathia*: A delayed and explosive pain response to a stimulus applied to the symptomatic area.

In cancer patients, neuropathic pain may result from the effects of cancer on surroundings tissues or the cancer treatment itself, for example, radiation, chemotherapy, and surgery (Martin and Hagen, 1997; Amato and Collins, 1998; Katz, 2000). Cancer-treatment-related mechanisms linked to the development of chronic pain include, for example, the use of antineoplastic therapeutic agents such as cisplatinum, taxoids, and vincristine. Further, postradiation plexopathies may arise when radiation more than 60 Gy (6,000 rad) of irradiation is given to the patient. Surgical resection of cancers may result in traumatic injuries to peripheral nerves, with development of painful neuromas. Cancer-related mechanisms of neuropathic pain include compression, mechanical traction, inflammation, or infiltration of nerve trunks or plexi caused by the progression of the primary or metastatic cancer (Martin and Hagen, 1997; Amato and Collins, 1998; Katz, 2000).

Successful treatment of neuropathic pain is highly important, because it can severely impair patients' daily functioning, and substantially decrease the quality of patients' lives. There is a wide spectrum of pharmacological agents that are used for the pain management of neuropathic pain, for example, antidepressants, anticonvulsants, muscle relaxants, steroids, and in selected cases, opioids. Nonpharmacologic treatment strategies, including neuromodulatory brain stimulation techniques, may represent a promising option to explore, especially in patients that do not respond to pharmacologic treatment, or who experience dose-limiting side effects and remain with excruciating pain and severe functional impairment despite multiple treatment cycles with a variety of pharmacologic agents.

Recent applications of both invasive and noninvasive techniques of central neuromodulation, in chronic neuropathic pain populations, have yielded promising results. Although research data are still very limited, some evidence on central neuromodulation, specifically in cancer patients, does exist.

10.2   NEUROMODULATORY TECHNIQUES

The major invasive brain stimulation methods are deep brain stimulation and motor cortex stimulation. The noninvasive approach includes mainly transcranial magnetic stimulation and transcranial direct current stimulation, though other neuromodulatory techniques, such as motor imagery or sensory motor training, are also available.

10.2.1   INVASIVE APPROACH

10.2.1.1   Deep Brain Stimulation (DBS)

DBS is an electrical stimulation performed after stereotactic implantation of thin stick leads into subcortical areas such as the thalamus or basal ganglia. DBS was first used for the treatment of chronic pain in the 1950s, and targeted the hypothalamus (Pool et al., 1956). Later, DBS expanded to other targets, such as thalamic nuclei and adjacent structures (Mazars et al., 1960, 1973, 1974; Mark et al., 1960; Mark and Ervin, 1965; Ervin et al., 1966; White and Sweet, 1969, Hosobuchi et al., 1973; Mazars, 1975), the internal capsule (Adams et al., 1974; Fields and Adams, 1974; Hosobuchi et al., 1975), and the periventricular and periaqueductal gray (PVG/PAG) regions (Hosobuchi et al., 1977; Richardson and Akil, 1977a, 1977b, 1977c). It is estimated that about 1,300 cases of DBS for chronic pain have been reported (Kringelbach et al., 2010), yielding promising results in patients with neuropathic pain of various origins, including cancer and cancer-treatment-related neuropathic pain (Gybels and Kupers, 2000; Krauss et al., 2002; Levy, 2003; Tronnier, 2003, Hamani et al., 2006; Owen et al., 2006). For example, Mundinger and Salomão (1980) reported results of 32 cases, including cancer pain, plexus lacerations, and other lesions. DBS in that study demonstrated a reduction in pain of over 50%, in 53% of patients. Barraquer-Bordas and colleagues (1999) reported a case of a patient with central pain associated with a subinsular hematoma followed by parieto-occipital tumor.

The patient suffered from constant burning and lancinating pain with allodynia, both of which were successfully managed by DBS of the thalamic VPL nucleus for 5 months. Kumar and colleagues (1985, 1990) reported their experience with DBS in 48 patients followed for up to 10 years, 30 of whom achieved long-term pain control. The authors noted that their cancer patients fared better than patients with thalamic pain, cauda equina injury, or phantom limb pain, but worse than patients treated for failed-back syndrome following multiple disc operations. A meta-analysis of overall DBS success (Bittar et al., 2005) indicated that the effects of DBS are parameter dependent, and factors such as the targeted brain structure and the type of pain play a significant role in outcomes. The three sites most commonly targeted for stimulation were the periventricular/periaqueductal gray matter (PVG/PAG), with a long-term effectiveness rate of 79%, the internal capsule (IC) (84% effective when targeted in conjunction with PVG/PAG), and the sensory thalamus (ST) (less effective, about 58%). It should also be noted that the effectiveness of DBS correlates strongly with the type of pain; nociceptive pain is more responsive (63% long-term success) than deafferentation (47% effective). In cancer patients, DBS has become a part of the treatment ladder in carefully selected cases with terminal cancer pain, when all other modalities have failed (Pagni and Franzini, 1981).

As with all other invasive procedures, DBS carries some risk for the patient, and can lead to intracranial bleeding, usually in about 2.0 to 2.5% of DBS implants (Benabid et al., 1996; Beric et al., 2001). Other potential complications include hardware-related problems such as dislocation, lead fracture, and infection (6%) (Hariz, 2002). Stimulation-induced side effects (3%), such as paresthesia, dyskinesia, or tonic muscle contractions, have also been noted (Bejjani et al., 1999, 2002; Krack et al., 2001; Kulisevsky et al., 2002; Temel et al., 2004).

Nevertheless, DBS, as the last-resort treatment, can benefit patients who fail to respond to other treatment strategies. The optimal patient selection for DBS should include a multidisciplinary assessment. Medical contraindications to DBS include uncorrectable coagulopathy (obviating neurosurgery), and ventriculomegaly sufficient to preclude direct electrode passage to the surgical target (Kringelbach et al., 2010). Patients considered for DBS are those demonstrating quantitatively severe pain refractory to medication for a long period of time, with significantly impaired quality of life, and likely neuropathic etiology without predominantly spinal involvement. When successfully applied, DBS can be very beneficial for the patient, as it enables the stimulation in a long-term mode (several hours on, several hours off) for months or even years, and thus provides long-term pain relief.

10.2.1.2 Motor Cortex Stimulation (MCS)

MCS is an electrical stimulation of the precentral gyrus using epidural surgical leads and subthreshold stimulation (Brown and Barbaro, 2003) (Figure 10.1).

The first results of MCS were published by Tsubokawa in patients with poststroke pain (PSP) in the early 1990s (Tsubokawa et al., 1991, 1993). Subsequently, case report series, studies, and reviews on MCS in chronic pain include treatment of pain of central origin, involving pain pathways in the central nervous system and also neuropathic pain following peripheral nerve injury (cranial nerves, brachial plexus, nerve roots) (Nguyen et al., 1998; Cioni and Megglio, 2007; Friedland et al., 2007;

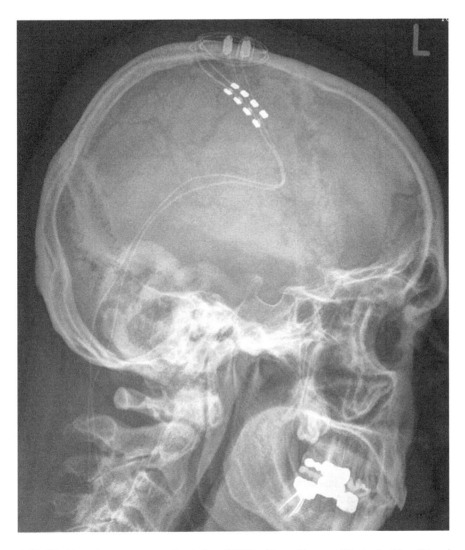

FIGURE 10.1   Motor cortex stimulation (MCS). (From Nguyen JP. et al., *Mov Disord* 13:84–88, 1998. With permission.)

Arle et al., 2008; Arle and Shils, 2008; Lima and Fregni, 2008). For example, Nguyen and colleagues (1998) reported a case of a patient with a voluminous mass in the left cerebellopontine space (an acoustic neuroma) that required nine surgical operations for excision and esthetic corrections. Resulting severe pain was resistant to all tested drugs. Remarkably, addition of MCS produced complete pain relief. Three months after MCS, the patient withdrew from analgesics and the pain relief persisted throughout the 32-month follow-up. Lefaucheur and colleagues (2009) reported the results of the first randomized controlled trial (*n* =16) for treating peripheral nerve lesions with MCS. Clinical assessment and follow-up continued for up to 1 year after MCS, at which time MCS efficacy was considered good or satisfactory in 60% of patients.

Esfahani et al. (2011) reported a series of three cases that demonstrated near-complete resolution of pain following MCS in three types of neuropathic facial pain: postherpetic neuralgia, trigeminal deafferentation, and deafferentation pain secondary to meningioma. All three patients had a pain score of 8 out of 10 for 8 years or longer prior to MCS. After receiving the MCS treatment, all three patients experienced pain relief, with pain intensity scores reduced to 0 to 2 out of 10.

MCS is, like DBS, reserved for patients who do not respond to any pharmacologic or conservative treatment, usually at the end of the patient treatment course as a last-resort treatment strategy. Therefore, the indication for MCS is limited to a small group of carefully selected patients with intractable chronic pain conditions. Well-located neuropathic pain syndromes resulting from peripheral nerve injury seem to respond more favorably than pain syndromes after central lesions.

10.2.2 Noninvasive Approach

10.2.2.1 Transcranial Magnetic Stimulation (TMS)

TMS applied over the scalp exerts its effects on brain structures via electrical currents induced by a powerful magnetic field. It can be delivered as a single pulse or a repeated train of pulses (repetitive TMS (rTMS)). The first trial exploring TMS for the treatment of pain dates to 1995 (Migita et al., 1995). Since then, numerous studies have been published (e.g., Rollnik et al., 2002; Kanda et al., 2003; Lefaucheur, 2004; Pleger et al., 2004; Summers et al., 2004; Tamura et al., 2004; Khedr et al., 2005; Andre-Obadia et al., 2006). The findings suggest that the efficacy of TMS pain relief is highly dependent upon the parameters of the treatment (Pascual-Leone et al., 1994; Chen et al, 1997; Wassermann and Lisanby, 2001). For example, studies using stimulation of 1 Hz or less either failed to demonstrate a long-lasting, significant antinociceptive effect or resulted in pain exacerbation (Lefaucheur et al., 2001b; Tamura et al., 2004). Application of higher frequencies (10 or 20 Hz) resulted in pain relief in most studies (Canavero et al., 2002; Khedr et al., 2005; Andre-Obadia et al., 2006; Zaghi et al., 2009). Andre-Obadia and colleagues reported immediate pain relief after 20 Hz as well as after 1 Hz stimulation, but only 20 Hz TMS elicited lasting beneficial effects 1 week later (Andre-Obadia et al., 2006). Overall, the studies indicate that both the frequency of stimulation and the characteristics of the patient population are significant in determining outcomes. Lefaucheur (2004) assessed the efficacy of rTMS in 60 patients with drug-resistant intractable pain with variable characteristics of pain quality, location, and level of sensory loss. Although the overall pain reduction was significantly greater in the rTMS group than in the sham group (22% versus 7.8% of overall pain reduction, effect size 2.8/10), the efficacy of rTMS was significantly influenced by the location of the pain, type of lesion, and level of sensory loss. The best results were obtained in patients with trigeminal nerve lesions and facial pain, and in those without sensory loss.

Promising results from rTMS studies have facilitated further exploration of other noninvasive neuromodulation techniques, such as transcranial direct current stimulation.

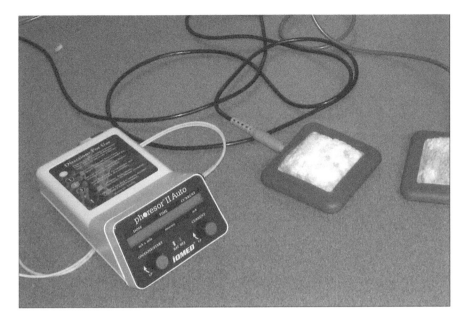

FIGURE 10.2 Transcranial direct current stimulation (tDCS) device. A battery-operated main unit and two saline-soaked sponge electrodes. (Courtesy of Helena Knotkova and Ricardo Cruciani.)

10.2.2.2 Transcranial Direct Current Stimulation (tDCS)

In comparison with TMS, tDCS devices are portable, battery operated, and easy to apply (Figure 10.2).

TDCS exerts its effects via low-intensity direct current penetrating through the scalp to the brain, influencing neuronal excitability and modulating the firing rate of individual neurons. The nature of tDCS-induced changes of cortical excitability depends on the polarity of the current. Anodal (facilitatory) tDCS increases cortical excitability, whereas cathodal (inhibitory) tDCS decreases it (Nitsche and Paulus, 2001; Nitsche et al., 2003). Evidence up to date suggests that the analgesic effect can be elicited by either tDCS of cathodal polarity applied over the somatosensory cortex (Antal et al., 2008; Knotkova et al., 2009) or tDCS of anodal polarity applied over the primary motor cortex (Fregni et al., 2006a, 2006b; Fenton et al., 2008; Kühnl et al., 2008; Knotkova et al., 2008). Some of tDCS-induced changes occur immediately during the stimulation (so-called intra-tDCS changes), whereas others occur later as short-lasting and long-lasting aftereffects (Nitsche and Paulus, 2000, 2001; Nitsche et al., 2003, 2004; Lang et al., 2004, 2005; Paulus, 2004).

As suggested by recent pharmacologic studies (Liebetanz et al., 2002; Nitsche et al., 2004, 2005), intraeffects depend on the activity of sodium and calcium channels, but not on the efficacy changes of NMDA and GABA receptors. Thus, intraeffects are probably generated solely by polarity-specific shifts of resting membrane potentials. Although the aftereffects (to some degree) also depend on membrane potential changes (Nitsche at al., 2003), they mostly result from modulations of

NMDA receptor efficacy. It has been shown that the aftereffects are accompanied by modifications of intracellular cAMP and calcium levels (Hattori et al., 1990; Islam et al., 1995) and depend on modifications of NMDA receptor efficacy (Liebetanz et al., 2002; Nitsche et al., 2003, 2004). Interestingly, modification of the NMDA receptor is a mechanism known to be involved in brain neuroplasticity.

Research studies in patients with chronic pain and healthy subjects with experimentally induced pain, as well as clinical experience from tDCS in patients with various pain syndromes, indicate the following:

1. The analgesic effect can be elicited either by tDCS of cathodal polarity applied over the somatosensory cortex (Antal et al., 2008; Knotkova et al., 2009) or by tDCS of anodal polarity applied over the primary motor cortex (Fregni et al., 2006a, 2006b; Fenton et al., 2008; Kühnl et al., 2008; Knotkova et al., 2009).
2. The analgesic effects of tDCS are cumulative. Independent observations (e.g., Fregni et al., 2006a, 2006b; Knotkova et al., 2008; Kühnl et al., 2008) suggest that repeated tDCS sessions on several (usually five) consecutive days can yield significantly better pain relief than a single application.
3. Analgesic effects are not permanent, but outlast the tDCS stimulation (Fregni et al., 2006a, 2006b; Roizenblatt et al., 2007; Knotkova et al., 2008; Kühnl et al., 2008). However, the durability of the effect shows high interindividual variability, ranging from several days to 4 months after the stimulation.
4. Besides pain control, tDCS results in secondary benefits. The study by Roizenblatt and colleagues (2007) in patients with fibromyalgia indicates a beneficial effect from anodal tDCS delivered over the motor cortex on patients' sleep pattern: tDCS treatment increased sleep efficiency by 11.8% and decreased arousal by 35%. Other secondary benefits observed after tDCS treatment include decrease of pain medication intake and improvement of patients' quality of life (Knotkova et al., 2009, 2010).

To date, tDCS has been successfully used to alleviate pain related to various chronic pain syndromes, such as central pain due to spinal cord injury, pelvic pain, fibromyalgia, trigeminal pain, multiple-sclerosis-related pain, and pain in complex regional pain syndrome (CRPS) (Fregni et al., 2006a, 2006b; Roizenblatt et al., 2007; Knotkova et al., 2008, 2010; Kühnl et al., 2008). Further, there is preliminary evidence of analgesic effect of tDCS in cancer pain (Silva et al., 2007). Silva and colleagues (2007) reported a sham-controlled use of tDCS to examine whether tDCS can produce clinically meaningful analgesia in a patient (65 years old, female) with pain due to pancreatic cancer. Surgical treatment was not considered due to local and metastatic invasion, and the patient was started on chemotherapy with gemcitabine, which helped with her pain to some extent. After 6 months of treatment, her pain returned and she was started on 180 mg of codeine and up to 2 g of acetaminophen per day. During the study, the patient received a session of active anodal tDCS over the motor cortex and a session of sham stimulation in a crossover randomized order. The patient was blinded to the treatment condition and withheld from her medication.

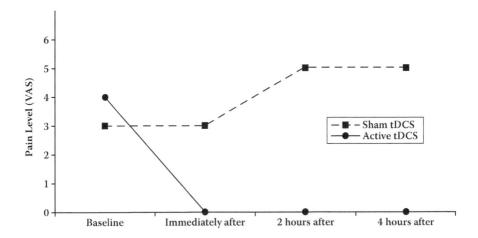

FIGURE 10.3   Pain relief induced by tDCS in a patient with pancreatic cancer as determined by pain levels during treatment with sham and active tDCS. During treatment with tDCS, medications were withheld. (From Silva G. et al., *J Pain Symptom Manage* 34(4):342–345, 2007. With permission.)

After active stimulation, not only did the patient's pain score significantly decrease from 4 to 0, but pain relief lasted for several hours even though the patient did not take any medication during the study treatment (Figure 10.3).

Prior to the study, the patient could not tolerate missing one dose of her medication for more than 4 hours. In contrast to active tDCS, sham stimulation did not result in pain relief. These findings are promising and justify larger tDCS studies in patients with cancer pain.

10.3   CONCLUSION

Despite their novelty, both the invasive and noninvasive neuromodulatory approaches in the treatment of chronic pain have yielded promising results in various patient populations. Although the mechanisms underlying the analgesic effects of the neuromodulatory methods have not yet been fully ellucidated, evidence gained from recent studies facilitates further explorations of the clinical potential of each available neuromodulatory method.

REFERENCES

Adams JE, Hosobuchi Y, Fields HL. (1974). Stimulation of internal capsule for relief of chronic pain. *J Neurosurg* 41:740–44.

Amato AA, Collins MP. (1998). Neuropathies associated with malignancy. *Semin Neurol* 18:125–44.

Andre-Obadia N, Peyron R, Mertens P, Mauguiere F, Laurent B, Garcia-Larrea L. (2006). Transcranial magnetic stimulation for pain control. Double-blind study of different frequencies against placebo, and correlation with motor cortex stimulation efficacy. *Clin Neurophysiol* 117:1536–44.

Antal A, Brepohl N, Poreisz C, Boros K, Csifcsak G, Paulus W. (2008). Transcranial direct current stimulation over somatosensory cortex decreases experimentally induced acute pain perception. *Clin J Pain* 24(1):56–63.

Antal A, Nitsche MA, Paulus W. (2003). Transcranial magnetic and direct current stimulation of the visual cortex. *Suppl Clin Neurophysiol* 56:291–304.

Arle JE, Apetauerova D, Zani J, VedranDeletis D, Penney DL, Hoit D, Gould C, Shils JL. (2008). Motor cortex stimulation in patients with Parkinson disease: 12-months follow-up in 4 patients. *J Neurosurg* 109:133–39.

Arle JE, Shils JL. (2008). Motor cortex stimulation for pain and movement disorders. *Neurotherapeutics* 5(1):37–49.

Banati RB, et al. (2002). Brain plasticity and microglia: Is transsynaptic glial activation in the thalamus after limb denervation linked to cortical plasticity and central sensitization? *J Physiol Paris* 96:289–99.

Barraquer-Bordas L, Molet J, Pascual-Sedano B, Catala H. (1999). Retarded central pain associated with a subinsular hematoma followed by a parietoccipitaltumour. The favourable effect of chronic stimulation of the VPL thalamic nucleus. *Rev Neurol* 29:1044–47.

Bejjani BP, Damier P, Arnulf I, Thivard L, Bonnet AM, Dormont D, Cornu P, Pidoux B, Samson Y, Agid Y. (1999). Transient acute depression induced by high-frequency deep-brain stimulation. *N Engl J Med* 340:1476–80.

Bejjani BP, Houeto JL, Hariz M, Yelnik J, Mesnage V, Bonnet A, Pidoux B, Dormont D, Cornu P, Agid Y. (2002). Aggressive behavior induced by intraoperative stimulation in the triangle of Sano. *Neurology* 59:1425–27.

Benabid AL, Pollak P, Gao D, Hoffmann D, Limousin P, Gay E, Payen I, Benazzouz A. (1996). Chronic electrical stimulation of the ventralis intermedius nucleus of the thalamus as a treatment of movement disorders. *J Neurosurg* 84:203–14.

Beric A, Kelly PJ, Rezai A, Sterio D, Mogilner A, Zonenshayn M, Kopell B. (2001). Complications of deep brain stimulation surgery. *Stereotactic Funct Neurosurg* 77:73–78.

Birbaumer N, Lutzenberger W, Montoya P, Larbig W, Unertl K, Töpfner S, Grodd W, Taub E, Flor HJ. (1997). Effects of regional anesthesia on phantom limb pain are mirrored in changes in cortical reorganization. *Neuroscience* 17:5503–8.

Bittar RG, Otero S, Carter H, Aziz TZ. (2005). Deep brain stimulation for phantom limb pain. *J Clin Neurosci* 12:399–404.

Brown JA, Barbaro NM. (2003). Motor cortex stimulation for central and neuropathic pain: Current status. *Pain* 104:431–35.

Canavero S, Bonicalzi V, Dotta M, Vighetti S, Asteggiano G, Cocito D. (2002). Transcranial magnetic cortical stimulation relieves central pain. *Stereotact Funct Neurosurg* 78:192–96.

Chen R, Classen J, Gerloff C, Celnik P, Wassermann EM, Hallett M, Cohen LG. (1997). Depression of motor cortex excitability by low frequency transcranial magnetic stimulation. *Neurology* 48:1398–403.

Chen R, Cohen LG, Hallett M. (2002). Nervous system reorganization following injury. *Neuroscience* 111:761–73.

Cioni B, Megglio M. (2007). Motor cortex stimulation for chronic non-malignant pain: Current state and future prospects. *Acta Neurochir Suppl* 97(2):45–49.

Cohen LG, Bandinelli S, Findley TW, Hallett M. (1991). Motor reorganization after upper limb amputation in man. *Brain* 114:615–27.

Drewes AM, Rossel P, Le Pera D, Arrendt-Nielsen L, Valeriani M. (2005). Cortical neuro-plastic changes to painful colon stimulation in patients with irritable bowel syndrome. *Neuroscience* 375:157–61.

Eisenberg E, Chystiakov AV, Yudashkin M, Kaplan B, Hafner H, Feinsod M. (2005). Evidence for cortical hyperexcitability of the affected limb representation area in CRPS: A psychophysical and transcranial magnetic stimulation study. *Pain* 113:99–105.

Elbert T, Flor H, Birbaumer N, Hampson S, Taub E. (1994). Extensive reorganization of the somatosensory cortex in adult humans after nervous system injury. *NeuroReport* 5:2593–97.

Ervin FR, Brown CE, Mark VH. (1966). Striatal influence on facial pain. *Confin Neurol* 127:75–90.

Esfahani DR, Pisansky MT, Dafer RM, Anderson DE. (2011). Motor cortex stimulation: Functional magnetic resonance imaging-localized treatment for three sources of intractable facial pain. *J Neurosurg* 114(1):189–95.

Fenton B, Fanning J, Boggio P, Fregni F. (2008). A pilot efficacy trial of tDCS for the treatment of refractory chronic pelvic pain. *Brain Stimulation* 1(3):260.

Fields HL, Adams JE. (1974). Pain after cortical injury relieved by electrical stimulation of the internal capsule. *Brain* 97:169–78.

Flor H. (2000). The functional organization of the brain in chronic pain. In *Progress in brain research*, Sandkühler J, Bromm B, Gebhart GF (eds.), 313–22. Elsevier Science, Amsterdam.

Flor H. (2002). The modification of cortical reorganization and chronic pain by sensory feedback. *Appl Psychophysiol Biofeedback* 27:215–27.

Flor H. (2003). Cortical reorganization and chronic pain: Implications for rehabilitation. *J Rehabil Med* 41:66–72.

Flor H, Braun C, Elbert T, Birbaumer N. (1997). Extensive reorganization of primary somatosensory cortex in chronic back pain patients. *Neurosci Lett* 22:5–8.

Flor H, Elbert T, Knecht S, Wienbruch C, Pantev C, Birbaumer N, Larbig W, Taub E. (1995). Phantom limb pain as a perceptual correlate of massive cortical reorganization in upper extremity amputees. *Nature* 357:482–84.

Fregni F, Boggio PS, Lima MC, Ferreira MJ, Wagner T, Rigonatti SP, Castro AW, Souza DR, Riberto M, Freedman SD, Nitsche MA, Pascual-Leone A. (2006b). A sham-controlled, phase II trial of transcranial direct current stimulation for the treatment of central pain in traumatic spinal cord injury. *Pain* 122(1–2):197–209.

Fregni F, Gimenes R, Valle AS, Ferreira MJ, Rocha RR, Natalle L, Bravo R, Rigonatti SP, Freedman SD, Nitsche MA, Pascual-Leone A, Boggio PS. (2006a). A randomized, sham-controlled, proof of principle study of transcranial direct current stimulation for the treatment of pain in fibromyalgia. *Arthritis Rheum* 54(12):3988–98.

Friedland DR, Gaggl W, Runge-Samuelson C, Ulmer JL, Kopell BH. (2007). Feasibility of auditory cortical stimulation for the treatment of tinnitus. *Otol Neurotol* 28:1005–12.

Garcia-Larrea L, Peyron R, Mertens P, Gregoire MC, Lavenne F, LeBars D. (1999). Electrical stimulation of motor cortex for pain control: A combined PET-scan and electrophysiological study. *Pain* 83:259–73.

Gybels J, Kupers RC. (2000). Brain stimulation in the management of persistent pain. In *Schmidek and Sweet operative neurosurgical techniques*, Schmidek HH (ed.), 1639–51. Saunders, Philadelphia.

Hamani C, Schwalb JM, Rezai AR, Dostrovsky JO, Davis KD, Lozano AM. (2006). Deep brain stimulation for chronic neuropathic pain: Long-term outcome and the incidence of insertional effect. *Pain* 125:188–96.

Hariz MI. (2002). Complications of deep brain stimulation surgery. *Mov Disord* 17:162–66.

Hattori Y, Moriwaki A, Hori Y. (1990). Biphasic effects of polarizing current on adenosine-sensitive generation of cyclic AMP in rat cerebral cortex. *Neurosci Lett* 116:320–24.

Hosobuchi Y, Adams JE, Linchitz R. (1977). Pain relief by electrical stimulation of the central gray matter in humans and its reversal by naloxone. *Science* 197:183–86.

Hosobuchi Y, Adams JE, Rutkin B. (1973). Chronic thalamic stimulation for the control of facial anesthesia dolorosa. *Arch Neurol* 129:158–61.

Hosobuchi Y, Adams JE, Rutkin B. (1975). Chronic thalamic and internal capsule stimulation for the control of central pain. *Surg Neurol* 4:91–92.

Islam N, Aftabuddin M, Moriwaki A, Hattori Y, Hori Y. (1995). Increase in the calcium level following anodal polarization in the rat brain. *Brain Res* 684:206–8.

Johnson S, Summers J, Pridmore S. (2006). Changes to somatosensory detection and pain thresholds following high frequency repetitive TMS of the motor cortex in individuals suffering from chronic pain. *Pain* 123:187–92.

Kanda M, Tatsuya M, Oga T. (2003). Transcranial magnetic stimulation of the sensorimotor and medial frontal cortex modifies human pain perception. *Clin Neurophysiol* 114:860–66.

Karl A, Birbaumer N, Lutzenberg W, Cohen LG, Flor H. (2001). Reorganization of motor and somatosensory cortex in upper extremity amputees with phantom limb pain. *J Neurosci* 21:3609–18.

Katz N. (2000). Neuropathic pain in cancer and AIDS. *Clin J Pain* 16:S41–48.

Khedr EM, Kotb H, Kamel NF, Ahmed MA, Sadek R, Rothwell JC. (2005). Long-lasting antalgic effects of daily sessions of repetitive transcranial magnetic stimulation in central and peripheral neuropathic pain. *J Neurol Neurosurg Psychiatry* 76:833–38.

Knotkova H, Esteban S, Sibirceva U, Das D, Cruciani RA. (2010). Non-invasive brain stimulation therapy for the management of complex regional pain syndrome (CRPS). In *Brain stimulation for the treatment of pain*, Knotkova H, Cruciani RA (eds.), 143–57. Nova Publishers, New York.

Knotkova H, Feldman D, Dvorkin E, Cruciani RA. (2008). Transcranial direct current stimulation (tDCS): A novel strategy to alleviate neuropathic pain. *J Pain Manage* 1(3):257–67.

Knotkova H, Homel P, Cruciani RA. (2009). Cathodal tDCS over the somatosensory cortex relieved chronic neuropathic pain in a patient with complex regional pain syndrome (CRPS/RSD). *J Pain Manage* 2(3):365–68.

Krack P, Kumar R, Ardouin C, Dowsey PL, McVicker JM, Benabid AL, Pollak P. (2001). Mirthful laughter induced by subthalamic nucleus stimulation. *Mov Disord* 16:867–75.

Krauss JK, Pohle T, Weigel R, Burgunder JM. (2002). Deep brain stimulation of the centre median-parafascicular complex in patients with movement disorders. *J Neurol Neurosurg Psychiatry* 72:546–48.

Kringelbach L, Pereira E, Green A, Owen S, Aziz T. (2010). Deep brain stimulation for chronic pain. In *Brain stimulation for the treatment of pain*, Knotkova H, Cruciani RA (eds.), 65–78. Nova Science Publishers, New York.

Kühnl S, Terney D, Paulus W, Antal A. (2008). The effect of daily sessions of anodal tDCS on chronic pain. *Brain Stimulation* 1(3):281.

Kulisevsky J, Berthier M, Gironell A, Pascual-Sedano B, Molet J, Pares P. (2002). Mania following deep brain stimulation for Parkinson's disease. *Neurology* 59:1421–24.

Kumar K, Wyant GM. (1985). Deep brain stimulation for alleviating chronic intractable pain. *Can J Surg* 1:20–22.

Kumar K, Wyant GM, Nath R. (1990). Deep brain stimulation for control of intractable pain in humans, present and future: A ten-year follow-up. *Neurosurgery* 5:774–82.

Lang N, Nitsche MA, Paulus W, Rothwell JC, Lemon RN. (2004). Effects of transcranial direct current stimulation over the human motor cortex on cortical and transcallosal excitability. *Exp Brain Res* 156:439–43.

Lang N, Siebner HR, Ward NS, Lee L, Nitsche MA, Paulus W, Rothwell JC, Lemon RN, Frackowiak RS. (2005). How does transcranial DC stimulation of the primary motor cortex alter regional neuronal activity in the human brain? *Eur J Neurosci* 22:495–504.

Lefaucheur JP. (2004). Transcranial magnetic stimulation in the management of pain. *Suppl Clin Neurophysiol* 57:737–48.

Lefaucheur JP, Drouot X, Cunin P, Bruckert R, Lepetit H, Créange A, Wolkenstein P, Maison P, Keravel Y, Nguyen JP. (2009). Motor cortex stimulation for the treatment of refractory peripheral neuropathic pain. *Brain* 132(6):1463–71.

Lefaucheur JP, Drouot X, Keravel Y, Nguyen JP. (2001b). Pain relief induced by repetitive transcranial magnetic stimulation of precentral cortex. *Neuroreport* 12:2963–65.

Lefaucheur JP, Drouot X, Nguyen JP. (2001a). Interventional neurophysiology for pain control: Duration of pain relief following repetitive transcranial magnetic stimulation of the motor cortex. *Neurophysiol Clin* 31:247–52.

Levy RM. (2003). Deep brain stimulation for the treatment of intractable pain. *Neurosurg Clin N Am* 14:389–99.

Liebetanz D, Nitsche MA, Tergau F, Paulus W. (2002). Pharmacological approach to the mechanisms of transcranial DC-stimulation-induced after-effects of human motor cortex excitability. *Brain* 125:2238–47.

Lima MC, Fregni F. (2008). Motor cortex stimulation for chronic pain: Systematic review and meta-analysis of the literature. *Neurology* 70:2329–37.

Maihöfner CCA, Handwerker HO, Neundorfer B, Birklein F. (2004). Cortical reorganization during recovery from complex regional pain syndrome. *Neurology* 63:693–701.

Mark VH, Ervin FR. (1965). Role of thalamotomy in treatment of chronic severe pain. *Postgrad Med* 37:563–71.

Mark VH, Ervin FR, Hackett TP. (1960). Clinical aspects of stereotactic thalamotomy in the human. Part I. The treatment of chronic severe pain. *Arch Neurol* 3:351–67.

Martin LA, Hagen NA. (1997). Neuropathic pain in cancer patients: Mechanisms, syndromes, and clinical controversies. *J Pain Symptom Manage* 14:99–117.

Mazars G, Merienne L, Ciolocca C. (1973). Intermittent analgesic thalamic stimulation. Preliminary note. *Rev Neurol* 128:273–79.

Mazars G, Merienne L, Cioloca C. (1974). Treatment of certain types of pain with implantable thalamic stimulators. *Neurochirurgie* 20:117–24.

Mazars G, Roge R, Mazars Y. (1960). Results of the stimulation of the spinothalamic fasciculus and their bearing on the physiopathology of pain. *Rev Prat* 103:136–38.

Mazars GJ. (1975). Intermittent stimulation of nucleus ventraliposterolateralis for intractable pain. *Surg Neurol* 4:93–95.

Migita K, Tohru U, Kazunori A, Shuji M. (1995). Transcranial magnetic coil stimulation of motor cortex in patients with central pain. *Neurosurgery* 36:1037–40.

Mundinger F, Salomão JF. (1980). Deep brain stimulation in mesencephalic lemniscus medialis for chronic pain. *Acta Neurochir Suppl* 30:245–48.

Nguyen JP, Lefaucher JP, Le Guerinel C, Eizenbaum JF, Nakano N, Carpentier A, Brugieres P, Pollin B, Rostaining S, Keravel Y. (2000). Motor cortex stimulation in the treatment of central and neuropathic pain. *Arch Med Res* 31:263–65.

Nguyen JP, Pollin B, Feve A, Geny C, Cesaro P. (1998). Improvement of action tremor by chronic cortical stimulation. *Mov Disord* 13:84–88.

Nitsche MA, Fricke K, Henschke U. (2003). Pharmacological modulation of cortical excitability shifts induced by transcranial direct current stimulation in humans. *J Physiol* 553:293–301.

Nitsche MA, Jaussi W, Liebetanz D, Lang N, Tergau F, Paulus W. (2004). Consolidation of human motor cortical neuroplasticity by D-cycloserine. *Neuropsychopharmacology* 29:1573–78.

Nitsche MA, Paulus W. (2000). Excitability changes induced in the human motor cortex by weak transcranial direct current stimulation. *J Physiol* 527:633–39.

Nitsche, MA, Paulus W. (2001). Sustained excitability elevations induced by transcranial DC motor cortex stimulation in humans. *Neurology* 57:1899–901.

Nitsche MA, Seeber A, Frommann K. (2005). Modulating parameters of excitability during and after transcranial direct current stimulation of the human motor cortex. *J Physiol* 568:291–303.

Owen SLF, Green AL, Nandi D, Bittar RG, Wang S, Aziz TZ. (2006). Deep brain stimulation for neuropathic pain. *Neuromodulation* 9:100–6.

Pagni CA, Franzini A. (1981). Therapeutic strategy in cancer pain. *Minerva Med* 72(1):1–16.

Pascual-Leone A, Valls Sole J, Wassermann EM, Hallett M. (1994). Responses to rapid-rate transcranial magnetic stimulation of the human motor cortex. *Brain* 117:847–58.

Paulus W. (2004). Outlasting excitability shifts induced by direct current stimulation of the human brain. *Suppl Clin Neurophysiol* 57:708–14.

Pleger B, Janssen F, Schwenkreis P, Volker B, Maier C, Tegenthoff M. (2004). Repetitive transcranial magnetic stimulation of the motor cortex attenuates pain perception in complex regional pain syndrome type I. *Neurosci Lett* 356:87–90.

Pleger B, Tegenthoff M, Ragert P, Forster AF, Dinse H, Nicolas PV, Maier C. (2005). Sensorimotor returning in complex regional pain syndrome parallels pain reduction. *Ann Neurol* 57:425–29.

Pool JL, Clark WD, Hudson P, Lombardo M. (1956). Steroid hormonal response to stimulation of electrodes implanted in the subfrontal parts of the brain. In *Hypothalamic-hypophysial interrelationships*, Fields WS, Guillemin R, Carton CA, Charles C (eds.), 114–24. Charles C. Thomas, Springfield, IL.

Richardson DE, Akil H. (1977a). Long term results of periventricular gray self-stimulation. *Neurosurgery* 1:199–202.

Richardson DE, Akil H. (1977b). Pain reduction by electrical brain stimulation in man. Part 1: Acute administration in periaqueductal and periventricular sites. *J Neurosurg* 47:178–83.

Richardson DE, Akil H. (1977c). Pain reduction by electrical brain stimulation in man. Part 2: Chronic self-administration in the periventricular gray matter. *J Neurosurg* 47:184–94.

Roizenblatt S, Fregni F, Gimenez R, Wetzel T, Rigonatti SP, Tufik S, Boggio PS, Valle AC. (2007). Site-specific effects of transcranial direct current stimulation on sleep and pain in fibromyalgia: A randomized, sham-controlled study. *Pain Pract* 7(4):297–306.

Rollnik JD, Wustefeld S, Dauper M, Karst M, Fink M, Kossev A, Dengler R. (2002). Repetitive transcranial magnetic stimulation for the treatment of chronic pain—A pilot study. *Eur Neurol* 48:6–10.

Silva G, Miksad R, Freedman SD, Pascual-Leone A, Jain S, Gomes DL, Amancio EJ, Boggio PS, Correa CF, Fregni F. (2007). Treatment of cancer pain with noninvasive brain stimulation. *J Pain Symptom Manage* 34(4):342–45.

Summers J, Johnson S, Pridemore S, Oberoi G. (2004). Changes to cold detection and pain thresholds following low and high frequency transcranial magnetic stimulation of the motor cortex. *Neurosci Lett* 368:197–200.

Tamura Y, Okabe S, Ohnishi T, Saito D, Arai N, Mochio S, Inoue K, Ugawa Y. (2004). Effects of 1-Hz repetitive transcranial magnetic stimulation on acute pain induced by capsaicin. *Pain* 107:107–15.

Temel Y, Van Lankveld J, Boon P, Spincemaille G, Van der Linden C, Visser-Vandewalle V. (2004). Deep brain stimulation of the thalamus can influence penile erection. *Int J Impot Res* 16:91–94.

Tinazzi M, Fiaschi A, Rosso T, Faccioli F, Grosslercher J, Aglioti SM. (2000). Neuroplastic changes related to pain occur at multiple levels of human somatosensory system: A somatosensory-evoked potentials study in patients with cervical radicular pain. *J Neurosci* 20:9277–83.

Tronnier VM. (2003). *Deep brain stimulation*. Elsevier, Amsterdam.

Tsubokawa T, Katayama Y, Yamamoto T, Hirayama T, Koyama S. (1991). Chronic motor cortex stimulation for the treatment of central pain. *Acta Neurochir (Wien) Suppl* 52:137–39.

Tsubokawa T, Katayama Y, Yamamoto T, Hirayama T, Koyama S. (1993). Chronic motor cortex stimulation in patients with thalamic pain. *J Neurosurg* 93:393–401.

Wassermann EM, Lisanby SH. (2001). Therapeutic application of repetitive transcranial magnetic stimulation: A review. *Clin Neurophysiol* 112:1367–77.

White JC, Sweet WH. (1969). *Pain and the neurosurgeon*. Charles C. Thoms, Springfield, IL.

Zaghi S, DaSilva AF, Acar M, Lopes M, Fregni F. (2009). One-year rTMS treatment for refractory trigeminal neuralgia. *J Pain Symptom Manage* 38(4):1–5.

11 Nerve Decompression for Chemotherapy-Induced Neuropathic Pain

Michael I. Rose

CONTENTS

11.1 Introduction 195
11.2 Nerve Decompression 196
    11.2.1 Background 196
    11.2.2 Basic Science and Clinical Data 197
    11.2.3 Human Data 198
11.3 Diagnosis 198
11.4 Surgical Treatment 200
11.5 Conclusion 203
References 203

11.1 INTRODUCTION

Despite the limited efficacy of current medical treatments, and the fact that they only treat the pain component of chemotherapy-induced peripheral neuropathy (CIPN), until recently there has been little interest in exploring surgical therapies for this condition. This is not at all surprising, because at first blush, it would seem that there is no rationale for a surgical approach to a systemic side effect of a medication (neurotoxicity). Similar reasoning had previously been applied to other forms of systemic-disease-induced neuropathy, such as diabetic neuropathy. This resulted in a long lag between the recognition of the cause of diabetic neuropathy and the application of a successful surgical treatment to alleviate its effects on the extremities. The lessons learned from the success in the treatment of diabetic neuropathy allowed for investigations into the feasibility of transferring similar techniques into the realm of chemotherapy-induced neuropathy. These surgical techniques have proven to be valuable adjuncts to available medical therapies for this disabling and painful condition.

Chemotherapy-induced neuropathy affects a large percentage of patients who receive chemotherapeutic agents. Not all chemotherapy agents cause neuropathy, but platin-based compounds, taxanes, and vinca alkaloids are the most common offenders, among many (Quastohoff et al., 2002). Even the more rarely used thalidomide, and several other atypical chemotherapeutic agents, have a strong correlation with the development of painful neuropathy. For all of these agents, the affect appears

195

to be dose dependent and is typically a sensory neuropathy, although a motor component is not unheard of (Rosson, 2006). The neuropathic effects for most of these drugs tend to abate slowly after cessation of therapy, but in many cases they persist long after the drug is discontinued. There is even a clinical phenomenon known as coasting, where a previously asymptomatic patient develops neuropathic symptoms weeks or months after the cessation of therapy. These patients with persistent neuropathic symptoms are in a confusing clinical situation: although they have successful cancer outcomes, the severity of their neuropathy symptoms prevents them from returning to work or partaking in activities they enjoyed prior to their cancer treatment. Further dampening these patients' outlook is the following: for all intents and purposes, there is no current medical treatment of CIPN, but rather, there are only ways to ameliorate the pain. Even when successful at relieving the pain of CIPN, the current medical treatments have troublesome adverse effects.

Like most systemic problems, initial treatments are aimed at systemic amelioration of symptoms. Medicinal treatments such as gabapentin and pregabalin are commonly prescribed along with selective serotonin reuptake inhibitors (SSRIs) such as duloxetine. Opioids are frequently needed. While many of these treatments offer some degree of symptomatic efficacy, they also have attendant adverse effects or potential for misuse and abuse. What they all have in common is that they simply manage, cover-up or make tolerable the pain. They do little or nothing to reverse or treat the underlying cause. Furthermore, while pain is the main symptom that drives the patient to seek help, it is not in fact the symptom that is most threatening to the patient. The resulting lack of protective sensation in the neuropathic extremity is a major cause of ulcers, infections, and subsequent amputations (Aszmann et al., 2004).

11.2   NERVE DECOMPRESSION

11.2.1   BACKGROUND

Dellon published the seminal paper demonstrating the efficacy of nerve decompression on both the symptoms and the natural course of diabetic neuropathy (Dellon, 1992). Not only were the symptoms improved in 85% of treated patients, but treated extremities—unlike the remaining untreated extremities—were no longer experiencing ulcers, infections, and subsequent amputations. This indicated that the decompression was protective against future neuropathy-derived morbidity. This phenomenon was further discussed in a paper in 2004 (Aszmann et al., 2004). To date there are 13 clinical studies demonstrating the efficacy of the nerve decompression approach to the treatment of diabetic neuropathy (reviewed by Melenhorst et al., 2009). Nevertheless, the surgical approach to the treatment of diabetic peripheral neuropathy has its critics (Therapeutics and Technology Assessment Subcommittee, 2006).

Over time, clinicians with experience with the surgical approaches to diabetic neuropathy began to expand their indications for this treatment. First, it was diabetic neuropathy, then it was idiopathic neuropathy, and eventually chemotherapy-induced neuropathy became a valid target for this treatment (Dellon et al., 2003; Valdivia et al., 2005). In fact, this approach has been successfully applied to alcoholic neuropathy, lead neuropathy, and the neuropathy of Hanson's disease (A.L. Dellon, personal communication). It would seem that the cause of the neuropathy is somewhat irrelevant, as there is some degree of a common pathologic pathway that renders the nerves susceptible to compression at known sites of anatomic narrowing. This allows for nerve decompressions to treat the effects of many variations of neuropathy.

The crux of the problem, and the reason that surgery can be effective, relates to the double-crush phenomenon (Upton and McComas, 1973). The double-crush hypothesis is that separate insults to the peripheral nervous system—neither of which would have caused symptoms on their own—are additive and thus cause significant symptoms, even when the separate insults are relatively minor. This phenomenon has been clearly elucidated in animal models and explains clinically why diabetic patients are more susceptible to compression neuropathies such as carpal tunnel syndrome (Dellon and MacKinnon, 1991).

While the exact mechanism for the development of neuropathy after chemotherapy is not known, there is evidence for direct neuronal toxicity as well as a component of intracellular and extracellular edema as a response to that neurotoxicity. The slow component of axoplasmal transport appears diminished in most forms of CIPN, a pathophysiogic mechanism that is also found in diabetes-induced peripheral neuropathy (Tassler et al., 2000). The resulting stiffening and swelling of the nerves may result in neurocompressive symptoms caused at the known sites of anatomic narrowing (carpal tunnel, tarsal tunnel, etc.). So the direct effect of the toxic agent causes decreased function of the nerve, but more importantly, decreased function leads to stiffness and swelling of the nerve, and in predisposed individuals that results in nerve compression at the anatomic tunnels. This is precisely what the double-crush hypothesis predicts.

A loose analogy would be if a man who wore the same suit and tie every day gained 30 pounds. He would certainly be less healthy for the weight gain, but it would be his belt and his collar (sites of fixed anatomic narrowing) that would be most likely to cause him pain and distress. After loosening his belt, and unbuttoning his collar, he will feel considerably better, even though the underlying problem is still there. So the weight gain is one crush, but the presence of fixed-diameter tunnels provides the second crush that ultimately leads to the distress. Neither crush alone would have caused the problem, but together they result in disease.

11.2.2 BASIC SCIENCE AND CLINICAL DATA

Most of the work in the surgical treatment of neuropathy has been done in the diabetes model, with some additional study in a chemotherapy-induced model. Dellon et al. (1994) found that rats made diabetic with streptozotocin developed a neuropathic walking tract pattern. This pattern could be prevented by pretreating the rats with decompression of their tarsal tunnels. By eliminating one of the "crushes" the animals were rendered asymptomatic. This study was duplicated by Kale et al. (2003). Similar studies were performed in a model of cisplatin neuropathy in adult rats. In that study, rats administered cisplatin developed neuropathic walking patterns, yet rats that had tibial nerve decompressions concurrent with the commencement of cisplatin therapy did not develop these abnormal walking patterns.

This indicated that similar to the diabetic model, tibial nerve decompressions were protective against the development of neuropathic walking patterns in the adult rat (Tassler et al., 2000).

11.2.3 HUMAN DATA

Human clinical data remain sparse despite the fact that the two known papers were published 6 and 8 years ago, respectively (Dellon et al., 2003; Rose et al., 2006). There is one case series of nine patients and one double case report of two additional patients with CIPN who were successfully treated with nerve decompressions. In the case series, six of the nine patients fit the World Health Organization's clinical definition of chemotherapy-induced neuropathy and are the basis of the results and conclusions of the paper. All six of these patients had statistically significant reductions in the visual analog scale (VAS) for pain, and all had varying degrees of improvement in 2-point discrimination in the treated extremity. The second paper is a double case report of two patients with CIPN from thalidomide. Both were treated with nerve decompressions and both had measurable decreases in their VAS pain score and improvement in their 1-point pressure thresholds and 2-point discrimination thresholds. Due to the novelty of this approach to treat the symptoms of CIPN, there remains significant clinical resistance to applying it to patients. Furthermore, third-party payers might not reimburse for such treatment, which in some cases further hinders its application clinically.

11.3 DIAGNOSIS

Chemotherapy-induced neuropathy is fairly obvious and straightforward to diagnose clinically, but in fact there is no test for neuropathy. It is thus a diagnosis of exclusion and a clinical diagnosis. However, the symptom cluster for CIPN varies so much from patient to patient that the only thing consistent is that there is no consistency. Not all patients report pain, and every patient with pain reports it to varying degrees. Some complain of numbness and tingling while others have cramping pain or shooting pains. Some are affected at night, others during the day. Some feel better lying down, some standing up and walking. Some feel like there is something stuck in their shoe (like walking on sand, or that their sock is bunched up) while others notice that they cannot feel all or part of their foot—despite the pain they feel. What drives the diagnosis is that there is a clearly definable cause (chemotherapy) and a clearly correlated onset of symptoms after the commencement of therapy.

Typically the patient will be sent for expensive and painful electromyograms (EMGs) and nerve conduction studies. Unfortunately, electrodiagnostic studies are notoriously unreliable in distal extremity neuropathy diagnosis (Perkins et al., 2002; Quasthoff and Hartung, 2002; Dellon, 2005). Furthermore, expense and patient discomfort preclude these modalities as a screening test, or one that can be used repeatedly to follow the course of disease over time. Dellon and others advocate non-invasive neurosensory testing as a modality to quantify and follow the progression of disease over time, and after surgical therapy (Tassler and Dellon, 1995; Rosson,

2006). Since many CIPN patients do improve over 3 to 6 months following the cessation of the offending treatment, surgical intervention is ideally postponed until this time unless symptom severity dictates a more aggressive timetable. Painless, inexpensive, noninvasive neurosensory testing is an excellent way to follow these patients and document progression, or regression of disease. One clear indication for early consideration of surgery would be significant motor weakness in the affected extremities. Both peripheral sensory and motor nerves can regenerate at any time after injury; however, the motor nerves terminate at motor endplates on the muscle that irreversibly disappear sometime between 6 and 12 months after impulses stop being received at the motor endplate. This physiologic fact makes the timing of intervention with motor neuropathy more critical. Since there is a lag between the time of nerve decompression and the resumption of motor impulses on the order of several months, it behooves the surgeon to consider surgery for motor symptoms well prior to the 6- to 12-month window where the endplates begin to stop functioning forever.

Once a patient is clinically diagnosed with CIPN, he or she may be sent for electrodiagnostic tests to rule out another cause, and possibly illuminate the current disease process, but in most cases clinical examination coupled possibly with noninvasive sensory threshold testing is adequate to make a decision to move forward with treatment, including surgery. One issue that remains is the ability to reliably predict outcomes from surgery preoperatively. Multiple factors determine who will or will not be helped by the surgical decompressions, but currently no reliable test exists to select the best candidates for the procedure. Interestingly, the diabetic neuropathy literature presents evidence that the presence of a positive Tinel-Hoffman sign is a strongly positive predictor of a good outcome (Lee and Dellon, 2004). Anecdotal evidence in the two published human papers regarding the surgical treatment of CIPN indicates that a positive Tinel-Hoffman sign is a good predictor of outcomes in this population as well, but more studies are needed to confirm this (Rose et al., 2006).

Typically, a patient will have a stocking-and-glove distribution of his or her symptoms, but isolated mononeuropathies are reported. A Tinel sign should be present at the site of anatomic narrowing to establish a high chance of clinical success after surgery. The typical sites on the upper extremity to be examined are cubital tunnel, carpal tunnel, Guyon's canal at the wrist, and the radial nerve in the dorsal forearm. On the lower extremity, it is typical to examine the tarsal tunnel, the common peroneal nerve's tunnel just below the lateral condyle of the fibular neck, and the deep peroneal nerve as it passes underneath the extensor halucis brevis tendon in the mid-dorsum of the foot. If Tinel signs are positive at these sites, with symptoms in the distribution covered by that nerve, then surgical decompression has a high likelihood of success.

Prior to surgery, the patient should be examined and worked up to eliminate more central causes for the neuropathic symptoms (e.g., disk compressions, spinal stenosis, etc.). Furthermore, vascular compromise of the lower extremity can alter healing capacity, and can also mimic neuropathy symptoms and should be ruled out prior to surgical intervention. The patients' general health should be evaluated prior to surgery as well.

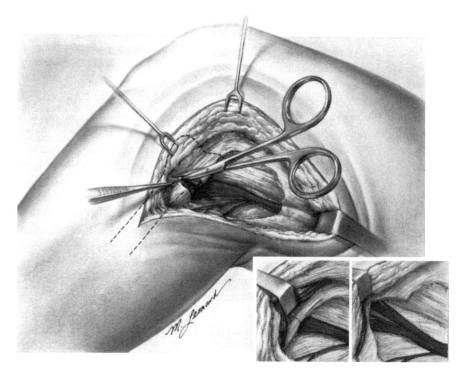

FIGURE 11.1 In the lower extremities common peroneal nerve compression is treated by release of the nerve as it passes through the peroneous longus fascia just inferior to the lateral fibular neck. (Schematic provided by A. Lee Dellon, M.D., Ph.D., Dellon.com. With permission.)

11.4 SURGICAL TREATMENT

In the upper extremity, compressions of the nerves occur in well-described anatomic points, and surgical treatment of the upper extremity is a bit more studied and understood. Neuropathy decompression includes release of the cubital tunnel, carpal tunnel, Guyon's canal, and the radial nerve in the distal forearm. For a glove distribution, all of the sites will be decompressed. If symptoms are more localized, then a focused approach should be used. Whether endoscopic releases offer any benefit in the setting of neuropathy decompressions remains to be demonstrated. Similarly, in the lower extremities common peroneal nerve compression is treated by release of the nerve as it passes through the peroneous longus fascia just inferior to the lateral fibular neck (Figure 11.1).

Deep peroneal nerve decompression is executed by resecting a segment of the extensor halucus brevis tendon as it passes over the deep peroneal nerve in the dorsum of the foot (Figure 11.2).

There is no functional consequence to sacrificing this tendon as the extensor halucus longus tendon is the primary extensor of the great toe. Finally, the tarsal tunnel as well as the four medial ankle tunnels should be decompressed to improve symptoms attributable to the tibial nerve (Figure 11.3).

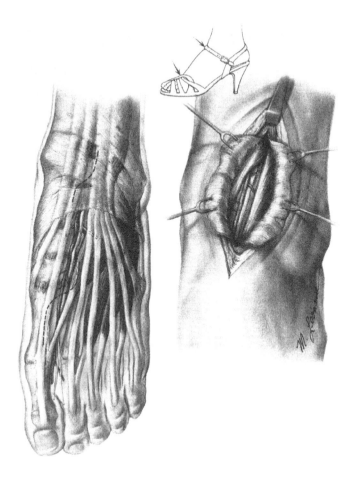

FIGURE 11.2   Deep peroneal nerve decompression is executed by resecting a segment of the extensor halucus brevis tendon as it passes over the deep peroneal nerve in the dorsum of the foot. (Schematic provided by A. Lee Dellon, M.D., Ph.D., Dellon.com. With permission.)

Traditionally, tarsal tunnel release is the simple opening of the flexor retinaculum over the tibial neurovascular bundle. Results tend to be much more predictable if the T-shaped roof and septum between the medial and lateral plantar nerves (see Figure 11.3, inset) are excised. This results in a common tunnel into the porta pedis of the foot. Surgery is generally performed as an outpatient procedure, with follow-up typically 1 week after the surgery when the bulky but soft dressing is to be removed. To avoid wound healing issues, the patient is instructed to elevate the extremity postoperatively, but he or she is allowed to bear weight and use the extremity gingerly during the healing phase to minimize scarring and reentrapment of the nerves during the healing process. Sutures are removed 3 weeks after surgery since these incisions are over high-stress, active-motion areas.

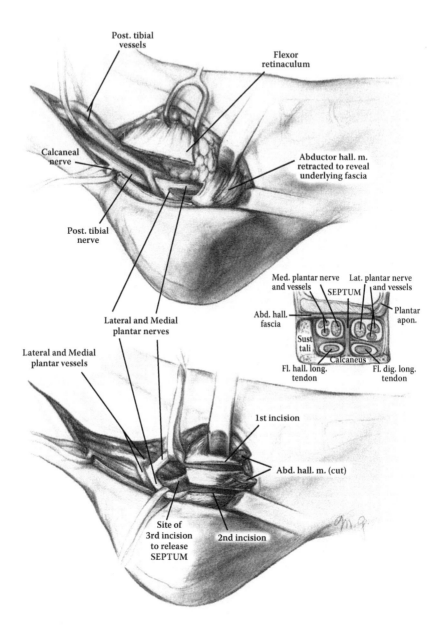

FIGURE 11.3 The tarsal tunnel as well as the four medial ankle tunnels should be decompressed to improve symptoms attributable to the tibial nerve. (Schematic provided by A. Lee Dellon, M.D., Ph.D., Dellon.com. With permission.)

11.5   CONCLUSION

While data are still sparse, there is a small body of human and animal data that support the application of nerve decompression surgery for the relief of CIPN. Patients should be chosen carefully to maximize the chance of a good outcome and minimize complications. Further clinical and basic science studies are needed to confirm definitively the efficacy of this approach and to cement it as a weapon in the armamentarium of the surgeon against this debilitating effect of chemotherapy.

REFERENCES

Aszmann O, Tassler PL, Dellon AL. (2004). Changing the natural history of diabetic neuropathy: Incidence of ulcer/amputation in the contralateral limb of patients with a unilateral nerve decompression procedure. *Ann Plast Surg* 53(6):517–22.

Dellon AL. (1992). Treatment of symptomatic diabetic neuropathy by surgical decompression of multiple peripheral nerves. *Plast Reconstr Surg* 89(4):689–97.

Dellon AL. (2005). Measuring peripheral nerve function: Electrodiagnostic versus neurosensory testing. *Atlas Hand Clin* 10(1):1–31.

Dellon AL, Dellon ES, Seiler WA. (1994). Effect of tarsal tunnel decompression in the streptozotocin-induced diabetic rat. *Microsurgery* 15:265–68.

Dellon AL, MacKinnon SE. (1991). Chronic nerve compression model for the double crush hypothesis. *Ann Plast Surg* 26:259–64.

Dellon AL, Swier P, Maloney CT Jr, Livengood MS, Werter S. (2003). Chemotherapy-induced neuropathy: Treatment by decompression of peripheral nerves. *Plast Reconstr Surg* 114(2):478–83.

Kale B, Yuksel F, Celikoz B, Sirvanci S, Ergun O, Arbak S. (2003). Effect of various nerve decompression procedures on the functions of distal limbs in streptozotocin-induced diabetic rats: Further optimism in diabetic neuropathy. *Plast Reconstr Surg* 111(7):2265–72.

Lee CH, Dellon AL. (2004). Prognostic ability of Tinel sign in determining outcome for decompression surgery in diabetic and nondiabetic neuropathy. *Ann Plast Surg* 53(6):523–27.

Melenhorst WB, Overgoor ML, Gonera EG, Tellier MA, Houpt P. (2009). Nerve decompression surgery as treatment for peripheral diabetic neuropathy: Literature overview and awareness among medical professionals. *Ann Plast Surg* 63(2):217–21.

Perkins BA, Olaleye D, Bril V. (2002). Carpal tunnel syndrome in patients with diabetic polyneuropathy. *Diabetes Care* 25(3):565–69.

Quasthoff S, Hartung HP. (2002). Chemotherapy-induced peripheral neuropathy. *J Neurol* 249(1):9–17.

Rose MI, Rosson GD, Elkwood AL, Dellon AL. (2006). Thalidomide-induced neuropathy: Treatment by decompression of peripheral nerves. *Plast Reconstr Surg* 117(7):2329–32.

Rosson GD. (2006). Chemotherapy-induced neuropathy. *Clin Podiatr Med Surg* 23(3):637–49.

Tassler PL, Dellon AL. (1995). Correlation of measurements of pressure perception using the pressure-specified sensory device with electrodiagnostic testing. *J Occup Med* 37(7):862–66.

Tassler PL, Dellon AL, Lesser GJ, Grossman S. (2000). Utility of decompressive surgery in the prophylaxis and treatment of cisplatin neuropathy in adult rats. *J Reconstr Microsurg* 16(6):457–63.

Therapeutics and Technology Assessment Subcommittee of the American Academy of Neurology; Chaudhry V, Stevens JC, Kincaid J, So YT. (2006). Practice advisory: Utility of surgical decompression for treatment of diabetic neuropathy: Report of the Therapeutics and Technology Assessment Subcommittee of the American Academy of Neurology. *Neurology* 66(12):1805–8.

Upton AR, McComas AJ. (1973). The double crush in nerve entrapment syndromes. *Lancet* 2:359–62.

Valdivia JM, Dellon AL, Weinand ME, Maloney CT Jr. (2005). Surgical treatment of peripheral neuropathy: Outcomes from 100 consecutive decompressions. *J Am Podiatr Med Assoc* 95(5):451–54.

Bibliography

Peripheral neuropathy induced by oxaliplatin-based chemotherapy. *J Support Oncol* 2006; 482–83.

CI-PERINOMS: Chemotherapy-induced peripheral neuropathy outcome measures study. *J Peripher Nerv Syst* 2009; 14: 69–71.

Alford M. Chemotherapy-induced peripheral neuropathy was described as background noise affecting daily life. *Evid Based Nurs* 2008; 11: 62.

Almadrones L, McGuire DB, Walczak JR, Florio CM, Tian C. Psychometric evaluation of two scales assessing functional status and peripheral neuropathy associated with chemotherapy for ovarian cancer: A Gynecologic Oncology Group study. *Oncol Nurs Forum* 2004; 31: 615–23.

Alvarez P, Ferrari LF, Levine JD. Muscle pain in models of chemotherapy-induced and alcohol-induced peripheral neuropathy. *Ann Neurol* 2011; 70: 101–9.

Amara S. Oral glutamine for the prevention of chemotherapy-induced peripheral neuropathy. *Ann Pharmacother* 2008; 42: 1481–85.

Argyriou AA, Kalofonos HP. Vitamin E for preventing chemotherapy-induced peripheral neuropathy. *Support Care Cancer* 2011; 19: 725–6; author reply, 7–8.

Argyriou AA, Polychronopoulos P, Iconomou G, Koutras A, Makatsoris T, Gerolymos MK, Gourzis P, Assimakopoulos K, Kalofonos HP, Chroni E. Incidence and characteristics of peripheral neuropathy during oxaliplatin-based chemotherapy for metastatic colon cancer. *Acta Oncol* 2007; 46: 1131–37.

Argyriou AA, Polychronopoulos P, Koutras A, Iconomou G, Gourzis P, Assimakopoulos K, Kalofonos HP, Chroni E. Is advanced age associated with increased incidence and severity of chemotherapy-induced peripheral neuropathy? *Support Care Cancer* 2006; 14: 223–29.

Argyriou AA, Polychronopoulos P, Koutras A, Iconomou G, Iconomou A, Kalofonos HP, Chroni E. Peripheral neuropathy induced by administration of cisplatin- and paclitaxel-based chemotherapy. Could it be predicted? *Support Care Cancer* 2005; 13: 647–51.

Argyriou AA, Polychronopoulos P, Koutras A, Xiros N, Petsas T, Argyriou K, Kalofonos HP, Chroni E. Clinical and electrophysiological features of peripheral neuropathy induced by administration of cisplatin plus paclitaxel-based chemotherapy. *Eur J Cancer Care (Engl)* 2007; 16: 231–37.

Armstrong T, Almadrones L, Gilbert MR. Chemotherapy-induced peripheral neuropathy. *Oncol Nurs Forum* 2005; 32: 305–11.

Bakitas MA. Background noise: The experience of chemotherapy-induced peripheral neuropathy. *Nurs Res* 2007; 56: 323–31.

Barton DL, Wos EJ, Qin R, Mattar BI, Green NB, Lanier KS, Bearden JD 3rd, Kugler JW, Hoff KL, Reddy PS, Rowland KM Jr., Riepl M, Christensen B, Loprinzi CL. A double-blind, placebo-controlled trial of a topical treatment for chemotherapy-induced peripheral neuropathy: NCCTG trial N06CA. *Support Care Cancer* 2011; 19: 833–41.

Bashir RM, Bierman P, McComb R. Inflammatory peripheral neuropathy following high dose chemotherapy and autologous bone marrow transplantation. *Bone Marrow Transplant* 1992; 10: 305–6.

Binner M, Ross D, Browner I. Chemotherapy-induced peripheral neuropathy: Assessment of oncology nurses' knowledge and practice. *Oncol Nurs Forum* 2011; 38: 448–54.

Cata JP, Weng HR, Lee BN, Reuben JM, Dougherty PM. Clinical and experimental findings in humans and animals with chemotherapy-induced peripheral neuropathy. *Minerva Anestesiol* 2006; 72: 151–69.

Cavaletti G, Bogliun G, Marzorati L, Zincone A, Piatti M, Colombo N, Parma G, Lissoni A, Fei F, Cundari S, Zanna C. Grading of chemotherapy-induced peripheral neurotoxicity using the Total Neuropathy Scale. *Neurology* 2003; 61: 1297–300.

Cavaletti G, Frigeni B, Lanzani F, Piatti M, Rota S, Briani C, Zara G, Plasmati R, Pastorelli F, Caraceni A, Pace A, Manicone M, Lissoni A, Colombo N, Bianchi G, Zanna C. The Total Neuropathy Score as an assessment tool for grading the course of chemotherapy-induced peripheral neurotoxicity: Comparison with the National Cancer Institute-Common Toxicity Scale. *J Peripher Nerv Syst* 2007; 12: 210–15.

Cavaletti G, Jann S, Pace A, Plasmati R, Siciliano G, Briani C, Cocito D, Padua L, Ghiglione E, Manicone M, Giussani G. Multi-center assessment of the Total Neuropathy Score for chemotherapy-induced peripheral neurotoxicity. *J Peripher Nerv Syst* 2006; 11: 135–41.

Chaudhry V, Rowinsky EK, Sartorius SE, Donehower RC, Cornblath DR. Peripheral neuropathy from taxol and cisplatin combination chemotherapy: Clinical and electrophysiological studies. *Ann Neurol* 1994; 35: 304–11.

Cundari S, Cavaletti G. Thalidomide chemotherapy-induced peripheral neuropathy: Actual status and new perspectives with thalidomide analogues derivatives. *Mini Rev Med Chem* 2009; 9: 760–68.

Cunningham JE, Kelechi T, Sterba K, Barthelemy N, Falkowski P, Chin SH. Case report of a patient with chemotherapy-induced peripheral neuropathy treated with manual therapy (massage). *Support Care Cancer* 2011; 19: 1473–76.

Davis ID, Kiers L, MacGregor L, Quinn M, Arezzo J, Green M, Rosenthal M, Chia M, Michael M, Bartley P, Harrison L, Daly M. A randomized, double-blinded, placebo-controlled phase II trial of recombinant human leukemia inhibitory factor (rhuLIF, emfilermin, AM424) to prevent chemotherapy-induced peripheral neuropathy. *Clin Cancer Res* 2005; 11: 1890–98.

De Grandis D. Acetyl-L-carnitine for the treatment of chemotherapy-induced peripheral neuropathy: A short review. *CNS Drugs* 2007; 21 (Suppl 1): 39–43; discussion, 5–6.

Dellon AL, Swier P, Maloney CT Jr., Livengood MS, Werter S. Chemotherapy-induced neuropathy: Treatment by decompression of peripheral nerves. *Plast Reconstr Surg* 2004; 114: 478–83.

Donald GK, Tobin I, Stringer J. Evaluation of acupuncture in the management of chemotherapy-induced peripheral neuropathy. *Acupunct Med* 2011; 29: 230–33.

Donofrio PD, Albers JW, Greenberg HS, Mitchell BS. Peripheral neuropathy in osteosclerotic myeloma: Clinical and electrodiagnostic improvement with chemotherapy. *Muscle Nerve* 1984; 7: 137–41.

Dunlap B, Paice JA. Chemotherapy-induced peripheral neuropathy: A need for standardization in measurement. *J Support Oncol* 2006; 4: 398–99.

Ferrari G, Gemignani F, Macaluso C. Chemotherapy-associated peripheral sensory neuropathy assessed using *in vivo* corneal confocal microscopy. *Arch Neurol* 2010; 67: 364–65.

Gent P, Massey K. An overview of chemotherapy-induced peripheral sensory neuropathy, focusing on oxaliplatin. *Int J Palliat Nurs* 2001; 7: 354–59.

Gidoh M. The control leprous peripheral neuropathy and chemotherapy. *Nihon Hansenbyo Gakkai Zasshi* 1999; 68: 83–86.

Griffith KA, Merkies IS, Hill EE, Cornblath DR. Measures of chemotherapy-induced peripheral neuropathy: A systematic review of psychometric properties. *J Peripher Nerv Syst* 2010; 15: 314–25.

Gutierrez-Gutierrez G, Sereno M, Miralles A, Casado-Saenz E, Gutierrez-Rivas E. Chemotherapy-induced peripheral neuropathy: Clinical features, diagnosis, prevention and treatment strategies. *Clin Transl Oncol* 2010; 12: 81–91.

Hausheer FH, Schilsky RL, Bain S, Berghorn EJ, Lieberman F. Diagnosis, management, and evaluation of chemotherapy-induced peripheral neuropathy. *Semin Oncol* 2006; 33: 15–49.

Hilkens PH, Pronk LC, Verweij J, Vecht CJ, van Putten WL, van den Bent MJ. Peripheral neuropathy induced by combination chemotherapy of docetaxel and cisplatin. *Br J Cancer* 1997; 75: 417–22.

Hilkens PH, ven den Bent MJ. Chemotherapy-induced peripheral neuropathy. *J Peripher Nerv Syst* 1997; 2: 350–61.

Hohmann AG. A cannabinoid pharmacotherapy for chemotherapy-evoked painful peripheral neuropathy. *Pain* 2005; 118: 3–5.

Hughes R. NCI-CTC vs TNS: Which tool is better for grading the severity of chemotherapy-induced peripheral neuropathy? *Natl Clin Pract Neurol* 2008; 4: 68–69.

Kaley TJ, Deangelis LM. Therapy of chemotherapy-induced peripheral neuropathy. *Br J Haematol* 2009; 145: 3–14.

Kassem LA, Yassin NA. Role of erythropoeitin in prevention of chemotherapy-induced peripheral neuropathy. *Pak J Biol Sci* 2010; 13: 577–87.

Kautio AL, Haanpaa M, Kautiainen H, Leminen A, Kalso E, Saarto T. Oxaliplatin Scale and National Cancer Institute-Common Toxicity Criteria in the assessment of chemotherapy-induced peripheral neuropathy. *Anticancer Res* 2011; 31: 3493–96.

Kirchmair R, Tietz AB, Panagiotou E, Walter DH, Silver M, Yoon YS, Schratzberger P, Weber A, Kusano K, Weinberg DH, Ropper AH, Isner JM, Losordo DW. Therapeutic angiogenesis inhibits or rescues chemotherapy-induced peripheral neuropathy: Taxol- and thalidomide-induced injury of vasa nervorum is ameliorated by VEGF. *Mol Ther* 2007; 15: 69–75.

Kiser DW, Greer TB, Wilmoth MC, Dmochowski J, Naumann RW. Peripheral neuropathy in patients with gynecologic cancer receiving chemotherapy: Patient reports and provider assessments. *Oncol Nurs Forum* 2010; 37: 758–64.

Kottschade L, Loprinzi C, Rao R. Vitamin E for the prevention of chemotherapy-induced peripheral neuropathy: Rationale for an ongoing clinical trial. *Support Cancer Ther* 2007; 4: 251–53.

Kottschade LA, Sloan JA, Mazurczak MA, Johnson DB, Murphy BP, Rowland KM, Smith DA, Berg AR, Stella PJ, Loprinzi CL. The use of vitamin E for the prevention of chemotherapy-induced peripheral neuropathy: Results of a randomized phase III clinical trial. *Support Care Cancer* 2011; 19: 1769–77.

Kuroi K, Shimozuma K, Ohashi Y, Hisamatsu K, Masuda N, Takeuchi A, Aranishi T, Morita S, Ohsumi S, Hausheer FH. Prospective assessment of chemotherapy-induced peripheral neuropathy due to weekly paclitaxel in patients with advanced or metastatic breast cancer (CSP-HOR 02 study). *Support Care Cancer* 2009; 17(8): 1071–80.

Kuroi K, Shimozuma K, Ohashi Y, Takeuchi A, Aranishi T, Morita S, Ohsumi S, Watanabe T, Bain S, Hausheer FH. A questionnaire survey of physicians' perspectives regarding the assessment of chemotherapy-induced peripheral neuropathy in patients with breast cancer. *Jpn J Clin Oncol* 2008; 38: 748–54.

Malik B, Stillman M. Chemotherapy-induced peripheral neuropathy. *Curr Pain Headache Rep* 2008; 12: 165–74.

Markman M. Can we do a better job preventing clinically-relevant peripheral neuropathy resulting from carboplatin/paclitaxel chemotherapy? *Cancer Invest* 2004; 22: 471–73.

Markman M. Chemotherapy-induced peripheral neuropathy: An increasing concern for oncologists. *Curr Oncol Rep* 2005; 7: 159–60.

Markman M. Chemotherapy-induced peripheral neuropathy: Underreported and underappreciated. *Curr Pain Headache Rep* 2006; 10: 275–78.

Nurgalieva Z, Xia R, Liu CC, Burau K, Hardy D, Du XL. Risk of chemotherapy-induced peripheral neuropathy in large population-based cohorts of elderly patients with breast, ovarian, and lung cancer. *Am J Ther* 2010; 17: 148–58.

Ocean AJ, Vahdat LT. Chemotherapy-induced peripheral neuropathy: Pathogenesis and emerging therapies. *Support Care Cancer* 2004; 12: 619–25.

Oestreicher P. Put evidence into practice to treat chemotherapy-induced peripheral neuropathy. *ONS Connect* 2007; 22: 24–25.

Osborne WL, Holyoake TL, McQuaker IG, Parker AN. Fatal peripheral neuropathy following FLA chemotherapy. *Clin Lab Haematol* 2004; 26: 295–96.

Pachman DR, Barton DL, Watson JC, Loprinzi CL. Chemotherapy-induced peripheral neuropathy: Prevention and treatment. *Clin Pharmacol Ther* 2011; 90: 377–87.

Paice JA. Clinical challenges: Chemotherapy-induced peripheral neuropathy. *Semin Oncol Nurs* 2009; 25: S8–19.

Park JW, Jeon JH, Yoon J, Jung TY, Kwon KR, Cho CK, Lee YW, Sagar S, Wong R, Yoo HS. Effects of sweet bee venom pharmacopuncture treatment for chemotherapy-induced peripheral neuropathy: A case series. *Integr Cancer Ther* (in press).

Parra R, Fernandez JM, Garcia-Bragado F, Bueno J, Biosca M. Successful treatment of peripheral neuropathy with chemotherapy in osteosclerotic myeloma. *J Neurol* 1987; 234: 261–63.

Polomano RC, Bennett GJ. Chemotherapy-evoked painful peripheral neuropathy. *Pain Med* 2001; 2: 8–14.

Postma TJ, Aaronson NK, Heimans JJ, Muller MJ, Hildebrand JG, Delattre JY, Hoang-Xuan K, Lanteri-Minet M, Grant R, Huddart R, Moynihan C, Maher J, Lucey R. The development of an EORTC quality of life questionnaire to assess chemotherapy-induced peripheral neuropathy: The QLQ-CIPN20. *Eur J Cancer* 2005; 41: 1135–39.

Postma TJ, Heimans JJ. Grading of chemotherapy-induced peripheral neuropathy. *Ann Oncol* 2000; 11: 509–13.

Postma TJ, Heimans JJ, Muller MJ, Ossenkoppele GJ, Vermorken JB, Aaronson NK. Pitfalls in grading severity of chemotherapy-induced peripheral neuropathy. *Ann Oncol* 1998; 9: 739–44.

Quasthoff S, Hartung HP. Chemotherapy-induced peripheral neuropathy. *J Neurol* 2002; 249: 9–17.

Rao RD, Flynn PJ, Sloan JA, Wong GY, Novotny P, Johnson DB, Gross HM, Renno SI, Nashawaty M, Loprinzi CL. Efficacy of lamotrigine in the management of chemotherapy-induced peripheral neuropathy: A phase 3 randomized, double-blind, placebo-controlled trial, N01C3. *Cancer* 2008; 112: 2802–8.

Rao RD, Michalak JC, Sloan JA, Loprinzi CL, Soori GS, Nikcevich DA, Warner DO, Novotny P, Kutteh LA, Wong GY. Efficacy of gabapentin in the management of chemotherapy-induced peripheral neuropathy: A phase 3 randomized, double-blind, placebo-controlled, crossover trial (N00C3). *Cancer* 2007; 110: 2110–18.

Renn CL, Carozzi VA, Rhee P, Gallop D, Dorsey SG, Cavaletti G. Multimodal assessment of painful peripheral neuropathy induced by chronic oxaliplatin-based chemotherapy in mice. *Mol Pain* 2011; 7: 29.

Reyes-Gibby CC, Morrow PK, Buzdar A, Shete S. Chemotherapy-induced peripheral neuropathy as a predictor of neuropathic pain in breast cancer patients previously treated with paclitaxel. *J Pain* 2009; 10: 1146–50.

Roelofs RI, Hrushesky W, Rogin J, Rosenberg L. Peripheral sensory neuropathy and cisplatin chemotherapy. *Neurology* 1984; 34: 934–38.

Siau C, Bennett GJ. Dysregulation of cellular calcium homeostasis in chemotherapy-evoked painful peripheral neuropathy. *Anesth Analg* 2006; 102: 1485–90.

Smith EM, Beck SL, Cohen J. The Total Neuropathy Score: A tool for measuring chemotherapy-induced peripheral neuropathy. *Oncol Nurs Forum* 2008; 35: 96–102.

Smith EM, Cohen JA, Pett MA, Beck SL. The reliability and validity of a modified Total Neuropathy Score-reduced and neuropathic pain severity items when used to measure chemotherapy-induced peripheral neuropathy in patients receiving taxanes and platinums. *Cancer Nurs* 2010; 33: 173–83.

Smith TJ, Coyne PJ, Parker GL, Dodson P, Ramakrishnan V. Pilot trial of a patient-specific cutaneous electrostimulation device (MC5-A Calmare(R)) for chemotherapy-induced peripheral neuropathy. *J Pain Symptom Manage* 2010; 40: 883–91.

Stillman M, Cata JP. Management of chemotherapy-induced peripheral neuropathy. *Curr Pain Headache Rep* 2006; 10: 279–87.

Storey DJ, Colvin LA, Mackean MJ, Mitchell R, Fleetwood-Walker SM, Fallon MT. Reversal of dose-limiting carboplatin-induced peripheral neuropathy with TRPM8 activator, menthol, enables further effective chemotherapy delivery. *J Pain Symptom Manage* 2010; 39: e2–4.

Takemoto S, Ushijima K, Honda K, Wada H, Terada A, Imaishi H, Kamura T. Precise evaluation of chemotherapy-induced peripheral neuropathy using the visual analogue scale: A quantitative and comparative analysis of neuropathy occurring with paclitaxel-carboplatin and docetaxel-carboplatin therapy. *Int J Clin Oncol* (in press).

Tofthagen C. Patient perceptions associated with chemotherapy-induced peripheral neuropathy. *Clin J Oncol Nurs* 2010; 14: E22–28.

Tofthagen C, Overcash J, Kip K. Falls in persons with chemotherapy-induced peripheral neuropathy. *Support Care Cancer* 2012; 20(3): 583–89.

Tofthagen CS, McMillan SC, Kip KE. Development and psychometric evaluation of the chemotherapy-induced peripheral neuropathy assessment tool. *Cancer Nurs* 2011; 34: E10–20.

Velasco R, Bruna J. Chemotherapy-induced peripheral neuropathy: An unresolved issue. *Neurologia* 2010; 25: 116–31.

Visovsky C. Chemotherapy-induced peripheral neuropathy. *Cancer Invest* 2003; 21: 439–51.

Visovsky C, Collins M, Abbott L, Aschenbrenner J, Hart C. Putting evidence into practice: Evidence-based interventions for chemotherapy-induced peripheral neuropathy. *Clin J Oncol Nurs* 2007; 11: 901–13.

Visovsky C, Daly BJ. Clinical evaluation and patterns of chemotherapy-induced peripheral neuropathy. *J Am Acad Nurse Pract* 2004; 16: 353–59.

Wen PY. A randomized, double-blinded, placebo-controlled phase II trial of recombinant human leukemia inhibitory factor (rhuLIF, emfilermin, AM424) to prevent chemotherapy-induced peripheral neuropathy. *Clin Cancer Res* 2005; 11: 1685–86.

Wickham R. Chemotherapy-induced peripheral neuropathy: A review and implications for oncology nursing practice. *Clin J Oncol Nurs* 2007; 11: 361–76.

Wilkes G. Peripheral neuropathy related to chemotherapy. *Semin Oncol Nurs* 2007; 23: 162–73.

Wolf S, Barton D, Kottschade L, Grothey A, Loprinzi C. Chemotherapy-induced peripheral neuropathy: Prevention and treatment strategies. *Eur J Cancer* 2008; 44: 1507–15.

Wolf SL, Barton DL, Qin R, Wos EJ, Sloan JA, Liu H, Aaronson NK, Satele DV, Mattar BI, Green NB, Loprinzi CL. The relationship between numbness, tingling, and shooting/burning pain in patients with chemotherapy-induced peripheral neuropathy (CIPN) as measured by the EORTC QLQ-CIPN20 instrument, N06CA. *Support Care Cancer* 2011.

Wong R, Sagar S. Acupuncture treatment for chemotherapy-induced peripheral neuropathy—A case series. *Acupunct Med* 2006; 24: 87–91.

Xiao W, Boroujerdi A, Bennett GJ, Luo ZD. Chemotherapy-evoked painful peripheral neuropathy: Analgesic effects of gabapentin and effects on expression of the alpha-2-delta type-1 calcium channel subunit. *Neuroscience* 2007; 144: 714–20.

Xu WR, Hua BJ. Progress on the treatment of chemotherapy-induced peripheral neuropathy by Chinese and Western medicine. *Zhongguo Zhong Xi Yi Jie He Za Zhi* 2008; 28: 1049–52.

Yadav N, Philip FA, Gogia V, Choudhary P, Rana SP, Mishra S, Bhatnagar S. Radio frequency ablation in drug resistant chemotherapy-induced peripheral neuropathy: A case report and review of literature. *Indian J Palliat Care* 2010; 16: 48–51.

Yano T, Yamane H, Fukuoka R, Ninomiya T, Umemura S, Suzuki S, Saeki H, Hanaoka T, Katou T, Itoh K, Fujita T, Kamei H. Evaluation of efficacy and safety of adjuvant analgesics for peripheral neuropathy induced by cancer chemotherapy in digestive cancer patients—A pilot study. *Gan To Kagaku Ryoho* 2009; 36: 83–87.

Index

A

17-AAG; *See* 17-Allylamino-17-demethoxygeldanamycin
Acetyl L-carnitine (ALC), 153
Adenocarcinoma
　small bowel, 34
　stomach, 42
Ajani Sensory Scale, 12
ALC; *See* Acetyl L-carnitine
Allodynia, 7, 102, 140, 184
Allogeneic stem cell transplantation, 45
Allopregnanolone, 151
17-Allylamino-17-demethoxygeldanamycin
　(17-AAG), 53
Amitriptyline, 163–168
　CIPN management and prevention, 165–167
　　amitriptyline in CIPN prevention, 166–167
　　amitriptyline and nortriptyline in CIPN
　　　management, 165–166
　　efficacy of nortriptyline, 166
　　efficacy of tricyclic antidepressants, 165
　　future of, 167
　　pharmacology of tricyclic antidepressants,
　　　164–165
　　anticholinergic adverse effects, 165
　　clinical pharmacology, 165
　　CYP2D6-catalized metabolism, 165
　　glial cell line-derived neuropatrophic
　　　factor, 164
　　mechanisms of action, 164–165
　　sodium channel blockers, 164
Ampulla of Vater, 34
Anesthesia dolorosa, 99
APBSCT; *See* Autologous peripheral blood stem
　cell transplant
Assessment and grading of chemotherapy-induced
　neuropathic pain, 11–17
　assessment, 12, 13
　clinical conundrum, 11
　electromyography, 13
　future solutions, 15
　grading, 11, 12, 14
　identification of patients at risk, 15
　motor weakness, 12–13
　nerve conduction studies, 13
　physical examination and neurophysiologic
　　evaluation, 12–15
　risk factors, 11
　screening toolkit, 15

Auriculotemporal syndrome, 101
Autologous peripheral blood stem cell transplant
　(APBSCT), 63
Autologous stem cell transplantation, 49

B

BADT; *See* Bortezomib combined with epirubicin,
　dexamethasone, and thalidomide
B-cell lymphoma, 59
Biliary tract cancer, 32
Bisphosphonate-related osteonecrosis of jaws
　(BRONJ), 104
Bliss Independence, 179
BMS; *See* Burning mouth syndrome
Bortezomib, 49–61
　bortezomib in special populations, 60–61
　combination therapies, 50–55
　　bortezomib combined with thalidomide
　　　and dexamethasone, 50–51
　　bortezomib, cyclophosphamide,
　　　thalidomide, and dexamethasone, 51
　　bortezomib and dexamethasone combined
　　　with itraconazole or lansoprazole,
　　　54–55
　　bortezomib and dexamethasone and
　　　pegylated liposomal doxorubicin, 52
　　bortezomib and dexamethasone with
　　　romidepsin, 52
　　bortezomib and rituximab, 52–53
　　bortezomib and rituximab and
　　　cyclophosphamide and dexamethasone,
　　　53
　　bortezomib and tanespimycin, 53–54
　　bortezomib and temsirolimus, 54
　　bortezomib and tipifarnib, 54
　　bortezomib and vincristine,
　　　dexamethasone, pegylated
　　　L-asparaginase, and doxorubicin, 52
　comparative studies, 55
　　bortezomib and dexamethasone versus
　　　vincristine, doxorubicin, and
　　　dexamethasone, 56–57
　　bortezomib and dexamethasone
　　　versus vincristine, pirarubicin,
　　　dexamethasone, and melphalan, 57
　　bortezomib and dexamethasone with and
　　　without thalidomide, 55

bortezomib with melphalan and
prednisone versus bortezomib with
thalidomide and prednisone, 56
melphalan and prednisone with and
without bortezomib, 57–58
rituximab with and without bortezomib,
58–59
thalidomide and dexamethasone with and
without bortezomib, 55–56
dosing frequency of bortezomib, 59
monotherapy, 50
subcutaneous bortezomib, 60
Bortezomib combined with epirubicin,
dexamethasone, and thalidomide
(BADT), 68
Breast cancer, 23, 24, 36, 37, 38, 41, 44, 49, 81,
103, 156
BRONJ; *See* Bisphosphonate-related
osteonecrosis of jaws
Burning mouth syndrome (BMS), 108

C

Calcitonin gene-related peptide (CGRP), 125
CALYPSO study, 25
Cancer
adenocarcinoma
small bowel, 34
stomach, 42
ampulla of Vater, 34
B-cell lymphoma, 59
biliary tract, 32
breast, 23, 24, 36, 37, 38, 41, 44, 49, 81, 103, 157
central nervous system tumors, 70
colorectal, 30, 31, 34, 35, 102, 157
endometrial, 23, 39
esophageal, 27
Ewing sarcoma, 70
fallopian, 81
fibrosarcoma, 70
gastric, 28, 31, 33, 35, 123, 156
gastroesophageal, 28
glioblastoma, 64, 157
gynecological, 149
head and neck, 23, 37, 96, 98, 102
hematological, 49
hepatocellular, 32
Hodgkin's disease, 70
hormone-sensitive, 151
lung, 33, 97, 156
lymphoma, 156
lymphoplasmacytic lymphoma, 73
mantle cell lymphoma, 52
metastatic, 183
multiple myeloma, 15, 49, 57, 64
neuroblastoma, 70
non-small-cell lung, 23, 29, 33, 39, 43, 46, 47, 74

nonsolid, 98
oral, 96
osteosarcomas, 70
ovarian, 23, 25, 27, 38, 74, 81
pancreatic, 31, 32, 188, 189
peritoneal, 81
phobia, 108
prostate, 42, 64, 70, 79
renal cell, 54, 65
skin, 156
small-cell lung, 28, 75
squamous cell carcinoma of cervix, 46
testicular, 120
thyroid, 99, 101, 156
Waldenström macroglobulinemia, 73
Cannabis sativa, 153
Carbamazepine, 121, 151
Carboplatin, 22–27, 120
combination therapies, 22–25
carboplatin combined with docetaxel and
trastuzumab, 24
carboplatin and paclitaxel, 22–23
carboplatin and paclitaxel with
pegfilgrastim, 23–24
carboplatin and paclitaxel and trastuzumab,
24
carboplatin and thalidomide, 25
granulocyte colony stimulating factor, 23
comparative studies, 25–27
carboplatin and paclitaxel as maintenance
therapy, 26
carboplatin or paclitaxel plus belinostat,
26–27
carboplatin and paclitaxel versus
carboplatin and pegylated doxorubicin,
25–26
carboplatin and paclitaxel with or without
trastuzumab, 26
hydroxamic acid-type histone deacetylase
inhibitor, 26
Catharanthus roseus, 44
CDP; *See* Cisplatin, doxorubicin, and paclitaxel
Central nervous system (CNS) tumors, 70
Central neuromodulation; *See* Neuromodulation,
central
CFPS; *See* Complex regional pain syndrome
CGRP; *See* Calcitonin gene-related peptide
Chemotherapy-induced neuropathic pain (CIPN),
clinical features of, 1–9
additional tests and investigations, 8
clinical assessment, 4–5
chemotherapy-induced neuropathic pain, 5
factors, 4
neuropathic pain, 4–5
clinical features (examination), 6–7
allodynia, 7
chemotherapy-induced neuropathic pain, 7

hyperalgesia, 6
neuropathic pain, 6–7
sensory loss, 6
clinical features (history), 5–6
chemotherapy-induced neuropathic pain, 6
hyperalgesia, 5
neuropathic pain, 5–6
sensory loss, 5
visual analogue scale, 6
introduction to neuropathic pain, 1–4
examples of neuropathic pain syndrome
associated with malignancy, 3
neuropathic pain syndromes, 2
peripheral processes, 2
prevalence, 2
Cisplatin, 27–30, 116–120
combination therapies, 27–29
cisplatin and paclitaxel, 27–28
cisplatin and paclitaxel plus etoposide, 28
cisplatin and paclitaxel plus
5-fluorouracil, 28–29
comparative studies, 29–30
cisplatin versus carboplatin in
combination with paclitaxel, 29–30
liposomal cisplatin versus cisplatin in
combination with paclitaxel, 29
Cisplatin, doxorubicin, and paclitaxel (CDP), 39
Clinical studies, review of, 19–94
bortezomib, 49–61
bortezomib combined with thalidomide
and dexamethasone, 50–51
bortezomib, cyclophosphamide,
thalidomide, and dexamethasone, 51
bortezomib and dexamethasone combined
with itraconazole or lansoprazole,
54–55
bortezomib and dexamethasone and
pegylated liposomal doxorubicin, 52
bortezomib and dexamethasone with
romidepsin, 52
bortezomib and dexamethasone versus
vincristine, doxorubicin, and
dexamethasone, 56–57
bortezomib and dexamethasone
versus vincristine, pirarubicin,
dexamethasone, and melphalan, 57
bortezomib and dexamethasone with and
without thalidomide, 55
bortezomib with melphalan and
prednisone versus bortezomib with
thalidomide and prednisone, 56
bortezomib and rituximab, 52–53
bortezomib and rituximab and
cyclophosphamide and dexamethasone,
53
bortezomib in special populations, 60–61
bortezomib and tanespimycin, 53–54

bortezomib and temsirolimus, 54
bortezomib and tipifarnib, 54
bortezomib and vincristine,
dexamethasone, pegylated
L-asparaginase, and doxorubicin, 52
dosing frequency of bortezomib, 59
melphalan and prednisone with and
without bortezomib, 57–58
monotherapy, 50
rituximab with and without bortezomib,
58–59
subcutaneous bortezomib, 60
thalidomide and dexamethasone with and
without bortezomib, 55–56
carboplatin, 22–27
carboplatin combined with docetaxel and
trastuzumab, 24
carboplatin and paclitaxel, 22–23
carboplatin and paclitaxel as maintenance
therapy, 26
carboplatin and paclitaxel with
pegfilgrastim, 23–24
carboplatin or paclitaxel plus belinostat,
26–27
carboplatin and paclitaxel and trastuzumab,
24
carboplatin and paclitaxel with or without
trastuzumab, 26
carboplatin and paclitaxel versus
carboplatin and pegylated
doxorubicin, 25–26
carboplatin and thalidomide, 25
granulocyte colony stimulating factor, 23
hydroxamic acid-type histone deacetylase
inhibitor, 26
cisplatin, 27–30
cisplatin and docetaxel, 27
cisplatin and paclitaxel, 27–28
cisplatin and paclitaxel plus etoposide, 28
cisplatin and paclitaxel plus
5-fluorouracil, 28–29
cisplatin versus carboplatin in
combination with paclitaxel, 29–30
liposomal cisplatin versus cisplatin in
combination with paclitaxel, 29
docetaxel, 42–44
docetaxel and cisplatin, 43
docetaxel and dexamethasone, 42–43
docetaxel and gemcitabine, 43
docetaxel and mitomycin, 43
docetaxel and trastuzumab with and
without carboplatin, 44
docetaxel versus vinflunine, 43–44
monotherapies, 42
epothilones, 80–83
combination therapies, 82–83
monotherapies, 80–82

lenalidomide, 78–79
oxaliplatin, 30–36
    FOLFOX and erlotinib, 31
    FOLFOX and gemcitabine, 31–32
    FOLFOX4 with and without oxaliplatin,
        35–36
    oxaliplatin and capecitabine, 34–35
    oxaliplatin and capecitabine with
        epirubicin, 35
    oxaliplatin and dexamethasone and
        cytarabine and rituximab, 33
    oxaliplatin and doxorubicin, 32–33
    oxaliplatin and etoposide, l-leucovorin,
        and fluorouracil, 33
    oxaliplatin and fluoropyrimidine with and
        without cetuximab, 36
    oxaliplatin and 5-fluorouracil and
        leucovorin (FOLFOX), 30–31
    oxaliplatin and gemcitabine and
        bevacizumab, 32
    oxaliplatin and gemcitabine and
        cetuximab, 32
    oxaliplatin and gemcitabine and
        fluoropyramidine S-1, 32
    oxaliplatin and irinotecan, 33–34
    oxaliplatin and vinorelbine, 34
paclitaxel, 36–42
    monotherapies, 37–38
    nanoparticle albumin-bound (Nab)
        paclitaxel, 40–42
    paclitaxel and cisplatin plus doxorubicin, 39
    paclitaxel with cyclophosphamide and
        cisplatin, 38–39
    paclitaxel with epirubicin and
        vinorelbine versus cyclophosphamide,
        methotrexate, and 5-fluorouracil, 40
    paclitaxel and gemcitabine versus
        gemcitabine and pemetrexed, 39
    paclitaxel and lapatinib, 38
    paclitaxel and tosedostat, 38
platinum agents, 22–36
    carboplatin, 22–27
    cisplatin, 27–30
    oxaliplatin, 30–36
suramin, 79–80
    monotherapy, 79
    suramin and epirubicin, 80
    suramin and mitomycin C, 80
taxanes, 36–44
    docetaxel, 42–44
    paclitaxel, 36–42
thalidomide, 61–78
    carboplatin and epotoside with and
        without thalidomide, 75
    carboplatin and gemcitabine with and
        without thalidomide, 74–75

carboplatin with and without thalidomide,
    74
combination therapies, 66–74
comparative studies, 74–78
dexamethasone with and without
    thalidomide, 75
melphalan and prednisone with and
    without thalidomide, 77
monotherapies, 61–66
single nucleotide polymorphisms and
    thalidomide-induced peripheral
    neuropathy, 78
thalidomide and bortezomib, 67
thalidomide and bortezomib
    with chemotherapy (cisplatin,
    cyclophosphamide, etoposide, and
    dexamethasone), 68
thalidomide and bortezomib with
    epirubicin and dexamethasone, 68–69
thalidomide and capecitabine, 69–70
thalidomide and combination of
    bortezomib, melphalan, and
    dexamethasone, 69
thalidomide and cyclophosphamide, 70
thalidomide, cyclophosphamide, and
    dexamethasone, 70–71
thalidomide and dacarbazine, 71
thalidomide and dexamethasone, 66–67
thalidomide and dexamethasone and
    cyclophosphamide, 67
thalidomide and dexamethasone versus
    interferon-alpha and dexamethasone
    as maintenance therapy, 76–77
thalidomide and dexamethasone with and
    without bortezomib, 75–76
thalidomide and fludarabine, 71
thalidomide and granulocyte
    macrophage-colony stimulating factor,
    71–72
thalidomide and interleukin-2 plus
    granulocyte macrophage-colony
    stimulating factor, 72–73
thalidomide and melphalan and
    dexamethasone, 67–68
thalidomide and melphalan and
    lenalidomide and prednisone, 68
thalidomide and rituximab, 73
thalidomide and semaxanib, 73
thalidomide and vincristine with
    pegylated doxorubicin and
    dexamethasone, 73–74
thalidomide with and without interferon, 76
vincristine, liposomal doxorubicin, and
    dexamethasone with and without
    thalidomide, 77–78
vinca alkaloids, 44–49
    vincristine, 45

vindesine, 45
vinflunine, 46
vinorelbine, 46–49
vinorelbine, 46–49
    epirubicin with and without vinorelbine, 49
    monotherapy, 46
    vinorelbine and cisplatin, 46–47
    vinorelbine and gemcitabine, 47–48
    vinorelbine and gemcitabine compared to
        carboplatin and paclitaxel, 48–49
    vinorelbine and gemcitabine with and
        without cisplatin, 48
    vinorelbine and oxaliplatin, 47
    vinorelbine and paclitaxel, 47
CNS tumors; See Central nervous system tumors
COIN trial, 36
Colchicine, 138
Colorectal cancer, 30, 31, 34, 35, 102, 157
Complex regional pain syndrome (CRPS), 188
Cremophor EL, 37
Cytochrome P450 inhibitor, 55

D

Decreased-frequency dexamethasone (DVd), 74
Deep brain stimulation (DBS), 181, 183–184
Delta-9-tetrahydrocannabinol (THC), 153
Diamminocyclohexane (DACH), 122
DNA
    adduct formation, 114
    carboplatin interaction with, 22
    chromosomal fragmentation, 117
    damage, neurons, 116
    mitochondrial, 116
    -platinum binding, 118
    repair systems, 78
    synthesis inhibition, 71
Docetaxel, 42–44, 125
    combination therapies, 42–43
        docetaxel and cisplatin, 43
        docetaxel and dexamethasone, 42–43
        docetaxel and gemcitabine, 43
        docetaxel and mitomycin, 43
    comparative studies, 43–44
        docetaxel and trastuzumab with and
            without carboplatin, 44
        docetaxel versus vinflunine, 43–44
    monotherapies, 42
Dorsal root ganglia (DRG), 116
Dorsal root ganglia (research), 139–140
    hyperpolarization-activated cyclic nucleotide-
        gated channels, 140
    interleukin-1β, 140
    interleukin-6, 140
    matrix metallopeptidase-9, 140

    transient receptor potential vanilloid
        channels, 140
    tumor necrosis factor-α, 140
Double-crush hypothesis, 197
DRG; See Dorsal root ganglia
Drug treatment, example; See Amitriptyline
DVd; See Decreased-frequency dexamethasone

E

Eastern Cooperative Oncology Group scale, 12
EGFR; See Epidermal growth factor receptor
Electromyography (EMG), 13, 198
ELF; See Etoposide, l-leucovorin, and fluorouracil
Endometrial cancer, 23, 39
Epidermal growth factor receptor (EGFR), 38
EPO; See Erythropoietin
Epothilones, 80–83
    combination therapies, 82–83
    monotherapies, 80–82
Erythropoietin (EPO), 152, 157
Esophageal cancer, 27
Etoposide, l-leucovorin, and fluorouracil (ELF), 33
Ewing sarcoma, 70
EXE; See Oxaliplatin-capecitabine-epirubicin
Experimental design and analysis of drug
        combinations, 169–180
    agonist drugs, 169
    analysis on effect scale, 178–179
        Bliss Independence, 179
        response surface method, 178
    application (testing drugs for neuropathic pain),
        174–176
        anticonvulsants, 174
        isobologram, 175
        mu opioid agonist, 174
    curved isoboles, 176–178
    dose-effect analysis, 170–172
        potency value, 170
        smoothed curve, 170
    isoboles, 172–174
        description, 172
        isobologram, 173, 175
        linear isobole, 173
        standard error, 174
    methodology, 170
    nonsteroidal anti-inflammatory drugs, 179
    opioids, 179

F

Fallopian cancer, 81
Fibrosarcoma, 70
5-Flourouracil (5-FU), 157
FOLFOX; See Oxaliplatin and 5-fluorouracil and
        leucovorin
Frey syndrome, 98, 101

G

GABA-releasing neurons, 148
Gastric cancer, 28, 31, 33, 35, 123, 156
Gastroesophageal cancer, 28
GCSF; *See* Granulocyte colony stimulating factor
Glial cell line-derived neuropatrophic factor
        (GDNF), 164
Glioblastoma, 64, 157
Glossodynia, 108
Glutathione (GSH), 31
GM-CSF; *See* Granulocyte macrophage-colony
        stimulating factor
Graft versus host disease (GVHD), 98
Granulocyte colony stimulating factor (GCSF), 23
Granulocyte macrophage-colony stimulating
        factor (GM-CSF), 71–72
GSH; *See* Glutathione
GVHD; *See* Graft versus host disease
Gynecological cancer, 149

H

Hand-foot syndrome, 36
HCN channels; *See* Hyperpolarization-activated
        cyclic nucleotide-gated channels
HDAC; *See* Histone deacetylase
Head and neck cancer, 23, 37, 96, 98, 102
Heat shock protein 90 (HSP90), 53
Hematological cancers, 49
Hematopoietic stem cell transplantation (HSCT),
        105
Hepatocellular cancer, 32
Herpes simplex virus (HSV), 104
HER2 receptor; *See* Human epidermal growth
        factor receptor 2
Histone deacetylase (HDAC), 26
Hodgkin's disease, 70
Hormone-sensitive cancer, 151
HSCT; *See* Hematopoietic stem cell transplantation
HSP90; *See* Heat shock protein 90
HSV; *See* Herpes simplex virus
5-HT; *See* Serotonin
Human epidermal growth factor receptor 2
        (HER2 receptor), 24, 41
Hyperalgesia, 6, 102
Hypercalcemia, 104
Hyperpolarization-activated cyclic
        nucleotide-gated (HCN) channels, 140

I

IASP; *See* International Association for the
        Study of Pain
IENFs; *See* Intraepidermal nerve fibers
IFN-γ; *See* Interferon-gamma
IL-1β; *See* Interleukin-1β

IL-2; *See* Interleukin-2
IL-6; *See* Interleukin-6
Initiative on Methods, Measurement and
        Pain Assessment in Clinical Trials, 4
Interferon-alpha, 76
Interferon-gamma (IFN-γ), 154
Interleukin-1, 152
Interleukin-1β (IL-1β), 140
Interleukin-2 (IL-2), 72
Interleukin-6 (IL-6), 140
International Association for the Study of Pain
        (IASP), 1
Intraepidermal nerve fibers (IENFs), 138
In vivo models and assessment of
        pharmacotherapeutics, 147–162
        GABA-releasing neurons, 148
        models, 148–150
                CIPN-induced decrease in food
                        motivation procedure, 149
                CIPN-induced place conditioning
                        procedure, 150
        N-methyl-aspartic acid receptors, 148
        preclinical assessment, 150–157
                acetyl L-carnitine, 153
                Ca^{2+} and Na^+ channel blockers, 151–152
                cannabinoids, 153–157
                cytokines and glial modulators, 152–153
                glial cell modulation, 152
                interleukin-6, 152
                nerve growth factor, 153
                opioids, 150
                rostroventromedial medulla, 155
                tricyclic antidepressants, 150
                T-type calcium channels, 152
                tumor necrosis factor, 152
Isoboles, 172–174
        curved, 176–178
        description, 172
        isobologram, 173, 175
        linear isobole, 173
        standard error, 174

K

Kinase inhibitor, 54

L

Langerhans cell histiocytosis (LCH), 65
Lenalidomide, 78–79
Lung cancer, 33, 97, 156
Lymphoma, 156
Lymphoplasmacytic lymphoma, 73

M

Mantle cell lymphoma, 52
Matrix metallopeptidase-9 (MMP9), 140

MCS; *See* Motor cortex stimulation
Mitomycin C, 43, 80
Monoclonal antibody, 102, 104
    bevacizumab, 104
    cetuximab, 102
    denosumab, 104
    trastuzumab, 24
MOSAIC trial, 35
Motor cortex stimulation (MCS), 181, 184–186
Multiple myeloma, 15, 49, 57, 64
Mu opioid, 169, 174

N

National Cancer Institute Common Toxicity
        Criteria, 12, 166
Nerve conduction studies (NCS), 13, 198
Nerve decompression, 195–210
    analogy, 197
    background, 196–197
    basic science and clinical data, 197–198
    diagnosis, 198–199
    double-crush hypothesis, 197
    electromyograms, 198
    human data, 198
    nerve conduction studies, 198
    selective serotonin reuptake inhibitors, 196
    surgical treatment, 200–202
    Tinel sign, 199
Nerve electrophysiological studies (NES), 76
Nerve growth factor (NGF), 119, 153
Neuralgia-inducing cavitational osteonecrosis
        (NICO), 103
Neuroblastoma, 70
Neuromodulation, central, 181–194
    allodynia, 182
    complex regional pain syndrome, 188
    dysesthesia, 182
    hyperalgesia, 182
    hyperpathia, 182
    invasive techniques, 183–186
        deep brain stimulation, 183–184
        motor cortex stimulation, 184–186
    neuromodulatory techniques, 183–189
        invasive techniques, 183–186
        noninvasive techniques, 186–189
    noninvasive techniques, 186–189
        NMDA receptor efficacy, 188
        repetitive TMS, 186
        transcranial direct current stimulation,
            187–189
        transcranial magnetic stimulation, 186
    paresthesia, 182
    postradiation plexopathies, 182
NGF; *See* Nerve growth factor
NICO; *See* Neuralgia-inducing cavitational
        osteonecrosis

Nitrous oxide-cyclic guanosine monophosphate
        (NO/cGMP) pathway, 142
N-methyl-aspartic acid (NMDA) receptors, 148,
        188
NNH; *See* Number needed to harm
NNT; *See* Number needed to treat
NO/cGMP pathway; *See* Nitrous oxide-cyclic
        guanosine monophosphate pathway
Non-Hodgkin's lymphoma, 73
Non-small-cell lung cancer, 23, 29, 33, 39, 43, 46,
        47, 74
Nonsolid cancers, 98
Nonsteroidal anti-inflammatory drugs (NSAIDs),
        179
Norepinephrine, 148, 164, 169
NSAIDs; *See* Nonsteroidal anti-inflammatory drugs
Nuclear factor-kappa B ligand, 104
Numb chin syndrome, 98
Number needed to harm (NNH), 165
Number needed to treat (NNT), 165

O

Opioids, 150, 179, 183, 196
    mu, 169, 174
    short-acting, 103
Oral cancer, 96
Orofacial neuropathy and pain, 95–112
    cancer-related orofacial neuropathy, 98–99
        anesthesia dolorosa, 99
        facial palsy, 99
        Frey syndrome, 98
        mental nerve neuropathy, 98–99
        numb chin syndrome, 98
        painful trigeminal neuropathy, 99
        trigeminal neuralgia, 99
    cancer-related orofacial pain, 96–98
        head and neck malignancies, 96–97
        other malignancies, 97–98
    chemotherapy-related odontalgia, 104–108
        dental hypersensitivity, 105
        dental pain, 105–108
        hematopoietic stem cell transplantation,
            105
    chemotherapy-related orofacial neuropathy,
            102–107
        chemotherapy-related neurotoxicity,
            102–103
        drug-induced osteonecrosis of jaws, 104
        neuralgia-inducing cavitational
            osteonecrosis of jaws, 103
        neuropathies secondary to oral
            complications of chemotherapy, 104
        recurrent orofacial viral infections, 104
        vascular endothelial growth factor A, 104

other types of orofacial pain, 108
radiotherapy- and surgery-related
      neuropathies, 100–102
   auriculotemporal syndrome, 101–102
   Frey syndrome, 101
   postoperative neuropathies, 101
   taste dysfunction, 100–101
Osteosarcomas, 70
Ovarian cancer, 23, 25, 27, 38, 74, 81
Oxaliplatin, 30–36, 120–122
   combination therapies, 30–35
      FOLFOX and erlotinib, 31
      FOLFOX and gemcitabine, 31–32
      oxaliplatin and capecitabine, 34–35
      oxaliplatin and capecitabine with
         epirubicin, 35
      oxaliplatin and dexamethasone and
         cytarabine and rituximab, 33
      oxaliplatin and doxorubicin, 32–33
      oxaliplatin and etoposide, 1-leucovorin,
         and fluorouracil, 33
      oxaliplatin and 5-fluorouracil and
         leucovorin (FOLFOX), 30–31
      oxaliplatin and gemcitabine and
         bevacizumab, 32
      oxaliplatin and gemcitabine and cetuximab,
         32
      oxaliplatin and gemcitabine and
         fluoropyramidine S-1, 32
      oxaliplatin and irinotecan, 33–34
      oxaliplatin and vinorelbine, 34
   comparative studies, 35–36
      FOLFOX4 with and without oxaliplatin,
         35–36
      oxaliplatin and fluoropyrimidine with and
         without cetuximab, 36
Oxaliplatin-capecitabine-epirubicin (EXE), 35
Oxaliplatin and 5-fluorouracil and leucovorin
      (FOLFOX), 30–31

P

Paclitaxel, 36–42, 124–125
   combination therapies, 38–39
      paclitaxel and cisplatin plus doxorubicin, 39
      paclitaxel with cyclophosphamide and
         cisplatin, 38–39
      paclitaxel and lapatinib, 38
      paclitaxel and tosedostat, 38
   comparative studies, 39–40
      paclitaxel with epirubicin and
         vinorelbine versus cyclophosphamide,
         methotrexate, and 5-fluorouracil, 40
      paclitaxel and gemcitabine versus
         gemcitabine and pemetrexed, 39

monotherapies, 37–38
nanoparticle albumin-bound (Nab) paclitaxel,
      40–42
   Nab paclitaxel combined with
      bevacizumab and gemcitabine, 41
   Nab paclitaxel combined with carboplatin
      and trastuzumab, 42
Painful trigeminal neuropathy, 99
Pancreatic cancer, 31, 32, 188, 189
Pegylated liposomal doxorubicin (PLD), 52
Peripheral neuropathy, underlying, 113–135
   apoptosis, 117
   axonal refractoriness, 121
   carboplatin, 120
   chemotherapeutic drugs (classes and agents),
      116–127
      coasting, 116
      platinum-based chemotherapeutic agents,
         116–122
      presumed sites of cellular involvement, 116
      taxanes, 122–125
      vinca alkaloids, 125–126
   cisplatin, 116–120
   docetaxel, 125
   oxaliplatin, 120–122
   paclitaxel, 124–125
   peripheral nervous system vulnerability,
      115–116
   sodium channel dysfunction, 121
   some major unanswered questions, 127
   suramin, 126
   thalidomide, 126–127
Peritoneal cancer, 81
P-glycoprotein, 123
Pharmacotherapeutics, assessment of;
      See In vivo models and assessment
      of pharmacotherapeutics
Platinum agents, 22–36
   carboplatin, 22–27, 120
      carboplatin combined with docetaxel and
         trastuzumab, 24
      carboplatin and paclitaxel, 22–23
      carboplatin and paclitaxel as maintenance
         therapy, 26
      carboplatin and paclitaxel with
         pegfilgrastim, 23–24
      carboplatin or paclitaxel plus belinostat,
         26–27
      carboplatin and paclitaxel and
         trastuzumab, 24
      carboplatin and paclitaxel versus
         carboplatin and pegylated doxorubicin,
         25–26
      carboplatin and paclitaxel with or without
         trastuzumab, 26
      carboplatin and thalidomide, 25

granulocyte colony stimulating factor, 23
hydroxamic acid-type histone deacetylase
    inhibitor, 26
cisplatin, 27–30, 116–120
    cisplatin and docetaxel, 27
    cisplatin and paclitaxel, 27–28
    cisplatin and paclitaxel plus etoposide, 28
    cisplatin and paclitaxel plus
        5-fluorouracil, 28–29
    cisplatin versus carboplatin in
        combination with paclitaxel, 29–30
    liposomal cisplatin versus cisplatin in
        combination with paclitaxel, 29
oxaliplatin, 30–36, 120–122
    FOLFOX and erlotinib, 31
    FOLFOX and gemcitabine, 31–32
    FOLFOX4 with and without oxaliplatin,
        35–36
    oxaliplatin and capecitabine, 34–35
    oxaliplatin and capecitabine with
        epirubicin, 35
    oxaliplatin and dexamethasone and
        cytarabine and rituximab, 33
    oxaliplatin and doxorubicin, 32–33
    oxaliplatin and etoposide, 1-leucovorin,
        and fluorouracil, 33
    oxaliplatin and fluoropyrimidine with and
        without cetuximab, 36
    oxaliplatin and 5-fluorouracil and
        leucovorin (FOLFOX), 30–31
    oxaliplatin and gemcitabine and
        bevacizumab, 32
    oxaliplatin and gemcitabine and cetuximab,
        32
    oxaliplatin and gemcitabine and
        fluoropyramidine S-1, 32
    oxaliplatin and irinotecan, 33–34
    oxaliplatin and vinorelbine, 34
PLD; See Pegylated liposomal doxorubicin
Prostate cancer, 42, 64, 70, 79
Prostate-specific antigen (PSA), 42, 64, 80

Q

Quality of life (QoL), 167

R

Randomized and controlled trials (RCTs), 163
Renal cell cancer, 54, 65
Research, 137–146
    central sensitization, 140–142
        GLAST, 141
        GLT-1, 141
        nitrous oxide-cyclic guanosine
            monophosphate pathway, 142

chemotherapy-induced axon injury, 137–139
    colchicine, 138
    intraepidermal nerve fibers, 138
    mitochondrial dysfunction, 138
sensitization of primary sensory neurons in
        dorsal root ganglia, 139–140
    hyperpolarization-activated cyclic
        nucleotide-gated channels, 140
    interleukin-1β, 140
    interleukin-6, 140
    matrix metallopeptidase-9, 140
    transient receptor potential vanilloid
        channels, 140
    tumor necrosis factor-α, 140
RMPT therapy; See Thalidomide, melphalan,
        lenalidomide, and prednisone therapy
Rostroventromedial medulla (RVM), 155

S

Selective serotonin reuptake inhibitors (SSRIs), 196
Serotonin (5-HT), 148, 164, 169, 174
Single nucleotide polymorphisms (SNPs), 78
Skin cancer, 156
Small-cell lung cancer, 28, 75
SNPS; See Single nucleotide polymorphisms
Sodium channels
    blocker, 121, 151, 174
    dysfunction, 121
    nerve function and, 164
    oxalate and, 120
Squamous cell carcinoma of the cervix, 46
SSRIs; See Selective serotonin reuptake inhibitors
Streptozotocin, 197
Suramin, 79–80, 126
    combination therapy, 80
        suramin and epirubicin, 80
        suramin and mitomycin C, 80
    monotherapy, 79

T

Taxanes, 36–44, 122–125
    docetaxel, 42–44, 125
        combination therapies, 42–43
        comparative studies, 43–44
        docetaxel and cisplatin, 43
        docetaxel and dexamethasone, 42–43
        docetaxel and gemcitabine, 43
        docetaxel and mitomycin, 43
        docetaxel and trastuzumab with and
            without carboplatin, 44
        docetaxel versus vinflunine, 43–44
        monotherapies, 42
    paclitaxel, 36–42, 124–125
        combination therapies, 38–39
        comparative studies, 39–40

monotherapies, 37–38
nanoparticle albumin-bound (Nab)
    paclitaxel, 40–42
paclitaxel and cisplatin plus doxorubicin, 39
paclitaxel with cyclophosphamide and
    cisplatin, 38–39
paclitaxel with epirubicin and
    vinorelbine versus cyclophosphamide,
    methotrexate, and 5-fluorouracil, 40
paclitaxel and gemcitabine versus
    gemcitabine and pemetrexed, 39
paclitaxel and lapatinib, 38
paclitaxel and tosedostat, 38
TCAs; *See* Tricyclic antidepressants
tDCS; *See* Transcranial direct current stimulation
Testicular cancer, 120
Thalidomide, 61–78, 126–127
    combination therapies, 66–74
        thalidomide and bortezomib, 67
        thalidomide and bortezomib
            with chemotherapy (cisplatin,
            cyclophosphamide, etoposide, and
            dexamethasone), 68
        thalidomide and bortezomib with
            epirubicin and dexamethasone, 68–69
        thalidomide and capecitabine, 69–70
        thalidomide and combination of
            bortezomib, melphalan, and
            dexamethasone, 69
        thalidomide and cyclophosphamide, 70
        thalidomide, cyclophosphamide, and
            dexamethasone, 70–71
        thalidomide and dacarbazine, 71
        thalidomide and dexamethasone, 66–67
        thalidomide and dexamethasone and
            cyclophosphamide, 67
        thalidomide and fludarabine, 71
        thalidomide and granulocyte
            macrophage-colony stimulating factor,
            71–72
        thalidomide and interleukin-2 plus
            granulocyte macrophage-colony
            stimulating factor, 72–73
        thalidomide and melphalan and
            dexamethasone, 67–68
        thalidomide and melphalan and
            lenalidomide and prednisone, 68
        thalidomide and rituximab, 73
        thalidomide and semaxanib, 73
        thalidomide and vincristine with
            pegylated doxorubicin and
            dexamethasone, 73–74
    comparative studies, 74–78
        carboplatin and epotoside with and
            without thalidomide, 75
        carboplatin and gemcitabine with and
            without thalidomide, 74–75

carboplatin with and without thalidomide,
    74
dexamethasone with and without
    thalidomide, 75
melphalan and prednisone with and
    without thalidomide, 77
thalidomide and dexamethasone versus
    interferon-alpha and dexamethasone
    as maintenance therapy, 76–77
thalidomide and dexamethasone with and
    without bortezomib, 75–76
thalidomide with and without interferon, 76
vincristine, liposomal doxorubicin, and
    dexamethasone with and without
    thalidomide, 77–78
melphalan, lenalidomide, and prednisone
    therapy, 68
monotherapies, 61–66
single nucleotide polymorphisms and
    thalidomide-induced peripheral
    neuropathy, 78
THC; *See* Delta-9-tetrahydrocannabinol
Thyroid cancer, 99, 101, 156
TMS; *See* Transcranial magnetic stimulation
TNF; *See* Tumor necrosis factor
TNFα; *See* Tumor necrosis factor-α
Tramadol, 174, 176
Transcranial direct current stimulation (tDCS),
    187–189
Transcranial magnetic stimulation (TMS), 181, 186
Transient receptor potential vanilloid (TRPV)
    channels, 140
Tricyclic antidepressants (TCAs), 150, 163, 164;
    See also Amitriptyline
Tumor necrosis factor (TNF), 152
Tumor necrosis factor-α (TNFα), 61, 140, 154
Tyrosine kinase inhibitor, 38, 73

V

VAD-doxil; *See* Vincristine, liposomal
    doxorubicin, and dexamethasone
Varicella zoster virus (VZV), 104
VAS; *See* Visual analogue scale
Vascular endothelial growth factor (VEGF), 73, 104
VG; *See* Vinorelbine-gemcitabine
Vinca alkaloids, 44–49, 125–126
    suramin, 126
    thalidomide, 126–127
    vincristine, 45
    vindesine, 45
    vinflunine, 46
    vinorelbine, 46–49
        epirubicin with and without vinorelbine, 49
        monotherapy, 46
        vinorelbine and cisplatin, 46–47
        vinorelbine and gemcitabine, 47–48

vinorelbine and gemcitabine compared to
    carboplatin and paclitaxel, 48–49
vinorelbine and gemcitabine with and
    without cisplatin, 48
vinorelbine and oxaliplatin, 47
vinorelbine and paclitaxel, 47
Vincristine, liposomal doxorubicin, and
    dexamethasone (VAD-doxil), 77
Vincristine sulfate liposomes injection (VSLI), 45
Vinorelbine, 46–49
    combination therapies, 46–48
        vinorelbine and cisplatin, 46–47
        vinorelbine and gemcitabine, 47–48
        vinorelbine and gemcitabine with and
            without cisplatin, 48
        vinorelbine and oxaliplatin, 47
        vinorelbine and paclitaxel, 47

comparative studies, 48–49
    epirubicin with and without vinorelbine, 49
    vinorelbine and gemcitabine compared to
        carboplatin and paclitaxel, 48–49
monotherapy, 46
Vinorelbine-gemcitabine (VG), 48, 49
VISTA trial, 57, 58, 60
Visual analogue scale (VAS), 6
VSLI; *See* Vincristine sulfate liposomes injection
VZV; *See* Varicella zoster virus

W

Waldenström macroglobulinemia (WM), 73
Warfarin, 23
World Health Organization scale, 12